Errors in Medical Science Investigations

Hamid Soori

Errors in Medical Science Investigations

Springer

Hamid Soori
Faculty of Medicine
Cyprus International University
Nicosia, North Cyprus

School of Public Health and Safety
Shahid Beheshti University of Medical Sciences
Tehran, Iran

ISBN 978-981-99-8523-4 ISBN 978-981-99-8521-0 (eBook)
https://doi.org/10.1007/978-981-99-8521-0

Translation from the Persian language edition: "Common Errors in Medical Sciences and Their Control " by Hamid Soori, © Author 2006. Published by Shahid Beheshti University of Medical Sciences. All Rights Reserved.

This Springer imprint is published by the registered company Springer Nature Singapore Pte Ltd.
The registered company address is: 152 Beach Road, #21-01/04 Gateway East, Singapore 189721, Singapore

Paper in this product is recyclable.

To my family and honorable people who hold a candle in their hands to light the way for the misguided in this difficult and dark time.

Foreword

Biomedical research is a critical component of healthcare, providing the evidence base for the development of new treatments, therapies, and diagnostic tools. However, medical research is a complex and challenging field, with many potential sources of error that can affect the validity and reliability of research findings.

The book *Errors in Medical Science Investigations* is a timely and important contribution to the field of medical research. The book provides a comprehensive overview of the various types of errors that can occur in medical research, as well as the methods and techniques that can be employed to reduce or eliminate these errors.

The author of the book is an expert in epidemiology and research methodology.

Rector Cyprus International University
Nicosia, Cyprus

Halil Nadiri

Preface

The book *Errors in Medical Science Investigations* provides guidance on how to reduce or eliminate different types of errors in research. The book covers a variety of topics, including study design, data collection and analysis, statistical methods, and some other methodological considerations. The author draws on his experience to offer practical advice and insights into the most common types of errors and how to avoid them. The book is designed to be accessible and is an invaluable resource for biomedical students, researchers, and practitioners in the field of medical science.

Medical research is a crucial part of healthcare, providing the foundation for the development of new treatments, therapies, and diagnostic tools. However, the accuracy and validity of medical research depend on the quality of the research design, data collection, analysis, and interpretation.

The book *Errors in Medical Science Investigations* aims to help researchers identify, control, and avoid errors in medical research. It provides a comprehensive overview of the various types of errors that can occur in biomedical research, including bias, confounding variables, errors in data collection and analysis, and incorrect interpretation of results. The book is an essential resource for anyone involved in medical research, offering insights into the most common types of errors and providing strategies for avoiding or minimizing these errors. It is designed to be accessible and user-friendly, with clear explanations and examples that help readers understand complex concepts.

Nicosia, North Cyprus — Hamid Soori

Acknowledgments

I would like to thank our families and loved ones for their unwavering support and encouragement throughout the process of writing this book. Their patience and understanding have been greatly appreciated.

I am grateful to my colleague Professor R. Majdzadeh for his advice and checking the pre-print of the book.

Finally, I would like to extend my thanks to the team at the *Springer Nature* Group for their hard work and dedication in bringing this book to fruition. ....

I hope that this book will prove to be a valuable resource for researchers in the field of medical science and that it will contribute to the continued advancement of medical knowledge and healthcare for people.

Nicosia, North Cyprus
Tehran, Iran

Hamid Soori

Contents

Abbreviations

AIDS	Acquired immunodeficiency syndrome
ANOVA	Analysis of variance
AR	Attributable risk
AUC	Area under the curve
CDC	Centers for Disease Control and Prevention
CI	Confidence interval
COPD	Chronic obstructive pulmonary disease
CT	Computed tomography
CVD	Cardiovascular disease
DALY	Disability-adjusted life years
ECG	Electrocardiogram
FDA	Food and Drug Administration
HIV	Human immunodeficiency virus
HR	Hazard ratio
IQR	Interquartile range
IRB	Institutional Review Board
MRI	Magnetic resonance imaging
N	Sample size
NIH	National Institutes of Health
NNH	Number needed to harm
NNT	Number needed to treat
OR	Odds ratio
PAR	Population attributable risk
PET	Positron emission tomography
p-value	Probability value
RCT	Randomized controlled trial
ROC	Receiver operating characteristic
RR	Relative risk
SARS-CoV-2	Severe Acute Respiratory Syndrome Coronavirus 2 (causes COVID-19)
SD	Standard deviation
SE	Standard error
SMR	Standardized death ratio
WHO	World Health Organization
YLD	Years lived with disability
YLL	Years of life lost

Basic Concepts 1

Between the true knower and the blind imitator there are (great) differences, for the former is like David, while the other is (but) an echo. The purchaser of real knowledge is God: its market is always splendid. Conventional knowledge is (only) for sale (self-advertisement): when it finds a purchaser, it glows with delight. (http://www.masnavi.net/ Accessed: Feb 28, 2023)

—Rumi (The Persian Poet) (1207–1273)

1.1 Introduction

Having raw experiences is not enough to understand the truth, and the important thing is to have a correct and deep understanding of the reality (findings) and draw logical conclusions from them. This is considered a basic and important point in discovering scientific unknowns and producing science. When Isaac Newton was sitting under an apple tree and an apple fell from the tree, what led him to discover the gravity of the earth was this true and deep understanding of such a reality. Certainly, that apple was not the first apple that fell from the tree, and Newton was not the first to witness this happening. Millions of people watched such an event before him, but we consider Isaac Newton the discoverer of gravity. The main platform for a deep and accurate understanding of facts is thought. This is why thinking is considered the basis of research, and a researcher means someone who has reached a truth, who constantly thinks about the facts around him/her and tries to discover unknowns, and who understands truths so that it could facts from his/her specialized angle.

Another point in research is the courage to think, and the courage to express one's thoughts. According to what was said, the set of human scientific achievements is the result of the thoughts of past and present researchers—a fallible idea and an achievement that can be modified. What has caused the emergence and development of science throughout history has also been the result of the courage to think and express thoughts. Aristotle believed that the earth is the center of the universe, and all the celestial bodies revolve around the earth. But deeper thinking and research made this belief correct, because our understanding of the truth may be different from time to time. Innovation in tools, along with scientific discoveries and shifts in perspective, can reveal previously concealed dimensions of truth. A notable illustration of this is the invention of the MRI machine, which has empowered doctors to detect abnormalities during routine examinations, thereby uncovering previously unknown condi-

H. Soori, *Errors in Medical Science Investigations*, https://doi.org/10.1007/978-981-99-8521-0_1

tions. Similarly, the advent of the microscope has enabled researchers to observe and comprehend organisms that were once beyond human perception, leading to a concrete understanding of previously unexplored realms. These advancements exemplify how novel tools and fresh insights can unveil hidden truths and expand our knowledge.

In understanding the truth, perspective is also important. Because the truth is multifaceted, its understanding may be possible from different aspects, and everyone can infer it from a different point of view. Correcting the point of view, and perspective, and sometimes changing it can also be effective in our deeper understanding of the facts.

Based on the information presented thus far, it can be argued that there is a potential need to transition from a culture primarily focused on imitation to one that places greater emphasis on research. However, deep and accurate thinking, as well as choosing the right perspective for testing scientific hypotheses, solving problems, and answering unknowns and research questions, is indispensable. Because existing science is the result of human thought and this thought is fallible, science is also dynamic. If someone does not have a correct perspective on the research, his/her meaning will be associated with bias and error. This is sometimes unavoidable in scientific studies and therefore opens a door for us to criticize and review scientific materials.

Today, tens of thousands of scientific journal titles are published only in English worldwide, which contains scientific news and the result of research efforts of scientists and researchers from different countries. Of these, about 30,000 journals are related to medical sciences, which include about two million articles annually.[1] These articles have been able to be published after passing through various peer review and judging stages. Although many efforts have been made to minimize the errors related to the writing, research method, and other points, criticism and judgment are still open to the reader [1]. According to the investigations of the British Medical Association, more than two-thirds of the articles submitted to the BMJ series of journals are rejected for publication in the initial stages, from the rest; about 98% of the articles also need to be corrected, and only 15% of the experimental medical science articles published in these journals have a scientific basis.[2] They are firm, and the rest, despite repeated revisions before printing, have problems and errors, which are mainly due to methodological errors and due to the noncompliance of the research findings with the discussion and conclusions. One of the most important criteria for evaluating a valuable article is that this article has been used several times in other researchers' articles after being published. The above studies have shown that about two-thirds of the articles published in these journals have never been used or cited in other articles.[3]

In general, five features should be taken into account to express and present scientific materials, and any scientific material that benefits from these features will have more strength and credibility. A scientific article should:

1. Have the characteristics of being verifiable.
2. Have generality and can be generalized to all contents, or components that have similar characteristics.
3. Stay away from the personal, group, and ethnic feelings, emotions, prejudices, and theories.
4. Be dynamic and evolve.
5. Follow the proven scientific findings of previous researchers and not violate previous scientific axioms.

The practitioners of medical sciences for various reasons, such as using it to prepare educational texts; get familiar with scientific news; use it in planning and making decisions; compile, implement, or report a research plan; and sometimes judge an article at the request of a scientific journal with specialized articles, and they are engaged in research. Reading an article is done for any purpose, and writing scientific texts and organizing scientific articles require systematic and fundamental knowledge. To provide suitable conditions

[1] Abdalla SM, et al. BMJ Global Health 2020;5:e002884. doi:10.1136/bmjgh-2020-002884

[2] https://www.bmj.com/about-bmj/publishing-model

[3] https://www.nature.com/articles/d41586–017.08404-0

to fulfill the purpose of the reader, there are principles and regulations in scientific writing that are necessary to know. One of the most important tools for criticizing articles is recognizing research errors. No researcher can consider his/her research free of errors, and in any case, every study has a degree of error that the researcher tries to minimize by using the necessary measures [2].

Of course, it should be noted that clinical errors/mistakes are important topics that require serious attention and is beyond the scope of this book. Medical errors occur when part of what is planned for medical care is not achieved, or care is incorrectly planned from the beginning. Currently, such mistakes cause the death of hundreds of thousands of people every year and cause billions of tomans of damage in the world. Research clearly shows that many biomedical errors are preventable. Standardization of diagnostic and treatment protocols and quality control of these services are among the most important ways to prevent many of these errors.

In the context of medical research, the terms "mistake" and "error" are often used interchangeably, but they can have slightly different meanings. An error is an unintentional deviation from the truth, accuracy, or correctness. In medical research, this could be a miscalculation in statistical analysis or a measurement error in data collection.

On the other hand, a mistake is a failure to achieve a desired outcome even though the person has the knowledge, ability, and resources to perform the task correctly. In medical research, this could be a failure to control for confounding variables or a failure to follow ethical principles in conducting the study.

In summary, an error is unintentional and may be corrected with further analysis, while a mistake is a failure to achieve a desired outcome and may require changes in study design or methodology to correct.

1.2 Sources of Error in Biomedical Studies

Various factors are influential in estimating more, or less of a relationship, or basically (nonscientific) observation. These factors are divided into three important components, which are random errors, chance, and systematic errors (biases and confounders). We will discuss these errors in detail in the next chapter.

1.2.1 Random or Chance

In the context of medical research, the terms "random" and "chance" are often used to describe different phenomena. Random refers to a process that is unpredictable, with no identifiable pattern or order. In medical research, randomization is often used to assign participants to experimental or control groups, with the goal of minimizing bias and ensuring that the groups are comparable in terms of baseline characteristics. Random selection of participants is also important to ensure that the sample is representative of the population being studied.

Chance, on the other hand, refers to an occurrence that is attributable to probability or luck. In medical research, chance plays a role in statistical analysis and hypothesis testing. For example, the probability of obtaining a significant result by chance alone is often set at 5% ($p < 0.05$), meaning that there is a small likelihood that the observed effect is due to random variation rather than a true effect. In summary, random refers to a process that is unpredictable and/or used to minimize bias, while chance refers to the role of probability and statistical analysis in determining the likelihood of obtaining a particular result.

Suppose we want to determine the frequency of back pain in the employees of a large office. It is possible that it is not possible to examine all employees, and in practice, we are only able to determine the frequency of back pain in a sample with a certain volume of this population. In these conditions, it is possible that the sample population was selected from almost healthy employees completely randomly, which causes an underestimation of the number of people suffering from back pain. In other words, random error distorts the results. The smaller the selected sample size, the stronger the effect of coincidence in the results. Statistical methods are used to determine the impact of random errors on the observed results.

1.2.2 Bias

Another important factor is the presence of systematic errors in the design, guidance, or data analysis of each study. This factor is called bias.

An example of bias in medical investigation can occur when the researchers conducting the study have a financial interest in the outcome of the research. For example, a pharmaceutical company may fund a study on a new drug that they manufacture. The researchers may be pressured to produce results that show the drug is effective, or they may be hesitant to publish negative findings that could harm the company's financial interests. This creates a conflict of interest, which can lead to biased results and conclusions that may not be representative of the true effectiveness and safety of the drug. This can lead to potential harm to patients who rely on the drug for treatment.

In general, bias refers to a disproportionate weight given to one side of an argument opinion, or point of view over another. It is an unfair inclination toward certain people, ideas, or statements that affect the interpretation of information, leading to distorted or incomplete understanding of an issue or situation. For example, in a case-control study to investigate the effect of job exposure, with a specific agent, or condition (e.g., working in the country's automobile industry), if the examiner somehow cannot identify the cases and witnesses correctly, the results will be biased. It is known as the observer bias. There are two types of systematic biases, namely, selection bias and information bias. Selection bias occurs when the samples in a study are systematically different from the target population. Information bias is the deviation from the truth that arises in the collection, recall, recording, and handling of information in an investigation.

1.2.3 Confounder

The third factor in distorting scientific relations is the factor of confounder or confounding variable. Confounding occurs when a third factor (known as the confounder) is related to both the independent variable and the outcome variable. An example of confounding in a clinical investigation is when researchers are studying the effect of a new drug on blood pressure. They find that patients taking the drug have significantly lower blood pressure levels than those who did not take the drug. However, they failed to account for the fact that patients who were given the new drug also had a healthier lifestyle than the control group, resulting in a reduced risk of hypertension. In this case, the healthier lifestyle is the confounding variable because it is related to both the use of the new drug and the outcome (lower blood pressure) and affects the study's conclusion about the effectiveness of the new drug.

This situation occurs due to the multiple dependence between the exposure, the disease (outcome), and the third factor that is related to both of them and is effective separately in the development, or progression of the disease (confounding factor). For example, in the observed relationship between air pollution and mortality caused by respiratory system diseases, the existence of a causal relationship between pollution caused by fine particles suspended in the air and respiratory system diseases is a hypothesis whose validity is now questioned because the confounding factor is the ambient temperature. The phenomenon is effective. In general, when the air gets cold in winter, mortality increases, and this issue is also related to the phenomenon of airflow inversion, which causes an increase in air pollution. Considering this factor in the analysis of the findings, the relationship between air pollution and mortality caused by respiratory diseases becomes weaker. Using accurate and reliable equipment; using simple, accurate, and standard tests; repeating tests and using the average of several measurements or measurements; conducting completely random sampling; not using volunteers (even if possible); covering the entire area under investigation; and using tests appropriate statistics, selection of the appropriate number of samples (neither too low nor too low), and formulation of a suitable proposal and proper review and judgment are general measures to prevent errors in research. In the next chapters, we will go into more detail on identifying and controlling common errors in medical science research.

1.3 The Structure and Nature of Clinical Research

Research is a systematic and structured process of investigating a phenomenon or problem in order to gain new knowledge, solve problems, or improve existing understanding of a particular topic. It involves collecting, analyzing, and interpreting data to draw conclusions and create new knowledge. Research can be conducted in various fields, including the natural sciences, social sciences, humanities, and business.

The nature of research can vary depending on the particular goals of the study and the methods used. Some key characteristics of research include the following:

1. Systematic and structured: Research involves a systematic and structured approach to gather and analyze data, using methods that are appropriate for addressing the research question or hypothesis.
2. Objective and unbiased: Research strives to be objective and unbiased, using methods and procedures that do not systematically favor any particular outcome.
3. Rigorous and replicable: Research follows rigorous standards to ensure that the findings are valid and reliable and can be replicated by other researchers.
4. Ethical: Research is carried out in accordance with ethical principles, ensuring that the rights and welfare of human or animal participants are protected.
5. Cumulative: Research builds upon existing knowledge, contributing to the development of a body of knowledge that can inform future research studies.

Overall, the nature of research is characterized by a systematic, objective, and structured approach to investigating a problem or phenomenon, with the goal of advancing knowledge, solving problems, and improving understanding of the world around us.

Every clinical research can be divided into two main elements: the structure of the research and the nature of the research. The structure of the research includes the concrete elements of the study design, that is, the research question, the members under investigation, and the method of measuring the quantity of the sample size. One of the goals of the researcher is to design these elements in such a way that the project can be done cheaply, quickly, and easily. The nature of research includes the mechanism of research. In every research, firstly, what happens in the sample, and then its generalization to the larger society from which the sample was taken, valid inferences about these events are considered as the product, and benefit of each research [3, 4].

1.3.1 Research Structure

The structure of each research is stated in the proposal (protocol) of a study. The proposal is the written part of the research project. The correct arrangement of the proposal helps the researchers to design the analysis steps logically and to focus sufficiently on important and vital issues. Table 1.1 shows the main components of a proposal. In this part, we will give a brief description of each of the items mentioned in the proposed structure of a research project.

Preparing and organizing a regular and structured proposal form, in addition to having a very important role in finding financial resources and motivating officials to carry out the research, also helps the research group to better understand the research stages and find possible shortcomings and flaws in the different stages of the research. For this reason, preparing and organizing the proposal before starting the research project is necessary and helpful. Although every research institute has a special proposal form, the general framework and content of these forms are almost similar. Appendix A is dedicated to how to organize and complete the research proposal.

Table 1.1 An overview of research project proposals

Topic	Objective	Components
Research question	The research is related to which problem?	
Importance of the subject (background)	Why is this issue important to be considered?	
Proposing the problem and stating the issue	What is the study design?	Time frame Epidemiological method Selection criteria Sampling plan
Eligible members	Who are the eligible members for review, and how are they selected?	
Variables	Which factors should be measured, and recorded?	Dependent variables Confounding variables Response variable Hypotheses
Statistical Methods	What is the scope of the study, and how will it be analyzed?	Sample size Data analyzing methods

1.3.1.1 Research Question

The research question in a study is the key goal of that research. This question originates from a nondeterministic theory that the researcher wants to find the answer to. Usually, the initial question created in the minds of researchers is so broad that it is not possible to achieve it at once, and it is usually divided into smaller and simpler components, which are practical and feasible. For example, the initial question may be like this. "Do menopausal women need to take hormones?" This question can be broken down into the following components for implementation: How common is estrogen use in postmenopausal women? How common is the use of estrogen in menopausal women? Does estrogen use after menopause reduce the risk of developing coronary artery disease (CHD)? Are there any other benefits of using hormones?

An appropriate research question should possess the following five characteristics:

- Be applicable.
- Doing it should be attractive for researchers.
- Be novel.
- Be morally acceptable.
- Its benefits and applications are economical regarding the costs, time, and user consumed.

1.3.1.2 Applicability of the Study

One of the important things in designing a research question is for researchers to be aware of the limitations and problems in conducting the study. One of the important issues in this field is the possibility of access to the members of the predicted sample. The first step is to make initial estimates of the number of available samples. The next step is to determine the required sample size for the study. At this stage, the possibility of reducing the effective volume of the sample due to missing members of the sample, incomplete follow-up of the samples, and other such cases should also be taken into consideration. Even in very precise study designs, optimistic predictions are often made about the accessible members of the study. Sometimes, to avoid these inaccuracies in the estimation of study members, it is very appropriate to conduct a guided study.

Another issue is the practicality of the research in terms of technology and the existence of the necessary skills to carry out the research. Researchers should ensure the existence of co-investigator experts and skilled people and the availability of necessary equipment, supplies, sufficient experience, and expertise to motivate and encourage the sample members to participate in the study and continue it, collect research variables, manage the project, and analyze the results to represent [5]. Usually, the best strategy in this field is to use known resources and methods, because the process of creating or developing new methods and testing new skills are usually time-consuming, expensive, and uncertain. When using new methods, such as using a new questionnaire in a study, is unavoidable, researchers must have the ability to redesign and complete these methods successfully. Counseling is usually very useful in cases that are not in the researcher's field of expertise. The use of experts in the fields related to the research topic as project collaborators will have a more favorable effect. For example, it is often necessary to use an expert in biostatistics, or epidemiology from the beginning of the study design to the analysis stage of processing the results in the research group.

Accuracy and cost are also among the limitations that researchers should pay attention to in designing the research question. For expensive studies, it is necessary to provide sufficient financial resources before designing the study. Modifying and limiting the research question is also a suitable solution because low-cost research is done quickly and easily. Table 1.2 shows the possible shortcomings of the research question and study design and how to solve them.

1.3.1.3 Importance of the Subject

In this part, researchers should explain the importance of conducting such research to their audience and specify the benefits of this project and which part of the unknowns will be answered by conducting this research. Sometimes, in this section, researchers list only other studies related to this research that has been done in the past.

1.3.1.4 Study Design

The study design is one of the most complicated and technical parts of any study. This issue will be discussed in detail in the second and third chapters of this book. In Table 1.3, a general classification of types of research projects to conduct a hypothetical study to evaluate the effect of hormone therapy in postmenopausal women is presented.

Table 1.2 Shortcomings and ways to improve the research question and study design

Potential defect solution	Solution
A: The research question does not have one of the five mentioned characteristics	
1. The research question is not applicable because:	
– The research question is very broad	– Being limited to a set of fewer variables – Limiting the scope of the research question
– Inadequacy of population under study	– Expansion of study entry criteria – Removing, or modifying the exclusion criteria – Adding other sources, or centers to reach more samples – Increasing study time – Using solutions to reduce the sample size
– The methods in the study are beyond the scientific ability and experience of the research group	– Inviting experts, and experienced people to cooperate in research – Consulting or searching in specialized texts to find alternative methods
– Research is expensive	– Attention to the possibility of designing less expensive studies – Reduction of sample members, or measurements – Using cheaper tools and equipment – Shortening follow-ups
2. Research topic not being attractive, not new, or not applicable	– Changing, or improving the research question – Consultation with experienced people
3. Uncertainty of compliance with ethical standards	– Consultation with the ethics committee – Changing, or improving the research question
B: The study design is vague and imprecise.	– Revisiting the research question, and objectives – Rewriting the study design based on a standard style. – Accurate determination of sampling methods, measuring variables, conducting follow-ups, and collecting and analyzing results

Source with rewriting: https://writingcenter.unc.edu/tips-and-tools/research-questions/

Table 1.3 How to design clinical research to study the effect of hormone therapy after menopause to prevent CHD

Study design	The main feature	Examples
1. Observational studies		
Cohort study	Following a group over a certain period	Researchers examine a group of postmenopausal women annually for several years in terms of the occurrence of heart attacks, in two groups, those who use hormones and those who do not use hormones
Cross-sectional study	Examining a group in a short period	At one point in time, menopausal women are examined and classified in terms of the prevalence of heart attack and the use or nonuse of hormones
Case-control study	Examination of two groups based on the occurrence or nonoccurrence of the outcome	Researchers compare a group of postmenopausal women who have had a heart attack (cases) with a healthy group (without heart attacks) of postmenopausal women (controls) in terms of hormone use, or not
2. Interventional studies		
Randomized controlled clinical trials	Investigation of two groups who accidentally take hormones or placebo and are unaware of the type of treatment applied	Researchers randomly prescribe hormones or placebos to the population under study, and after following both groups for several years, they compare the incidence of heart attack between the two groups

1.3.1.5 Population under Study

One of the most important decisions in any research is to specify the desired criteria in selecting samples. In general, every design should have the following two criteria:

The inclusion criteria determine the target population, and the exclusion criteria determine which of the studied members do not have the necessary conditions for further follow-up and investigation and should be excluded from the study.

Entry criteria determine the main characteristics of the target community (Table 1.4). The process of determining clinical characteristics often includes making difficult judgments about the selection of important and influential factors in research and how to define them. For example, researchers have to decide, "how should the term 'good general condition' be defined in practice?" Suppose this term should be defined for research on osteoporosis. In this case, it is logical to exclude diseases that do not have much effect on this disease or cause quick death (such as high blood pressure), but diseases that cause osteoporosis, such as paralysis of both legs, or due to quick death. Let's classify those who disturb the follow-up (such as metastases) as sick people. In the case of demographic characteristics (such as age, gender, and race), a balanced state should always be taken into account, which brings the ability to generalize the results and the efficiency of the study. There is no right or wrong decision in this category. The important point is the meaningfulness of the decisions, the stability of the criteria during the study duration, and the comparability of the study with other previous research.

The exclusion criteria identify subgroups of the population that potentially have the possibility of participating in the study based on the research question but due to issues and problems such as the low quality of the data, the inadmissibility of random selection of samples, or the presence of complications. Side effects should be excluded from the study (Table 1.4).

The use of exclusion criteria by reducing the generalizability of the results increases the applicability and makes the interpretation of the results straightforward. For example, the study of a population who do not have a specific place of residence (homeless people) increases the generalizability of the results and makes it possible for researchers to compare the economic

Table 1.4 Setting the selection criteria for a clinical trial that examines the relationship between calcium stores and osteoporosis

	Considerations	Example
Inclusion criteria	The criteria determine the characteristics of the investigated community in terms of being related to the research question and making the study more efficient:	A trial with a five-year follow-up period to investigate the relationship between calcium stores and osteoporosis could include the following:
	Demographic characteristics	White women 50–60 years old
	Clinical features	Good general condition
	Geographical features	Those with a valid postcode
	Features specific to each study	Patients who visit the hospital between May and the end of February of the same year
Exclusion criteria	Determining the criteria determine which subgroups of society will not be examined in the study:	Osteoporosis study can include the following exclusion criteria:
	The possibility of missing patients in the follow-ups	The patient's decision to leave the city of residence
	Inability to provide high-quality data	Not being fluent in the English language
	Being exposed to side effects	Sarcoidosis due to high calcium in the blood
	The unethical nature of experiments on members	Corticosteroid use

and social status with the size of the prevalence in subgroups. However, the mentioned benefits are associated with problems such as increasing the sample size, increasing the missing rate, and complicating the follow-up process. For this reason, researchers can decide not to include homeless people in the study from the beginning. In this case, the separation of the population under study into people who have a fixed place of residence and those who do not have a fixed place to live will be another issue facing the researchers. In the case of clinical trials, the exclusion criteria can be somewhat different. For example, the existence of side effects caused by the use of drugs, ethical issues arising due to not taking the drug, the ineffectiveness of the drug used on the patients, the possibility of patients being lost in the follow-up, and the patient not being eligible to receive the drug are among the cases that can be the exclusion criteria. be from the study [6].

Appendix B examines two important methods of collecting information, namely, questionnaires and interviews.

1.3.1.6 Sampling Methods

Another important part of any research is deciding how to collect study units. These units can be people, hospitals, residential houses, pharmacies, or stores. The important part of how to collect the units is to decide on the use of the information in the files, registration data, and written records, or sampling and completing the information needed for the research through questionnaires or interviews. Researchers should consider issues such as the cost of sampling or collecting existing information, sampling error, registration statistics, project execution time, facilities, and experienced and trained staff in the proposal drafting stage and decide this issue.

In general, there are two sampling methods, which are known as the probability and the non-probability sampling method. Probability sampling is a term used by Deming in 1950. In probability sampling, each sample unit is extracted from the population with a certain probability. This method has expanded rapidly since 1940 and has replaced non-probability sampling in almost all applications.

In the non-probabilistic method, probabilities are not assigned to the selected units, and as a result, it is not possible to determine the accuracy of the sampling results. The non-probability sampling used in the 1920s and 1930s was mainly judgmental, purposive sampling and quota sampling.

Probability sampling includes methods such as random sampling, variable probability sampling, stratified sampling, cluster sampling (one-stage, two-stage, and multistage), and systematic sampling. The technical discussions related to the concepts, how to perform and calculate the desired estimates of these methods, are outside the scope of this book, and readers can read sources such as [7–9] and [5] for further study.

1.3.2 Variables

Usually, every research project includes measuring, observing, and recording some variables. The type of these variables, the method of measurement, the degree of accuracy, and the validity of the results are a topic that will be examined in the fifth chapter.

In general, the variables have a qualitative or quantitative scale. Qualitative variables are divided into two categories: nominal and ranked variables. Nominal variables are variables that do not have an ordering nature. Examples of this type of variable are different religions that can include Christian, Muslim, and Jewish and how to go to work by car, bicycle, bus, metro, and pedestrian. In nominal variables, the listing method does not have an ordering pattern.

Many variables have an ordering scale. These variables are called ranked variables. Examples of this type of scale are social class including prosperous, average, and poor and disease status including well, suitable, severe, and critical. Ordering variables have an order (ranking), but the distance between each rank is not known.

Quantitative variables have a numerical scale, and the distance between each of the values is known. For example, blood pressure, life expectancy, and monthly income are examples of this. Sometimes quantitative variables are also called ratio variables. In these types of variables, the ratio of two values is also meaningful.

The way to measure each variable determines its nature. For example, if education is classified as a public school, or a nonprofit school, it has a nominal scale, and if it is classified based on the level of education, that is, elementary, middle school, high school, post-graduate, and higher, it has a ranked scale, and when it is classified based on the number of years of education, that is, 1, 2, 3, etc., it has a quantitative scale.

Variables are divided into three groups based on their relationship with each other.

The response variable (dependent): These variables are the result of the final response or the effect of previous events. For example, in the relationship between intelligence and educational progress, educational progress is the response variable, and in the relationship between skin cancer and direct sunlight, skin cancer is the response variable.

Independent variable (exposure variable in observational studies, or intervention in experimental studies): These variables are responsible for the cause or justification of the consequences that happened and affect other variables in a way (which can be a cause and effect). In the above two examples, intelligence and direct sunlight are independent variables.

Confounding or background variable: Usually, when examining the relationship between two variables, other variables influence the strength of the relationship. For example, to investigate a new drug for lowering blood pressure, factors such as age, gender, race, diet, other diseases that a person is suffering from, the amount of daily activity, etc. can be effective. These variables can be associated, mediating, or confounding. In this case, observing the real relationship between blood pressure and drug consumption is only possible with special statistical methods that are mentioned in the next chapters.

1.3.2.1 Research Hypothesis

One of the elements of every study is the research question. In some studies, it is necessary to turn the research question into a technical version called a hypothesis so that the basis of the statistical tests appropriate to the research can be designed. Each hypothesis contains a summary of the elements of the study: sample, study design, response variable, and independent variable. It is not necessary to present a hypothesis in descriptive studies that show how the characteristics and traits of the population under study are distributed in society (such as prevalence studies), but it is necessary to make a hypothesis in analytical studies that aim to compare the findings in two, or more different groups (such as clinical trials). Since in most observational studies (such as cohort and case-control studies) the goal is to compare different groups with each other, we need to build at least one hypothesis.

If any of the following expressions are present in the research question, "greater than," "less than," "cause," "lead to," compared to "(compared with)," "more likely than," "associated with," "related to," "similar to," or "correlated with" (correlated with), the study will no longer be a simple descriptive study, and a hypothesis must be formulated for it.

1.3.2.2 Characteristics of a Good Hypothesis

Each of the hypotheses must be stated clearly and simply.

Simple or Complex In simple hypothesis, there is a dependent and an independent variable (a sedentary lifestyle is associated with an increased risk of protein in the urine in diabetic patients). In the complex hypothesis, there is more than one independent variable (inactivity lifestyle and alcohol consumption are related to increasing the risk of protein in the urine in diabetic patients), or dependent variable (alcohol consumption is related to increasing the risk of protein in the urine and neuropathy in diabetic patients). Complex hypotheses like the ones above are not suitable for investigation by a simple statistical test and can be easily separated into two or more simple hypotheses.

However, sometimes, independent or compound-dependent variables are also used (use of cigarettes, hookah, or pipe is associated with increasing the risk of protein in the urine in diabetic patients).

Clear, or Ambiguous Any specific hypothesis does not leave any vague and double-sided points about the subject, variables, and type of statistical test (the history of using tricyclic antidepressants, which is obtained by referring to the patient's medical records), in patients admitted to the hospital due to heart attack Modares Shahid Beheshti University of Medical Sciences last year is more common than the control group which includes patients admitted to the same hospital during this period due to pneumonia.

Usually, by the research hypothesis, the type of variable is determined in terms of nominal, continuous, or rank. In cases where this issue is not clear, the type of variable should be specified (alcohol consumption in mg/day). It is related to the increased risk of protein in the urine (>30 mg/dl) in diabetic patients).

If any of the definitions and corrections, units, and scales are defined elsewhere in the proposal, it is not necessary to include all of them in the hypothesis, which makes the sentences of the hypothesis longer.

Statistical Hypotheses

To perform statistical tests, the hypotheses must be stated in such a way that the expected differences between different study groups can be formulated.

The Null Hypothesis and Opposite Hypothesis The null hypothesis is formulated on the basis that there is no relationship between the independent variable and the response variable in society (there is no relationship between the frequency of consumption of healthy water and the presence of stomach ulcers). The null hypothesis is the basic basis for the formation of statistical tests. Assuming no dependence between the community groups, statistical tests calculate the probability of a chance relationship between the response variable and the independent variable.

The sentence that states the existence of a relationship between the response and independent variables is the opposite hypothesis (there is an inverse relationship between the frequency of consumption of safe and hygienic water and the presence of stomach ulcers).

Opposite One-Way and Two-Way Hypotheses In the one-way hypothesis, the direction of the relationship (direct, or inverse) between the response variable and the independent is specified. For example, the statement "Sanitary water consumption is different in people with peptic ulcers compared to healthy people" is a two-way hypothesis. In the two-way hypothesis, only the issue of the existence of communication (not its direction) is meant. For example, when we state that "the frequency of consumption of healthy and hygienic water in people with a gastric ulcer is different compared to healthy people," we have made a two-sided hypothesis.

The one-way hypothesis is used in special situations such as when the relationship is only important in one direction or is biologically meaningful. For example, in terms of the effectiveness of a new drug compared to a placebo, the possibility of a new drug being more effective than a placebo in improving the disease is not always correct. But the important issue is the efficiency of the new drug. Therefore, the one-sided hypothesis is a suitable choice. When based on previous studies, there is evidence and clues to confirm the relationship in one direction (such as investigating the relationship between smoking and increasing the risk of brain cancer), it is also appropriate to use a one-way hypothesis. However, researchers should note that many of the hypotheses that have been strongly supported (such as beta-carotene treatment in reducing the risk of lung cancer) have been strongly rejected in randomized trials. Choosing a one-sided hypothesis or a two-sided hypothesis is important in determining the sample size.

1.3.3 Calculation of Sample Size

After determining the research topic, type of study, and sampling method, the next step is to decide on the number of sample members. Even in very simple and clear plans in terms of content and implementation method, when the sample size is not enough, we are not able to scientifically and accurately investigate the research question. On the other hand, when the sample size is too large, time, cost, and facilities are wasted. The goal of determining the sample size is to estimate the optimal number of members needed in the study.

Although the issue of determining the sample size is considered a useful tool in research, another important goal in calculating the sample size is to achieve a clear perspective of the acceptability of the statistical tests used in the study. The validity of the obtained sample size is directly related to the validity of the information and data based on which the calculation was made (which usually remains speculative). The calculation of the sample size determines the feasibility of the study design. Calculating the sample size in the initial stage of study design, when there is still the possibility of making fundamental changes in the study design, helps researchers to change methods, control other variables, or limit the study if the number of required samples is too high. Therefore, the calculation of the sample size should be done in the initial stages of the study and during the design of the proposal, where there is still the possibility of fundamental changes.

In this part, we examine some basic statistical concepts to calculate the sample size.

1.3.3.1 The Minimal Clinically Significant Difference

The chance that a study based on sampling will reveal a relationship between the response variable and the independent variable depends to a great extent on the strength of the relationship in the target population. For example, if the average fasting blood sugar (FBS) in diabetic women who exercise is 20 mg/dl lower than in women who do not exercise, it is easier to demonstrate this difference (and as a result, infer the existence of a relationship between exercise and diabetes control) than when this difference is assumed to be 2 mg/dl.

Unfortunately, researchers are usually unaware of whether the real difference in society is large or small. One of the goals of the study is usually to estimate the effect size. For this reason, studies usually use the minimum amount of clinically important difference or the minimum amount of difference that the researcher wants to show in the study. This quantity is called effect size in clinical research. Choosing the appropriate effect size is the most difficult part of sample size estimation. For this purpose, the information obtained from previous studies should be reviewed first to obtain acceptable estimates of the effect size. When there is no acceptable information, it is probably necessary to conduct a pilot study.

1.3.3.2 Errors of Type I, Type II, and the Power of a Test

Sometimes, based on chance alone, the selected sample is not a suitable representative of the study population. In this case, the results obtained from the sample do not reflect the realities in society, and the inferences made are incorrect. Type 1 error occurs when the researcher rejects the null hypothesis (based on the sample at hand), but in the target population, the null hypothesis is true. Type II error occurs when the researcher does not reject the null hypothesis (based on the sample at hand) when the null hypothesis is not true in the target population. In this case, we are faced with four situations. Table 1.5 examines these modes.

Determining the maximum allowed value for the occurrence of each of the errors I and II is one of the important parts of any study. The probability of the first type of error is called a significance level.

Table 1.5 Different modes of statistical judgments and the realities of society

	The realities of society	
The results obtained from the sample	The existence of a relationship between response, and independent variables	Absence of relationship between response, and independent variables
Rejection of the null hypothesis	Correct	Error type I
Acceptance of the null hypothesis	Error type II	Correct

For example, in the study of the effect of exercise on diabetes control, if the alpha level is considered equal to 0.05, it means that the researcher has a maximum chance of 5% for rejecting the null hypothesis incorrectly (i.e., inferring that exercise and fasting blood sugar levels have are related if they are not related to each other), which has accepted.

The probability of the error type II is called beta, and based on this, the power of the test is defined as 1 minus beta. If we consider it equal to 0.1, in this case, we have accepted to ignore the relationship that exists in 10% of the cases with the size of the effect that has been determined in advance. This issue is equivalent to the test power of 0.9, which means that the inference is correct 90% of the time. For example, suppose that exercise lowers fasting blood sugar by 20 mg/dl in diabetics. Now, if the researcher takes several samples from society and repeats the same procedure for all the members of the samples every time, in 90 studies out of 100 studies, the researcher will be able to reject the null hypothesis that there is no relationship. However, this does not mean that the researcher can reveal smaller effects such as a reduction of 10 mg/dl with the same sample size under high conditions.

Ideally, alpha and beta should be zero, but in practice, these two errors should be made as small as possible. This issue is usually possible by enlarging the sample size. The main goal in calculating the sample size is to control alpha and beta at an acceptable level for the researcher, without making the study unnecessarily difficult, time-consuming, and expensive.

1.3.4 Response Variable Changes

Another important point that is considered in determining the sample size is the size of the changes (standard deviation) of the response variable. The greater the standard deviation of the response variable in the subjects under study, the more likely it is that there will be an overlap in

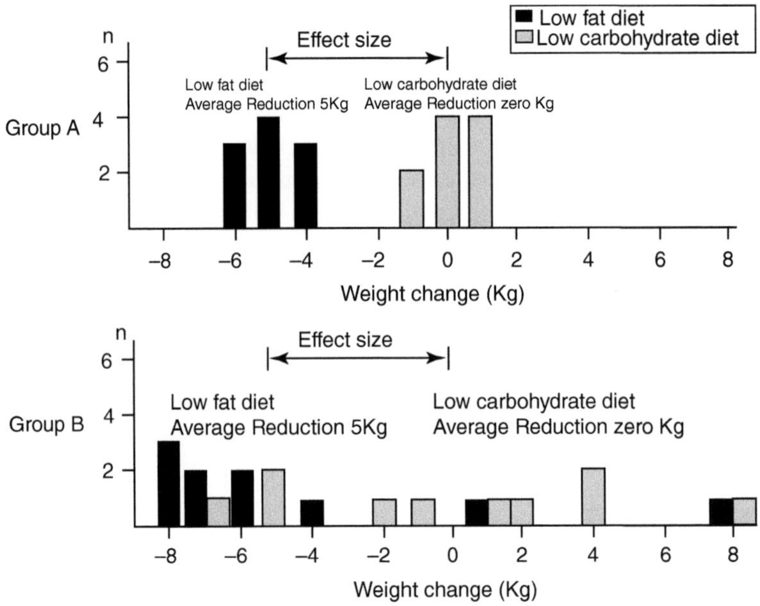

Fig. 1.1 A weight loss by following two types of diet is shown. The members of the low-fat diet group all lost between 4 and 6 kg, while the weight loss in the low-carbohydrate diet group fluctuated from −1 to 1 kg. Therefore, the effect size of these two diets is 5 kg, since a low-fat diet compared to a low-carbohydrate diet. Graph B also shows the weight loss there is no overlap between the two groups, it seems logical to conclude that there is superiority in the use of a low-fat diet compared to a low-carbohydrate diet. Graph B also shows the weight loss resulting from the two diets. In this figure, a wide overlap can be seen in the two groups, and some members in each group have gained weight. In this case, the size of the effect is 5 kg and in favor of the low-fat diet. However, the results of the study do not provide solid evidence that a low-fat diet is better than a low-carbohydrate diet

the response values of the groups. In this case, it is more difficult to reveal the differences in the groups, and naturally, a larger sample size is needed.

For example, consider a study to investigate two diets for weight loss in 20 volunteers. These diets include a low-fat diet and a low-carbohydrate diet. If all volunteers with a low-fat diet lose 5 kg on average and volunteer with a low-carbohydrate diet does not lose weight (effect size equal to 5 kg), it can be concluded that the low-fat diet is better (Fig. 1.1A). However, if the weight loss in the low-fat diet group is 5 kg and the low-carb group remains unchanged, there may be an overlap in the weight loss distribution of the two groups, as shown in Fig. 1.1B. In such situations, inference about the existence of a difference between the two regimes requires a larger sample size [9].

Appendix C is devoted to the study of sample size calculation methods for some statistical indicators.

1.3.4.1 *P*.Value

After collecting and analyzing the data, we need a standard criterion to reject the null hypothesis. This criterion is called probability value in statistical analysis. The probability value is a number between zero and one that specifies how likely the effect size is considered by the researcher or any effect size larger than this value is accepted by chance. When the null hypothesis is rejected and the opposite hypothesis (the existence of a relationship) is accepted, the numerical probability value is less than alpha (the value of which is determined before the test, e.g., 0.05 or 0.01). When the results are not statistically significant, that is, when the probability value is greater than alpha, it only means that the results observed in the sample are weaker than what could have happened based on chance (alpha value). For example, a researcher may conclude his research that people with high blood pressure are twice as likely to develop prostate cancer than normal

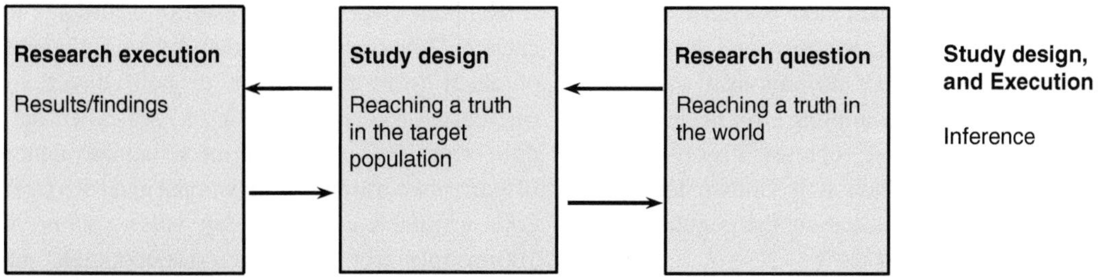

Fig. 1.2 The process of research design and implementation and the stage of making inferences and general conclusions

people. Only because the number of people with cancer in the study was relatively small and they were randomly placed in the group with high blood pressure, the probability value was equal to 0.18. This shows that even if blood pressure and prostate cancer have no relationship, in 18% of the cases, it is only possible to observe a significant relationship from a statistical point of view.

We must be very careful to interpret and draw scientific conclusions from the p-value. It should be noted that the p-value may sometimes be associated with misunderstanding and misinterpretation. For example, a lack of statistical significance does not indicate a small effect size, or a *P* value assumes that the test hypothesis is true—it is not a probability of the hypothesis and may be different from a logical association or non-association [10].

1.3.5 How to Statistically Analyze the Results

Setting up the research project, determining the sample size and statistical power of the tests, and determining how to carry out each of the inferences and appropriate statistical methods to achieve the desired goals in each research are measures that researchers should consider before implementing the plan and mention them in the research proposal.

1.3.5.1 Nature of Research

The goal of every clinical research is to make inferences from the results of the study about reality in the world. To achieve this issue, two separate steps must be designed and implemented. The first step of designing a clinical study includes the selection of sample units, measurement of the required variables, data collection, and analysis of the results to obtain the appropriate answer to the research question and its generalization to the target population.

The next step includes the correct conclusion of what happened in the study. In other words, it is a careful examination of the research process to achieve results that are as close to reality as possible. This process is presented in Fig. 1.2.

1.4 Sources of Error in the Design and Execution of the Study

Of course, no research is error-free. For this reason, the inferences made on this basis are never completely correct and valid. In general, one of the goals of designing any study is to maximize the validity of the study results.

There are several potential sources of error in study design, which can have significant impacts on the results and conclusions drawn from a research study. Some common sources of error include the following:

1. Bias: Bias occurs when there is a systematic deviation from the true value of a measurement, due to factors such as nonrandom sampling, measurement errors, or confounding variables. Bias can lead to inaccurate results and incorrect conclusions.
2. Confounding: Confounding occurs when two variables are associated in such a way that it is difficult to determine their individual effects.

This can occur when there is a third factor that influences both the exposure and the outcome, leading to incorrect attributions of causality.
3. Sampling error: Sampling error occurs when a study sample is not representative of the population from which it is drawn, leading to incorrect inferences about the population as a whole.
4. Measurement error: Measurement error occurs when the tools or methods used to measure a variable are not accurate or precise, leading to incorrect estimates or conclusions.
5. Selection bias: Selection bias occurs when the selection of study participants is not random or representative, leading to the over- or underrepresentation of certain groups and potentially biased results.
6. Information bias: Information bias occurs when there are errors or inaccuracies in the data collected or reported, leading to incorrect conclusions.

The best strategy to reduce errors in the study is a reflection and sufficient accuracy in the research design phase. Error prevention is more practical and cost-effective than any other action, although it should be noted that some errors are uncontrollable in the information analysis stage. Research errors are divided into random errors and systematic errors. Figure 1.3 shows the control methods of these errors.

Random errors are the result of errors due to chance. Unknown sources that distort the results obtained from the sample in both directions (increasing risk, or decreasing it) are called random errors. For example, if the actual prevalence of estrogen hormone use in women aged 50–69 is 20%, a suitable sampling plan with a volume of 100 people from the relevant population can include exactly 20 cases with this characteristic, although the possibility of having 18, 19, 20, or 22 cases is completely possible. It is possible. Chance or random error can rarely even produce results that are completely different from reality, such as 9 or 35. Among various proposed methods to reduce the effect of random error, the most obvious and simple one is to increase the sample size. Using more samples reduces the possibility of seeing wrong results by increasing the accuracy of the study.

Systematic errors are the result of errors due to bias. In systematic error, the results are directionally distorted. For example, choosing sample units from women visiting the clinic to estimate the prevalence of estrogen use will most likely cause an overestimation of the actual amount. Increasing the sample size has no effect in controlling or improving systematic error. The only way to reduce systematic errors is to increase the validity of the research. This issue is equivalent to knowing biased sources in the study and removing or modifying their work.

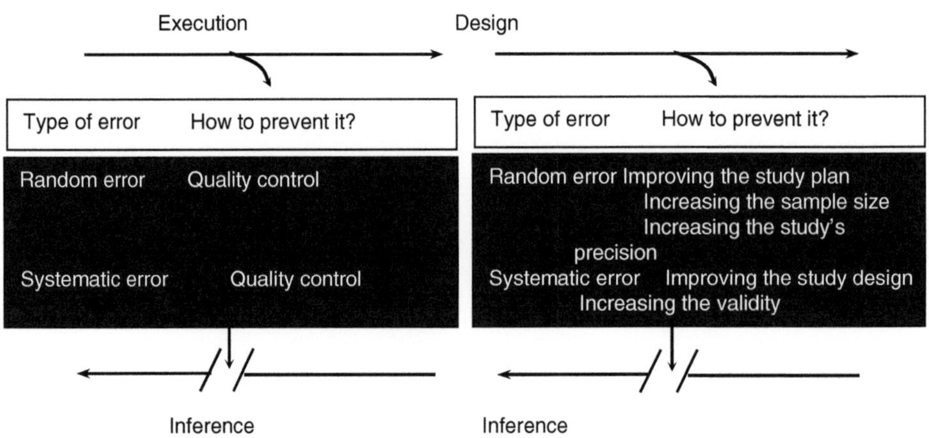

Fig. 1.3 How to control research errors

1.4.1 Study Design

The study design in medicine refers to the overall plan or structure of a research study that is designed to investigate a medical or healthcare-related question. There are several types of study designs used in medicine, each with its own strengths and weaknesses. Some common study designs used in medicine include the following:

1. Randomized controlled trial (RCT): This study design is considered one of the gold standards in medical research. In this design, participants are randomly assigned to either a treatment group or a control group, and outcomes are compared between the two groups. RCTs are particularly useful for testing new treatments and interventions.
2. Cohort study: In this study design, a group of individuals (the cohort) is identified and followed over a period of time, with data collected on various factors such as exposures, outcomes, and potential confounding variables. Cohort studies are useful for examining the association between an exposure and a particular outcome.
3. Case-control study: In this study design, individuals with a particular outcome or health condition (cases) are compared to individuals without the outcome (controls). Data is collected on various exposures and potential confounding variables to determine which factors may be associated with the outcome.
4. Cross-sectional study: In this study design, data is collected on a group of individuals at a single point in time. This type of study is useful for examining the prevalence of a particular health condition or risk factor within a population.
5. Systematic review and meta-analysis: These study designs involve the synthesis of data from multiple studies, usually RCTs, to draw conclusions about the effectiveness of a particular treatment or intervention.

Overall, the choice of study design in medicine depends on the research question, the type of data needed, and the available resources. Different study designs have different strengths and limitations, and careful consideration of these factors is important in order to ensure the validity and reliability of study findings.

The research question, as explained earlier, is a topic that researchers want to find answers about. To make things easier, we follow the topic with a simple example. Suppose we want to know the prevalence of using iron drops in one-year-old children.

It is impossible to answer this question with 100% accuracy because it is practically impossible to examine all children under 1 year old. For this reason, researchers should design another research question that can be checked. This question can be asked as follows: "What is the prevalence of using iron drops among one-year-old children who are taken to the health center for examination?"

One of the key components in turning the comprehensive research question into a researchable question is choosing a sample that will be a suitable substitute for society. For example, limiting the study to children taken to health centers is a debatable decision that was taken only because of the practical obstacles in choosing the subjects under study.

The next point is to select the variables that can be measured to check the status of the desired variable. Using a questionnaire to measure the prevalence of iron drop use is one of the quick and cheap methods to collect the necessary information, but using this method will not be completely accurate because some parents have given drops to their children, but now they have forgotten, or some may answer this question incorrectly because they did not understand the word "iron drop" in the questionnaire, or they do not know what kind of drop have been given to their children.

In general, the difference created between the comprehensive question of the research and the main design of the study is one of the sources of error that can lead to wrong findings [9, 11–13] Fig. 1.4 shows the common occurrence of these errors in the design of each study.

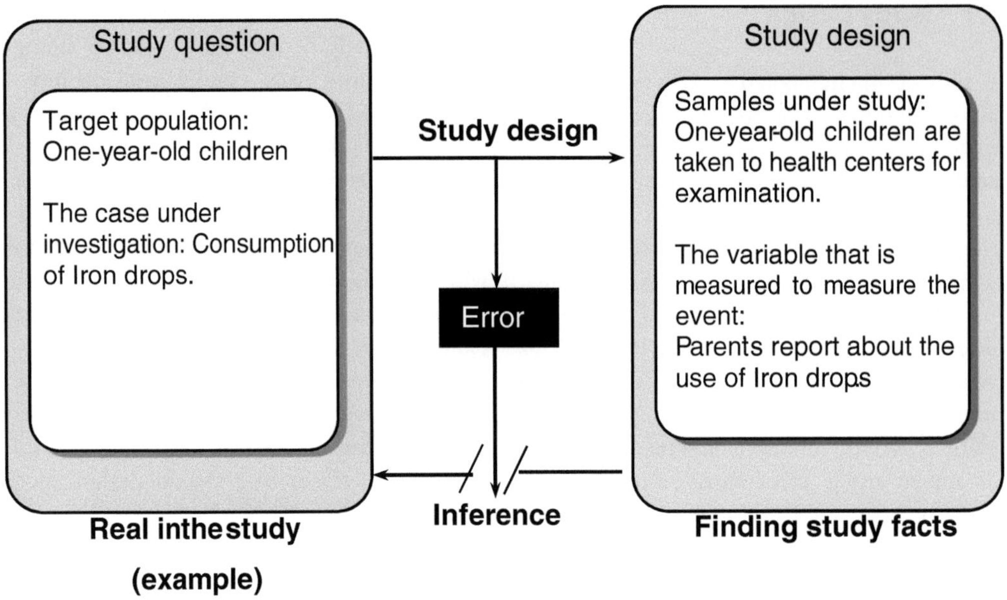

Fig. 1.4 Sources of error in the design of a hypothetical study

1.4.2 Implementation of Study

The actual members under study in any research are almost always different from the sample that should be collected. Consider the sampling design of one-year-old children taken to health centers.

Only 875 cases may be available from the 1000 samples previously selected to determine the prevalence. People who were not available or refused to cooperate may be different from others in some ways, and this issue will change the prevalence of using iron drops among them. Apart from this issue, things like the complexity of the questionnaire phrases and the illegibility of the sentences are also factors that can cause not answering a question, or giving wrong answers to questions. These obvious differences from the actual design of the study and its implementation cause changes or distortion of the answers. Figure 1.5 shows the role of other error sources that may occur during the execution phase.

A detailed explanation and more examples about random and systematic errors, how to increase the accuracy and validity of the study, and the methods of evaluating the accuracy and validity of the research results are the topics that are studied in the fourth chapter.

Appendix A provides more information about the regulation of research proposals.

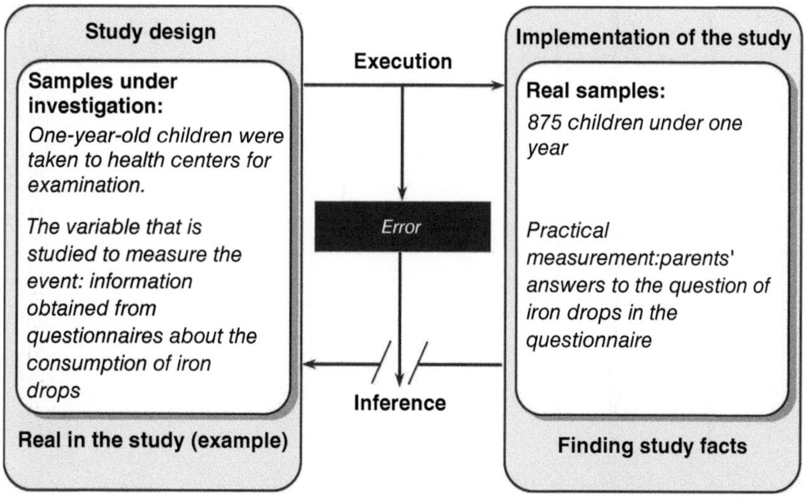

Fig. 1.5 Sources of error in the implementation of an unrealistic study

References

1. Greenhalgh T. How to read a paper: the basics of evidence-based medicine, and healthcare. 6th ed. Vancouver: John Wiley & Sons LTD; 2019.
2. Hall GM. How to write a paper. 5th ed. Vancouver: BMJ Publishing Group; 2012.
3. Kuhn TS. The structure of scientific revolutions: 50th anniversary edition. 4th ed. Vancouver: University of Chicago Press; 2012.
4. Hulley SB, et al. Designing clinical research: an epidemiologic approach. 2nd ed. Vancouver: Lippincott Williams & Wilkins; 2001.
5. Sakpal TV. Sample size estimation in a clinical trial. Perspect Clin Res. 2010;1(2):67.9.
6. United Nations Office on Drugs and Crimes (UNODC). Ethical challenges in drug epidemiology: issues, principles, and guidelines. Global Assessment Programme on Drug Abuse (GAP), Toolkit Module 7. Vancouver; 2004.
7. Latpate R, Kshirsagar J, Gupta VK, Chandra G. Advanced sampling methods. Singapore: Springer; 2021.
8. Basti M, Madadizadeh F. A beginner's guide to sampling methods in medical research. Crit Comments Biomed. 2021;2:2. https://doi.org/10.18502/ccb.v2i2.7397.
9. Amidi A. Theory of sampling, and its applications, first, and second volumes. Tehran: Academic Publishing Center; 2018.
10. Greenland S, Senn SJ, Rothman KJ, Carlin JB, Poole C, Goodman SN, Altman DG. Statistical tests, P values, confidence intervals, and power: a guide to misinterpretations. Eur J Epidemiol. 2016;31(4):337.350. https://doi.org/10.1007/s10654-016-0149-3.
11. Soori H. Evaluating and appraisal of epidemiological scientific papers. J Guilan Univ Med Sci. 2002;11(41):64–9.
12. Kulakowski E, Chronister LU. Research administration and management. United Kingdom: Jones & Bartlett Learning; 2006.
13. Chow SC, Shao J, Wang H, Lokhnygina Y. Sample size in clinical research. 2nd ed. Vancouver: CRC Press, Taylor & Francis Group, Chapman & Hall book; 2020.

2 Research Design Strategies in Medical Sciences and their Potential Specific Errors

2.1 Introduction

Choosing a study method to achieve research objectives can be seen as choosing a way to reach a destination. For example, if you want to go from Turin to Rome, you may choose a private car, bus, train, plane, or another vehicle, even bicycle or foot. This choice depends on various factors including the amount of money you want to spend, the amount of time you have for this trip, the safety of the vehicle, and so on. Choosing the most suitable vehicle can help you achieve your travel goals better. Various approaches to classify studies in medical sciences can be found in the literature. Qualitative–quantitative, basic–applied, observational–experimental, descriptive–analytical/causal and types of research methods such as ecological, cross-sectional, experimental, case-control, and cohort are among them.

When it comes to studying biomedical investigation, here are some tips for choosing a study method:

1. Read important papers: A lot of learning in biomedical investigation happens through reading scientific papers. Try to find papers related to the subject you're studying and read them thoroughly. Take notes and try to understand the concepts and methodologies presented.
2. Take notes during lectures: If you're attending lectures on biomedical investigation, make sure to take detailed notes. Pay attention to the key points the lecturer is emphasizing, and ask questions if you're unclear about anything.
3. Participate in group discussions: Discussing the topics with peers is a great way to deepen your understanding of biomedical investigation. By exchanging ideas and perspectives, you can gain new insights that you might not have considered before.
4. Use visualization tools: Creating diagrams, charts, and other visual aids can help you understand complex biochemical pathways and structures. This can be a useful study method for those who learn better through visual aids.
5. Use online resources: There are plenty of online resources available that provide further information on the subject of biomedical investigation. Online courses, webinars, and online communities can help you stay up-to-date with the latest developments in the field.
6. Practice problem-solving: Try to solve problems related to the subject of biomedical investigation. This could involve designing experiments, analyzing data, or interpreting results. This will help you develop your critical thinking skills and better understand the practical aspects of biomedical investigation.

H. Soori, *Errors in Medical Science Investigations*, https://doi.org/10.1007/978-981-99-8521-0_2

In general, studies in medical sciences can be divided into two major categories, observational and interventional; each of these two categories is based on attributes such as the data collection unit, time orientation, the method of collecting information or samples, and the role of researchers in the contact of the subjects under study with exposures. The studied items are divided into smaller subgroups. Choosing the correct research methodology can determine the success and quality of your study. This chapter is dedicated to the research design strategies in medical sciences and their potential specific errors. In this chapter, we focus on quantitative studies with some brief explanations of qualitative ones. In the quantitative research method, the data can be collected in many ways like experiments, surveys, existing data (such as publications or archival data), observations, and content analysis.

2.2 Basic Issues in Choosing a Research Approach

An important decision about study design involves the approach to be used to study a topic. The choice of study method and its design depends on various factors. Usually, researchers are interested in choosing an authentic study method with minimal errors in research, but practical limitations and obstacles make a study with a smaller scope, more limited goals, and less scientific ability to be designed and implemented [1]. In choosing the study method, first of all, one should have full knowledge of what is called the final goal of the study and pay attention to the advantages and limitations of each type of study plan, availability, and facilities, as well as the feasibility of the study. Some of the effective factors in choosing the study method are as follows:

- The purpose of the study.
- Measurement of events.
- Determining the relationship between risk factors and outcome.
- Study about the causes of disease.
- Ability to study.
- Accessibility to the study subjects.
- Tools and raw materials.
- Research personnel, time, and budget.
- Validity of the study.
- Sources of error (random and systematic).

Here are some indicators to consider when choosing an investigation study design:

1. Research question: The research question or hypothesis that will guide the study should be clear and concise. This will help determine the appropriate study design.
2. Study objectives: The study objectives should be clearly defined, such as the primary outcome measures and the secondary or exploratory ones.
3. Sample size: The sample size of the study will depend on the research question, the study design, and the statistical power required. The larger the sample size, the more accurate the results, but larger sample sizes may also be more expensive and time-consuming.
4. Study population: The population under study should be clearly defined along with any inclusion/exclusion criteria.
5. Ethics committee: Approval from an ethics committee or institutional review board may be required depending on the nature of the study with respect to participants, ethical considerations, and research methods.
6. Time frame: The timeframe of the study will depend on the research question, the study design, and the availability of resources. Some studies may extend over several years, while others may be completed within a few months.
7. Study design options: Different study designs can be chosen based on the research question and objectives, such as observational studies, cross-sectional studies, case-control studies, cohort studies, randomized controlled trials, and meta-analyses.

Ultimately, the appropriate study design depends on the research question, objectives, population under study, constraints, and ethical considerations. It is essential to consult with experts and special interest groups to determine the most appropriate study design for your research question.

2.3 Types of Biomedical Studies

There are several types of biomedical studies, including in general, biomedical studies, which can be divided into two categories (although other categorizations have been presented) [2].

The first category of studies is based on observations, and the second category is studies that are carried out by conducting interventions on the people under study. Based on this, the two main groups of medical studies are as follows:

- Observational studies.
- Intervention or experimental studies.

On the other hand, studies can be classified into two general categories: descriptive studies and analytical studies or quantitative and qualitative studies. Most medical science studies are quantitative. Qualitative studies are rooted in social sciences. The report of a qualitative study is full of text rather than the expression of numbers, and the qualitative study researcher accepts that the entire study can be done in an atmosphere with mental strain. Among the methods of data collection in qualitative studies, we can mention the Delphi method and the focused group discussion method.

Descriptive studies are focused on describing the distribution of the disease or event under study. For example, paying attention to the following cases in which populations or subgroups of the population the disease occurs or does not occur, in which geographical locations, there is the highest or lowest prevalence of the disease, or how the frequency of the disease changes over time, questions whose information is provided by using descriptive studies. Information about each of these characteristics can provide clues to formulate a hypothesis that is compatible with the existing knowledge about the occurrence of the disease [3].

Analytical studies are focused on the determinants of a disease with a hypothesis that is formulated in descriptive studies. These studies aim to identify the risk factors of the disease. Another category of analytical studies are intervention studies, in these studies, two or more treatment methods, diet, management method, and the like, which are called interventions (interventions are usually randomly assigned to the subgroups under study), with each other.

The design of each descriptive or analytical study has its unique strengths and limitations. Since this issue requires a general understanding of all types of studies and their internal relationships to provide a theoretical and scientific basis, in this chapter, we will have a brief look at all types of study plans. Table 2.1 shows an overview of the classification of medical study plans. More topics in this field will be presented in the third chapter.

2.3.1 Descriptive Studies

A descriptive study, as its name suggests, describes the characteristics and general characteristics of the distribution of a disease concerning person, place, and time [4]. Descriptive studies are divided into three categories of individual studies and correlation and cross-sectional studies in terms of comparing disease frequencies between different groups. Potential errors in descriptive studies are mainly:

- Population specification errors (occur when researchers don't know precisely who to survey. For example, who is the parent? mother? father? both? or guardian?).
- Survey sampling and sample frame errors. (These happen when the researcher does not know who should be questioned. For example, to answer the question, what is the common family breakfast? In a family, one person may prepare breakfast, which affects the choices of the whole family. He/she should be the respondent and not another family member!)

Table 2.1 Classification of some quantitative study designs in biomedicine

Type of study	Overall specifications
(a) Observational studies	It explores a wide range of goals, from studying the first hint of a potential cause of a disease to confirming the magnitude of previously reported associations. From clinical to biological and environmental observations
Descriptive	They describe: What is the intended event? (What), on whom is the study done and what are their characteristics? (Who), in what place? (where) and in what time frame? (when) They can be an introduction to analytical and interventional studies
Case study	Expressing the full details of a case or cases of a disease with unusual and remarkable features
Case-series	A descriptive report of a group of people (in aggregated form) who have a common disease with unusual symptoms, complications, or treatment
Normative	Normative research represents normal responses to stimuli in a defined population at a specific time.
Ecologic	They show the relationship (association) between two (or more) variables through the correlation coefficient, but association alone does not prove the causation. It is usually based on routinely collected information
Longitudinal	It is a type of correlational and descriptive research in which researchers observe some variables and collect them over time
Historical	By systematically collecting and evaluating data to describe and inform the public of actions or events that talks about a time that happened in the past. There is no intervention
KAP (Knowledge, Attitude, Practice)	It examines the knowledge, attitude, and practice of a group about a phenomenon. They are quantitative methods and a good way to evaluate healthcare services
(b) Research-based on existing data	
Secondary data analysis	Research data that has already been gathered can be accessed by researchers for more analyses. Common sources of existing secondary data include data collected by medical and health services department records, libraries, internet searches, and censuses
Ancillary	An independent study that uses samples from a primary study to expand knowledge in scientific areas beyond the primary scope of the primary study. Sometimes a side study needs additional data or sample collection, but it cannot interfere with the primary objectives of the main study
Systematic review and meta-analysis	They answer defined research questions by collecting and summarizing all empirical evidence with some criteria.
(c) Cross-sectional	A cross-sectional study determines the relationship between diseases and other desired variables in the conditions existing in a certain society and at a certain time. It is similar to a snapshot of an event
(d) Case-control	Subjects are examined as to whether they have the disease (cases) or not (controls). Then, cases and controls are compared concerning exposure to an agent
(e) Cohort	Subgroups of a certain population are divided based on having or not having exposure or different degrees of exposure that are assumed to affect the probability of disease. Groups do not have disease or complications in advance, and the occurrence of disease occurs over time
Prospective cohort	The exposure(s) and outcome(s)have not yet occurred, and the study begins in the present and ends in the future
Retrospective cohort	The exposure(s) and outcome(s) have already taken place and the study starts from the past and ends with the present
Historical cohort	The outcome(s) has not yet occurred and the study starts from the past and ends in the future
(f) Interventional	The researcher intervenes by administering an intervention to some or all of the participants in the study to determine the effect of exposure to the intervention on outcomes (e.g., clinical trials)

Table 2.1 (continued)

Type of study	Overall specifications
(g) Experimental	The experimental design of the research is conducted in an objective and maximally controlled manner. The goal is to determine the effect that an independent factor or variable has on a dependent variable
Parallel or concurrent experiment	A parallel design compares two or more interventions. Participants are randomly assigned to groups, treatments are administered, and outcomes are then compared
Cross-over design	A type of clinical trial in which all participants receive the same two or more treatments, but the order in which they receive them depends on the group to which they are randomly assigned
Field study	Refers to research that is undertaken in the real world, where the confines of a laboratory setting are abandoned in favor of a natural setting. This form of research generally prohibits the direct manipulation of the environment by the researcher
(h) Quasi-experimental	Like experimental designs, it tests causal hypotheses. Quasi-experimental designs identify a comparison group that is as similar as possible to the intervention group in terms of baseline (pre-intervention) characteristics. Unlike an experimental design, a quasi-experimental study lacks random assignment

- Selection error (sampling error). A common example is a survey of people who respond better and belong to only a small part of the target population. Survey results may change if the researcher attempts to follow up on nonrespondents.
- Nonresponse error. It occurs when people who participate in a study are systematically different from people who choose not to participate. For example, in determining the amount of participation in political elections, we usually go to the supporters and do not consider the opponents or do not participate in the survey themselves.
- Measurement error. It is an error that may occur due to any type of error in measurements. Inaccurate tools, the insufficient skill of the measurer, inappropriate measurement conditions, and measurement time and place errors are among the causes of measurement error.

Some types of descriptive studies are as follows:

2.3.1.1 Correlation Studies

Correlation study is different from other studies in that instead of measuring the desired characteristics for individual members of the society, the values of these characteristics are measured and reported for large groups of societies. These groups may be classes of a school or schools of a city, factories, cities, and countries. The only condition for conducting these studies is the availability of such information from the studied population. Disease prevalence and mortality are widely used in these studies to determine the occurrence of disease in groups, and exposed factors are measured and expressed with a set of general indicators. For example, the availability of information on the annual consumption of red meat and the number of deaths recorded from colon cancer, in different cities or countries, makes it possible to conduct a correlation study for the preliminary investigation of the existence of a relationship between the consumption of red meat and colon cancer. Since in correlation studies the sizes are measured based on the average value for each person, the size of the relationship calculated between exposure and disease cannot be attributed to each person in society. Error in inference is common in a correlational study. It can determine the association between exposure and outcomes but cannot predict causation.

2.3.1.2 Normative Studies

In these studies, quantitative characteristics or traits are determined in a population, and it becomes clear to what extent these characteristics or sizes differ from each other. Every society must carry out normative studies on the characteristics or sizes that may be different from one society to another due to various reasons (lifestyle, population characteristics, climatic characteristics, etc.). For example, the normal sizes of children's weight at birth should be determined for the same population due to differences related to this attribute in different populations in each society, and the same normal pattern cannot be considered for different populations. We need to measure them to identify the major health problems confronting society, contribute to the process of setting policy goals, and monitor the effectiveness of medical and health care. Health has a broad meaning, and its definition is influenced by the level of awareness and perception of societies with different geographical and cultural conditions. In addition, health is a dynamic process, and its concept will change over time. The World Health Organization defines it as *"A state of complete physical, mental and social. Well-being and not merely the absence of disease or infirmity."* Some see health on a spectrum, from perfect health to death, where each person falls somewhere on the spectrum, and some define it as the successful adaptation of humans to the environment. In another approach (normal distribution[1]people divide into two normal and abnormal groups (healthy vs. unhealthy) based on frequency distribution. It refers to the most frequent event or the most normal state. In the statistical model, all values less and more than two standard deviations from the mean are abnormal (assuming normal distribution).

The studies that define these normal and abnormal named normative studies. Errors due to this approach may occur because it must be determined for each community separately (characteristics such as height and weight). All attributes are not normally distributed. In this model, the assumption of normality must be made first, and if the distribution of the desired attribute is not normal, the conclusion will be wrong. Sometimes, the prevalence of an abnormal trait, especially in the psychological or social dimension, causes it to be considered a normal and natural situation. Small groups with their characteristics are considered abnormal if they are measured by the pattern of the large population in which they are located, which is not necessarily the case. In this model, we always have a number (5%) of abnormalities, which are not necessarily patients.

[1]Normal distribution or the Gaussian distribution is a probability distribution that is symmetric about the mean, showing that data near the mean are more frequent in occurrence than data far from the mean. In graphical form, the normal distribution appears as a "bell curve."

2.3.1.3 Longitudinal Studies

These studies are used to determine the pattern of an event over time. This type of study may be classified as an analytical study, but when the purpose of the research is not to determine the causal relationship, the longitudinal study is considered a descriptive study.

2.3.1.4 Historical Studies

Historical study is to describe and explain a problem that happened in the past. This study helps to make the situation of the current research problem clearer and clearer. The data relating to these studies are obtained by examining documents or interviewing knowledgeable people. Because they take a long time, longitudinal studies are costly and time-consuming, the participants may cease to take part, and a big attrition may occur. Measurement error is problematic in longitudinal data because it can create multiple types of errors that appear at different time points.

2.3.1.5 KAP Studies

These studies are conducted to investigate the knowledge, attitude, and practice of the people under study. This type of research is mostly used in medical education and health sciences [5]. For example, measuring the amount of information or information of students in the field of AIDS prevention, their views on this disease, and the measures they take to protect themselves from this disease is considered a KAP study. It is possible that the study of KAP is structurally considered the only subject of research and is not classified as a type of study. The value and strengths of the KAP survey depend upon the methods and strategy for collecting data (e.g., when you use a self-administered questionnaire, its results will differ when you use a group discussion and/or interview format). Furthermore, designing the questions (open vs. closed-ended questions) will also influence its results and conclusions. Also, the measurement scale and scoring to measure the knowledge and divided it into good, fair, and bad should be determined in detail by the methodology.

2.3.1.6 Existing Data Analyses

Many research questions can be answered quickly, efficiently, and economically by using the information that has already been collected. There are three general methods for designing this type of study. Data reanalysis is a method in which researchers examine and test a different research question using the information collected in a study, which is designed and implemented to answer a specific research question. A secondary study is a design in that by adding some questions to the questionnaire or measuring additional variables in the process of collecting information from the subjects under study, researchers can answer a separate research question. A systematic review is a composite study of all previous studies related to the research question. In this method, an estimate of the effective factors purified from all eligible studies is calculated. Creative use of methods based on available data, when we are faced with limited time and required resources, is one of the effective ways to answer some important research questions. An important disadvantage of using secondary data is that it has not been planned for research purposes and may not answer the specific research questions or contain specific information that the researcher would like to have.

2.3.1.7 Meta-Analysis

In medical science, about a subject, numerous studies are conducted in different parts of the world, which often bring contradictory results. To reach a single result, one of the methods is the integration of the results of these studies and their final analysis, which is called a meta-analysis. The term meta-analysis was first used by Glass, the president of the American Educational Research Association, in 1976. Glass said: meta-analysis is the integration of the findings of a large set of published single studies and their overall statistical analysis. Meta-analysis is the analysis of analyses in different studies. Meta-analysis methods are a set of techniques to statistically combine the results of several independent studies to find a general answer. The purpose of these methods is to provide a test with higher power than the power of individual independent studies. In a meta-analysis, the researcher uses statistical methods to integrate the findings of a set of studies and describes the results using numerical effect size estimates. Publication bias, bias caused by sampling error, errors related to heterogeneity, mistakes in choosing statistical models, significant testing, and errors related to subgroup analyses are common in meta-analyses [6, 7].

2.3.2 Analytical Studies

Most of the study plans are implicitly designed to compare the risk factors and to know the condition of the disease. For example, in a case report, when only one specific form of the disease is observed, a hypothesis is formulated based on an implicit comparison with common experience. In analytical studies, the comparison is made explicitly because the researcher regularly collects groups of people for a specific purpose to determine the difference in disease risk for people who have a particular exposure and those who do not slow. There are different ways to design analytical studies, based on the available conditions and facilities, and a certain type of them is used. Two general categories of analytical studies are observational studies and interventional studies. The main difference between these two strategies is in the role played by the researcher. In observational studies, the researcher simply observes the flow of natural events according to who is exposed or which healthy people are affected by the disease. In interventional studies, researchers select the exposure of the groups under study and then follow up with the individuals in terms of the incidence of disease or outcome. The main problem in observational studies is that usually the observed groups are different from each other in terms of some other characteristics in addition to the specific factor under study. Supposedly, different job groups are not only different in terms of exposure to job risks but also different in terms of past life events, because almost similar people are employed in similar jobs. This similarity can be due to personal interests, education, or suitability for the desired job. Because of these confounding factors, whose measurement is often associated with many difficulties, it becomes more difficult to show the role of the factor under investigation. Although experimental studies can show the causal relationship of a factor with a disease much better than observational studies, most of our information about diseases comes from observational studies.

In analytical studies, errors resulting from an increase in data variability due to instrument malfunction, failure to follow proper procedures, undetected failures in quality control, type one and two errors, sample misidentification, and/or test interference are common.

2.3.2.1 Observational Studies

The two main types of analytical observational studies are case-control studies and cohort studies. Theoretically, it is possible to investigate a hypothesis using any of these two methods. Each of these two types of studies has advantages and disadvantages that will be discussed in the third chapter. In general, the decision to use a strategy depends on factors such as the characteristics of the risk factor and disease at the current stage, the level of scientific awareness, and logical considerations such as resources and time.

Case studies include case investigations, case series, and controlled comparisons. Because of the absence of a control or comparison group case, investigation or case series are not able to make differences. A case-control method is a problem-solving tool. Case-control studies, like cohort studies, can show temporal relationships between exposure and outcome, and this strengthens the causal relationship. Temporality in case-control studies is demonstrated by assuring that exposure was present before the development of the disease. The main distinction between a case-control study and a cohort study is that cohort studies identify subjects based on their exposure status, whereas case-control studies identify subjects based on their outcome status. Case-control studies cannot estimate the actual incidence of a disease or outcome.

In case-control studies, the presence or absence of the desired disease is known, and the researcher examines the patient's history to discover the cause or possible risk factors raised in the study [8]. Cases are people who are sick or suffering from the desired outcome, and controls are healthy people or people without the desired disease. Researchers have identified the feature or risk factor that exists only in patients and not in healthy people and examined the history of the previous life events of patients and controls.

Possible sources of errors in case-control studies are as follows:

- Information on risk factor B (exposure) may be missing from the records or memories of the study subjects.
- Information on potentially important confounding variables may be missing or unavailable.
- Cases may seek to find the cause of their illness and thus be more likely to recall and report encounters with control subjects (recall bias).

In cohort studies, researchers select people at the beginning of the study and then determine the presence of the risk factor or the amount of contact with it. During a specific time, they study exposed or nonexposed people, taking into account the risk factor and future time orientation. Another type of cohort study is a historical cohort study. These studies are conducted using information collected from the past (available in files); however, the time orientation of the study is still future-oriented. That is, the beginning of the study is based on information about risk factors, and the consequences of risk factors are determined in the future. Potential sources of error in cohort studies can be the result of loss of follow-up (death, migration, and impossibility of follow-up), lack of access to subjects, and the effect of those who are no longer willing to continue cooperating with the research and measurement error such as incorrect definitions for cases of the disease.

2.3.2.2 Intervention Studies

Experiences are the strongest sources for testing any hypothesis. But it is rarely possible to use them in human societies. In medicine, those types of experimental studies that are performed on humans (randomization is performed on sick people) are called clinical trials. Interventions are divided into two groups: with control and without control (only treatment group). Controlled trials are divided into groups of randomized trials, non-randomized trials, and an intermediate state in terms of intervention (treatment) assignment. Those experimental studies in which the allocation of the intervention is done by chance, if using a sufficient sample size and taking into account some measures (such as blinding of the study, and control of environmental conditions), provide the strongest evidence in the study of studies between risk factors and disease. This is related to the unique power of randomization as a tool to determine and control the intervention. When participants are randomly selected to receive a drug or placebo, to be exposed to exposure or not, on average and in the long term, all other factors that may affect disease risk are controlled.

2.4 Study Design with a Causal Approach

Avicenna (Ibn Sina), the father of early modern medicine (980–1037 AD) believes that the origin (cause) is anything that has a complete and complete existence by itself or through another, and then it is the origin of the origin and consistency of other phenomena. He divides the cause into two types: complete cause, that is, a cause that does not need to be combined with other factors to create its effect, and incomplete cause, which means something that can be the source of creating something else, provided that it is combined with other factors. The traces of error in human history in identifying the causes and treatment of diseases and dealing with epidemics have been recorded many times. In analytical studies, an observed association may be due to the effects of chance (random error), bias (systematic error), confounding, reverse causality, and true causality [9, 10]. He is one of the pioneers of ethical consideration in research and a scientist that developed rules for the testing and experimental use of drugs[2] [9, 11].

---

[2]Avicenna's seven rules must be observed in finding out the potency of medicines through experimentation.

1. The drug must be free from any acquired quality: This may happen if the drug is temporarily exposed to heat or cold, causing a change like a drug, or if it is in the vicinity of another substance.
2. The experiment must be done on single conditions and not on combinations. In the latter case, if the condition involves two opposite diseases and the drug is tried and found to be beneficial in both, we cannot infer the true cause of the treatment. If a patient with more than one disease improves after receiving a drug, it cannot be concluded that that treatment was the cause of the improvement. Treatment should be tested in a controlled setting (such as excluding patients with complex and multiple diseases) to reduce the role of confounding factors. A drug can directly affect the disease itself and have a secondary and random effect.
3. The drug must be experienced in two opposite conditions. If it works on both, it is not possible to judge which disease directly benefited from the drug. The drug may act directly against one disease and the symptoms of another disease.
4. The strength of the medicine should be following the strength of the disease. So it is better to first experiment with the weakest [dose] and then gradually increase the dose until the strength of the medicine is known and there is no room for doubt.
5. The time required for the drug to take effect should be taken into account. If the medicine has an immediate effect, it means that it has worked against the disease itself. If the initial effect is not there at first, it shows itself later, leading to uncertainty and confusion. This uncertainty is related to the strength of the drug. This may be accidental, that is, their effect is hidden at first and becomes apparent later.
6. The effect of the drug should be the same in all or most cases. Otherwise, the effect is random.
7. Experiments must be done on the human body. If the experiment is done on the body of other animals, it

Understanding the causes of diseases is necessary not only for prevention but also for diagnosis and application of correct treatments. If we make a mistake in determining the causal relationship or make a mistake in inferring from raw and descriptive findings, we may be misled both in the diagnosis of the disease and in choosing the appropriate treatment methods and the appropriate choice of preventive interventions. Fallacy or false cause is assuming a causal relationship between two phenomena or events, which is not the case. An example of a spurious relationship can be seen by examining the relationship between the number of ice creams sold and the number of drownings in a city. When the rate of drownings in swimming pools in an area correlates with the highest rate of ice cream sales, concluding that ice cream sales cause drownings or vice versa implies a spurious relationship between the two. Warmer weather may have caused both (more ice cream sales and more swimming).[3] Here, heat wave is an example of a hidden or neglected variable and is also known as a confounding variable. Spurious correlations can result from small sample sizes or incomplete or arbitrary follow-up endpoints. Researchers use rigorous statistical analysis to determine spurious relationships. Confirming a causal relationship requires a study that controls all possible variables.

The explanation of causality using an imaginary or unrealistic model is simple in theory, but in practice, this model cannot be implemented in the real world. To prove causality, this model assumes that a single subject can be placed in the desired intervention group and the nonintervention group, that is, everyone can be under their control. If you can imagine these conditions, in this model, you can study and prove causality both at the individual level and at the group level, but as mentioned, this is an unrealistic model, and it is not possible to create and study it in the real world because only one of the two situations is conceivable and possible. Hence, real-world studies generate a series of missing data. Since in a randomized trial study, the allocation of people to two groups of intervention and nonintervention is done randomly, therefore, the missing data created in randomized trial studies are created randomly. This randomness of missing data makes intervention studies, whose randomization is done well, the best primary studies in proving causality.

To evaluate and prove the causal relationship, the study in question must establish conditions. These conditions are as follows:

- Ability to move.
- Being positive.
- The different levels of the investigated variable are well defined.

2.4.1 Ability to Move

Transferability means that when we intend to design and implement an analytical study to evaluate the relationship of an exposure variable such as prescribing a type of drug on an outcome such as preventing death from a specific type of disease, there is a difference in which of the target groups of the target drug and which of the groups receiving the compared intervention did not. When the ability to move between two groups is created when the distribution of confounding variables is the same between the two groups. In the ideal randomized trial study, this condition is met. When randomization is done well and the sample size is large enough, it results in the formation of groups that can move. Randomization controls for known and unknown confounding variables. Transferability in observational studies means that the intended intervention is transferable in two groups. In practice, such a thing is not possible in observational studies, and there is no ability to move in groups.

may fail for two reasons: the drug is hot compared to the human body and cold compared to the animal body. Another thing is that the quality of medicine may affect the human body differently than the animal body.

[3] https://en.wikipedia.org/wiki/Spurious_relationship. Accessed: Feb 20, 2023.

2.4.2 Being Positive

Being positive means that some subjects are placed in each group (intervention and nonintervention) so that the effect of the desired intervention can be evaluated on this group. In clinical trial studies, since the researcher assigns people to intervention and nonintervention groups by randomization and considers a chance greater than zero for each person to enter each group, positivity is guaranteed. Being positive in observational studies means that there is a certain number of subjects in different subgroups of confounding variables. In practice, positivity is not always present in observational studies.

2.4.3 The Different Levels of the Investigated Variable Are Well Defined

This condition means that both the desired intervention and the comparison group are well defined and applied without any ambiguity. Since, in interventional studies, the researcher himself applies this intervention, this condition is established in interventional studies, but in observational studies, it is one of the problems caused by defining and applying the studied variables. For example, if you intend to evaluate the effect of smoking in a cohort study, you must have a definition of smoking, which is usually not easily done. For example, you define smoking as smoking at least five cigarettes per day for a year. In contrast, anyone who smokes less than this limit can be included in the comparison group. Defining the variable and its levels is one of the problems in observational studies. This condition is easily applicable and controllable in ideal interventional studies where the design and implementation conditions are well implemented. For example, if you intend to study the effect of a drug on a treatment of a specific disease, after randomization, a group should receive the desired drug for the necessary time, and in contrast to the comparison group (if it is a placebo), no amount of the drug. Does not receive the desired If the control group is another dose of the same drug or another drug (intervention), its levels and amount are already known.

2.5 Clinical Investigations

Medical scientists have been trying to identify the cause of diseases for centuries. They have developed tools to obtain more precise measurements of variables related to health and disease, improved clinical examinations, and contributed to this with precise definitions of various diseases. New technologies have been used, and by referring to the data obtained from the state of health and disease in people, we have tried to gain more understanding. In the case of infectious diseases, the causes of diseases such as viruses, bacteria, fungi, parasites, arthropods, and prions have been identified. The behavior and biological nature of these pathogens are investigated at the cellular, molecular, and genetic levels. Although there are still errors in the diagnosis and cause of the disease, however these errors are decreasing day by day, and for this reason, the rate of recovery of diseases that were very fatal until a few years or decades ago has decreased or even reached zero. With the increase in the incidence and prevalence of noncommunicable diseases in the past few decades, the cause of identifying diseases became more complicated, and the criteria of causality affected by them changed. Risk factors are not necessarily the direct causes of disease, but they have been identified as factors that elevate the likelihood and probability of disease occurrence in individuals. In the field of medicine, etiology refers to the investigation and determination of the underlying causes of diseases or pathologies. Consequently, the etiology of nearly all known human diseases is extensively studied and researched.

2.5.1 Errors in Clinical Medicine

Humans make mistakes, and the medical community is no exception. It is important to learn from our mistakes and those of others, not to repeat the mistake, and try to minimize our mistakes as much as possible.

Clinical decisions can be complex, and errors can occur due to a variety of factors, including the following:

1. Confirmation bias: Clinicians may only look for evidence that confirms their initial diagnosis, leading them to miss other potential diagnoses.
2. Anchoring bias: Clinicians may fixate on a diagnosis, even if new evidence suggests a different conclusion.
3. Availability heuristic: Clinicians may overestimate the likelihood of particular diagnoses based on their recent experiences, rather than on clinical evidence.
4. Overconfidence: Clinicians may be overly confident in their diagnoses, leading them to dismiss alternative possibilities.
5. Systemic issues: Clinical decision-making can be affected by systemic issues, such as a lack of time to consider all relevant factors or insufficient resources to conduct necessary tests.

To reduce errors in clinical decision-making, clinicians need to be aware of these potential biases and errors and take steps to mitigate them. This includes continuing education, regular review of diagnoses, and the use of decision-making frameworks that prioritize evidence-based practices. Medical errors should be paid special attention, too because they may increase suffering, sometimes lead to death, sometimes cause irreparable damage to the patient, and in most cases increase the cost of treatment. The causes of mistakes in clinical medicine are diverse and numerous. From insufficient or incorrect training in the course of study to errors related to diagnostic tools, examinations, and incorrect communication between the patient and the doctor, all these can cause mistakes [12]. During the Arbaeen pilgrimage to Iraq, while visiting a hospital in Najaf, I examined the case of an Iranian patient. Due to the lack of proper language communication and the absence of a translator, the Arabic-speaking doctor cited drug addiction as the reason for hospitalization and prescribed methadone for the patient; however, the patient said that he did not take his heart medicine with him and did not take it! Due to the rapid scientific changes, having medical science up-to-date is a fundamental point in error prevention. Scientific medicine is practical, and its primary beneficiary is the patient. What is gained from medical knowledge should be used for the benefit of the patient? Whenever a doctor learns something or reads something, he should know how his knowledge will help the patient. Books and guides are edited every few years. Although old knowledge is not always useless, it is not possible to obtain modern knowledge from the latest editions of books. Sometimes, during the printing interval of two versions of a reference book, fundamental changes occur, which should be found in journals and reliable scientific websites.

2.5.2 Common Mistakes in Clinical Medicine

Diagnosis precedes treatment. Treatment without diagnosis and finding the cause of the disease is playing with the patient's life. Diagnosis is made with the help of history, general physical examination, examination of various body organs, and paraclinical tests. However, in some cases, even careful examination may not help in diagnosis. There are many conditions in which a patient dies without a clear diagnosis, and a pathological autopsy is needed to understand the course of the disease and the cause of death. History of a disease is the most important part of the diagnosis. The omission of some points in history can lead to a confusing clinical situation and unnecessary investigations.

Errors in the analysis of clinical symptoms, unusual manifestations of common diseases or common manifestations of uncommon diseases, insufficient or incorrect examination of the patient's family history, wrong information that the patient gives to the doctor for various reasons, forgetting about exposure to risk factors, errors in eliciting the symptoms of the disease (such as lack of relaxation of the patient during the examination or failure to respect the confidential issues of the patient), choosing the wrong examination method, missing or ignoring some obvious things, rushing to conclusions, and starting treatment are common mistakes in clinical medicine.

2.6 Common Errors in Nursing

It is estimated that more than one-third of medical errors are related to nurses [13]. In nursing, common errors could be operating errors (pharmaceutical, care, and equipment), precautionary errors (these errors occur due to carelessness and include medicine, symptoms, care, medicine, education, and equipment errors), diagnostic errors (misdiagnosis in the implementation of medication orders and clinical interventions and the identity of patients(, communication error, registration, and reporting errors [14].

Some of the errors in nursing services are caused by negligence. Failure to carefully examine the patient and take a history, wrong execution of treatment orders, mistake in identifying the patient, failure to measure or accurately record information, incorrect use of clinical tools and equipment, and medication errors are some of the most common errors in this job.

The National Coordinating Council for Medication Error Reporting and Prevention defines a medication error as "A medication error is any preventable event that may cause or lead to inappropriate medication use or harm to the patient or user. Such events may be related to professional practice, health care products, procedures, and systems, including prescribing, order communication, product labeling, packaging, and nomenclature, compounding, dispensing, distribution, administration, education, monitoring, and use.[4]" The frequency types of medication errors include wrong dose, wrong time, wrong drug, wrong route, omission of doses, wrong patient, lack of documentation, and technical errors.

[4]https://www.nccmerp.org/about-medication-errors. Accessed: Feb 20, 2023.

2.7 Qualitative Studies and their Potential Specific Errors

There are two general approaches to collecting information or data quantitative and qualitative research. Qualitative investigations have their importance and although there are many similar errors in both quantitative and qualitative studies. In general, in qualitative studies, the data are nonnumerical (so, usually they don't need statistical analyses), typically anthropological research methods use them.

Observations of a "natural" environment describe situations in depth and are interpretive and descriptive, and the six most common types are phenomenological, ethnographic, grounded theory, historical case study, and action research.

The findings of these types of studies fail to be representative of the target population because of some reasons. The limited number of respondents is too small to conclude. Because of these limitations, the data gathered does not result in a geographic or demographic representative sample of the whole population needed to draw broad, projectable conclusions. One of the common errors can be caused by the researcher trying to generalize the findings to other parts of the population. These studies have very little reproducibility or reliability. Observer bias is another potential error in these types of studies. Observer bias occurs when the researcher's beliefs, convictions, or prejudices influence what he or she perceives or records in a study. Researcher error could be due to confirmation bias (occurs when a researcher interprets the data in such a way to support his or her hypothesis or omit information that does not favor his/her hypothesis), question-order bias, and leading questions and wording bias.

Participant or subject bias also may occur. It happens when participants are not behaving how they normally would but are responding the way they think they are supposed to. The subject error could be due to social desirability bias or social acceptability bias, acquiescence or friendliness bias, habituation bias (occurs when participants provide the same answers in response to similarly-worded questions), and sponsor bias (can occur if a participant is opinionated about the sponsor of the research or gets influenced by the sponsor's reputation or mission statement).

2.7.1 Phenomenological Studies

Phenomenology consists of two parts: phenomenon and cognition (logy). It means studying phenomena of any kind and describing them considering how they occur, before trying to interpret them or judge them in terms of value (studying phenomena of any kind and describing them considering how they manifest, before any valuation, interpretation, or value judgment). Operational errors, such as problems with the analysis and interpretation of findings, usually result in lower levels of validity and reliability in these studies.

2.7.2 Ethnographic Studies

In ethnographic studies, the researcher observes and scientifically describes different cultures and interacts with the studied people in their natural and real-life environment. Ethnography is a method of studying people and cultures. This method relies on observation along with participation in the life of the studied community and is different from interviews and research questionnaires. In ethnographic research, the field of research and the human group should be limited and small so that a limited number of researchers can study the region in this way. This is why monograph study is very important in the field of anthropological studies. The results of ethnographic research can only be interpreted in the study environment, and it is a mistake to generalize the results to other societies. The pressure in the ethnographic research approach is due to the two principles of naturalism and its flexibility. The researcher is constantly involved in reconciling these two opposing elements. On the one hand, in reality, the research seeks a complete and detailed description of the phenomenon or culture, in a completely natural way, and on the other hand, because the flexibility is inevitably influenced by the researcher in the entire research, it creates a contradictory situation for the entire research. For this purpose, all the efforts of the researcher are aimed at adjusting these pressures to optimize the reflection of reality, which certainly causes errors in the research to some extent.

2.7.3 Grounded Theory Study

Grounded theory is a qualitative research method that is used to theorize about the topic of study. This method is used when the research literature around the topic is insufficient or ambiguous. It also aims to present a new theory that has been presented in research communities. The advantages of the grounded theory method are that the theory is formed regularly and based on real data, and it is suitable for a situation where our knowledge is limited, and there is no clear theory in which a hypothesis can be formulated for testing. Grounded theory develops during research and results from the continuous interaction between data collection and analysis. One of the possible errors in the grounded theory method is caused by the coding of the information obtained from the subjects.

2.7.4 Historical Case Study

A historical study is the kind of research that deals with a specific issue that happened in the past and at a specific point in time. In the historical method, researchers strive to uncover past events by collecting, evaluating, and verifying information. This involves employing a combination of logical reasoning and analysis to ensure the accuracy and validity of the gathered data. This approach stems from the understanding that events have occurred continuously in the past and that, with the aid of completed tools, researchers can diligently work towards revealing factual accounts of historical occurrences. The goal is to present this information in an orderly and objective manner, ultimately leading to defensible research results concerning the special assumption of the research. In these studies, to avoid errors, one should follow the principle of forgetfulness or self-forgetfulness and impartiality (the researcher should not impose the values of his time as well as his mental values on the time of research), the principle of reflection and positive skepticism (the researcher should reflect on the acceptance of data in different ways and in this way get help from common sense and self-knowledge), the principle of induction (researcher explores various documents and identifies the parts of the events to finally achieve a comprehensive knowledge), and paid attention to the principle of comprehensiveness (i.e., every event finds meaning within a set or a causal network).

2.7.5 Action Research

This type of research is the implementation of solutions obtained from previous studies to create change and solve problems. Being systematic, stating the problem, specific questions, documenting information, being critical, systematic control, and knowledge production are the characteristics of this type of study. The steps of the practical study include specifying the topic and title of the research, describing the current situation and diagnosing the problem, collecting evidence information, analyzing and interpreting data, temporarily choosing a new solution, implementing the new solution and monitoring it, collecting further evidence information, evaluating the impact of the new action, and determining its validity, revision, and presentation of the final report.

The researcher must be careful to control the potential errors in the research results and their interpretation. These errors include the time interval between two types of measurements (pre-test and post-test), changes that occur during the research in the subjects (maturation), changes in the measuring instrument, statistical regression, differential selection of subjects, experimental mortality effect, the mutual effect of factors, interaction of selection and experimental, reactive effect of testing, reactive effects of experiment, and multiple-treatment interference, which can endanger the internal and external validity.

References

1. Leavy P. Research design: quantitative, qualitative, mixed methods, arts-based, and community-based participatory research approaches. 2nd ed. New York: The Guilford Press; 2022.
2. Celentano D, Szklo M. Gordis epidemiology. 6th ed. Philadelphia: Elsevier; 2019.
3. Soori H, Asasi N. Descriptive study methods in methodology of applied research in medical sciences. Authors group. Tehran Medical Sciences Publications: Deputy of Research and Technology of the Ministry of Health, Treatment, and Medical Education; 2013.
4. Soori H. Generalities and principles of epidemiology, In Generalities of public health (3 Volumes), compiled by Hatami H. and colleagues (Authors group). Arjmand Publications; 2015.
5. Fos PJ, Fine DJ, Miguel A, Zúniga MA. Managerial epidemiology for health care organizations. Hoboken: John Wiley & Sons; 2018.
6. Schmid CH, White IR, Stijnen T. Handbook of meta-analysis. United Kingdom: Taylor & Francis Limited; 2022.
7. Borenstein M. Common mistakes in meta-analysis-and how to avoid them. Englewood: Biostat, Inc.; 2019.
8. Alastair Scott A, Wild CJ, Gail MH, Chatterjee N, Breslow N, Borgan Ø. Handbook of statistical methods for case-control studies. United Kingdom: CRC Press LLC; 2020.
9. Cox GS. Clinical trials handbook. Hoboken: John Wiley & Sons Inc.; 2009.
10. Jenicek M. How to think in medicine: reasoning, decision making, and communication in health sciences and professions. London: Taylor & Francis Limited; 2021.
11. Nasser M, Tibi A, Savage-Smith E. Ibn Sina's canon of medicine: 11th-century rules for assessing the effects of drugs. J R Soc Med. 2009;102(2):78–80.
12. Thibault GE. The appropriate degree of diagnostic certainty. N Engl J Med. 1994;331:1216–20.
13. Soozani A, Bagheri H, Poorheydari M. Investigating the factors affecting the incidence of drug mistakes from the viewpoints of nurses in different departments of imam Hossein Hospital in Shahroud. Knowledge and Health. 2007;3(2):8–13.
14. Ansari M, Sharifi S, Peikari HR, Etebarian KA. Types of nursing errors based on the Nurses' lived experience. Quarterly J Nurs Manag (IJNV). 2021;9(4):12–9. http://ijnv.ir/article-1-772-fa.html

3 The Method of Designing Studies in Medical Sciences

The scientific method is a way of thinking that emphasizes skepticism, testing, and evaluation of evidence.

—Carl Edward Sagan (1934–1996)

3.1 Introduction

In the previous chapter, different methods of designing medical science studies according to the possibilities and limitations and also how to classify these studies were discussed. In this chapter, the details related to the design and objectives of each of these studies are explained.

3.2 Methods of Descriptive Studies

Descriptive studies provide information about the frequency of occurrence of a specific situation or patterns of occurrence based on factors related to person, time, and place distribution. Commonly collected statistics, such as data related to death certificates, medical records, disease surveillance, and care programs, and data from sampling or census can be used in descriptive studies.

Descriptive studies are classified as nonexperimental studies. In these studies, the general characteristics of the distribution of a disease such as individual characteristics (e.g., age, sex, occupation, race, and marital status); characteristics related to lifestyle (e.g., eating habits, smoking, and drinking alcohol), climatic characteristics; the geographical distribution of factors and certain periods; and indicators of health, illness, or death in the studied people are described. The passage of time is ignored in these studies, and similar to a photograph, it only displays an image of a moment in time for the study audience. Descriptive research cannot be used to show a causal relationship.

3.2.1 Case Report or Case Study

A case report or study is a detailed description of a clinical case, careful attention, and investigation of an unusual case that investigates the how and possible mechanism of the desired event. Case studies often focus on a patient's diagnosis, treatment, and outcomes. These studies are cheap, convenient, and usually without problems caused by ethical considerations in study design. Case reports are typically published in medical journals and serve as a means of sharing clinical observations and experiences with other medical

H. Soori, *Errors in Medical Science Investigations*, https://doi.org/10.1007/978-981-99-8521-0_3

professionals. It is not possible to make a definite conclusion about the cause of the event in the case study, and the main goal of these studies is to describe the rare case of the disease. It usually involves describing the case history, including the patient's background symptoms, medical history diagnosis, treatment, and outcomes. It may include images to provide a visual representation of the case. Case studies are considered to be weaker than randomized controlled trials or other quantitative studies since they are based on a single case and are subject to bias and confounding factors. They should be interpreted with caution and used in conjunction with other forms of evidence.

3.2.2 Review of Cases (Case Series)

A case series is a type of medical study that involves a descriptive analysis of a group of patients who share a common characteristic or diagnosis. Browsing cases is expanding the case report or reporting several cases instead of one case. In the review of cases, usually, the characteristics of some patients are studied at a point or period, and the distribution of events in population subgroups is determined.

The case series has the following uses and benefits:

They can introduce signs, symptoms, and tests of a group of cases (patients) and help with case definitions, be applicable in clinical education and health services, audit, and research. Compared to the case study, it provides a more comprehensive picture of the disease pattern as a group (not individually). They can measure and track cases in terms of the date of illness or death, the person's place of residence and work, the characteristics of the population, and the possibility of collecting additional data from medical records. What is the answer to questions such as the size and characteristics of the population at risk? Who, what, why, when, and where the disease occurred? What is the condition of the disease being studied? Therefore, a description of the disease can be provided in case reports and case series. They can provide preliminary evidence to guide future research and can be useful for generating hypothesis. The limitation of this type of study is the impossibility of proving a causal relationship.

3.2.3 Correlation Studies (Ecological)

An ecological study is a type of epidemiological study that generates hypothesis and examines the correlation between a particular exposure or intervention and a health outcome in a specific population or geographical area. In correlation studies, instead of individuals, the main emphasis is on the comparison of groups. Ecological studies use aggregate data rather than individual-level data. The reason for conducting this type of study is the lack of information at the level of individual subjects. It is possible that at least for the joint distribution of two variables or even all variables, accurate and comprehensive information is not available. For this reason, in many fields, it seems justified to conduct these studies in medical sciences. However, it is very difficult to distinguish between individual sizes and macro (ecological) sizes and how to make inferences in this field.

Correlation studies are divided into three groups based on the content of measurements:

1. Summary measures: In this case, only a summary (e.g., mean or ratio) of the observations, which is related to the people under study, is available (e.g., the proportion of smokers and the average household income).
2. Environmental measures: Measuring physical characteristics in the place where the group under study lives or works, such as the amount of air pollution and hours of sunlight, constitute environmental measures. The remarkable point in this type of measurement is that for each person in the study group, separate measurements can be measured, and these individual exposures (or doses) are usually different in the studied subgroups. Some people may have no exposure at all.
3. Large dimensions: These dimensions are related to characteristics of groups, organiza-

tions, or places that no specific value can be calculated for the value of these characteristics at the individual level, such as population density, the existence of a set of specific laws, the type of medical service systems, and insurance coverage.

In the analysis of each study, one of the important points is the data collection unit. Usually, in data analysis, the smallest common level by which data can be expressed is used as the unit and basis of analysis. When the unit of measurement is individual subjects, there is one measurement for each member of the study. But when we are faced with ecological measures, there is no separate measure for each person in the society. For example, when the social status of people is determined based on their place of residence, all people who live in a certain area will have a common social class. Sometimes, when all the investigated variables (exposure, disease, and confounding variables) are of ecological type, the study is called a complete correlation study. At this time, the unit of analysis of the results is the groups. For example, these units can be different areas of a province or country, work environments, schools, or time intervals. In this case, there is no information available about the combined distribution of variables at the individual level (e.g., the frequencies of exposed cases, cases that are not exposed, exposed controls, and controls that are not exposed cannot be measured). In some other studies, it is possible to obtain additional information about some joint distributions, but complete knowledge of all joint distributions is not yet available. Such studies are called semi-correlation studies. For example, in a correlation study to investigate the incidence of cancer in different provinces, the age distribution (a covariate) and the occurrence or nonoccurrence of the disease in each province can be calculated from cancer registries in hospitals or death certificates [1, 2].

Advantages and disadvantages of correlation studies: There are various reasons that despite the structural and methodological limitations of correlation studies, their use is attractive and logical.

Ease of conducting and low cost of these studies: If secondary sources are available to collect the required data, it is easily possible to collect summary information for the desired indicators in the study. This issue makes the correlation studies low cost and can be done in a short time. The information sources of these studies can be registration statistics, censuses, data banks, and extensive field studies.

Existence of various limitations in individual measurements: In studies related to the effect of natural exposures and many other studies, individual measurements of exposure levels or doses on a wide scale were not practical, reliable, and valid, or at least without spending time, and a huge budget is not possible. In these cases, probably, the only practical method is macro measurement [3–5].

Existence of limitations in the design of individual studies: When the exposure under investigation has little changes in the investigated groups, designing a study based on the measurement of exposure for individual individuals is probably not practical. In such cases, it is possible to cover wide geographical areas by using correlation studies.

The purpose of the study: Sometimes, finding an ecological relationship in different societies is the main purpose of the study. For example, correlation studies are very suitable for investigating the effects of population interventions, such as new health policies [6–8]. Despite the practical advantages of correlation studies, there are methodological problems and difficulties in the design and interpretation of the results of these studies, which have severely limited the making of causal inferences from these studies. Some of these problems are as follows:

3.2.4 Ecological Pollution

The most important limitation of this study is the existence of ecological or cumulative pollution. Ecological bias may occur due to the existence of a relationship that is observed between variables at the macro level and between groups, while this relationship doesn't need to be true for each person at the individual level.

3.2.5 Misclassification Bias

Due to the structure of this study, which requires data collection on a large scale, the effect of misclassification in these studies is very serious.

3.2.6 Data Quality

The lack of required information or the low quality of recording and collecting ecological data is one of the practical problems of conducting these studies [9, 10] (Fig. 3.1).

One of the applications of cross-sectional studies is to evaluate the dependence and association between variables, but the calculated dependences do not necessarily mean a causal relationship, and basically, the naming of response and independent variables in this type of study is superficial and depends only on the initial hypotheses of the research. The main reason is that in this type of study, the logical process of moving from the cause of "exposure" to the effect of "disease" has not been observed, and no follow-up is done in a cross-sectional study (see Fig. 3.1). Of course, in variables such as age, sex, ethnicity, and genetic factors that are usually not affected by other factors, it is easy to determine the response and independent variable, but it is not always so easy to determine the response and independent variable. For example, when a cross-sectional study shows a relationship between obesity and watching television in children, it is almost impossible to determine which one was the other cause.

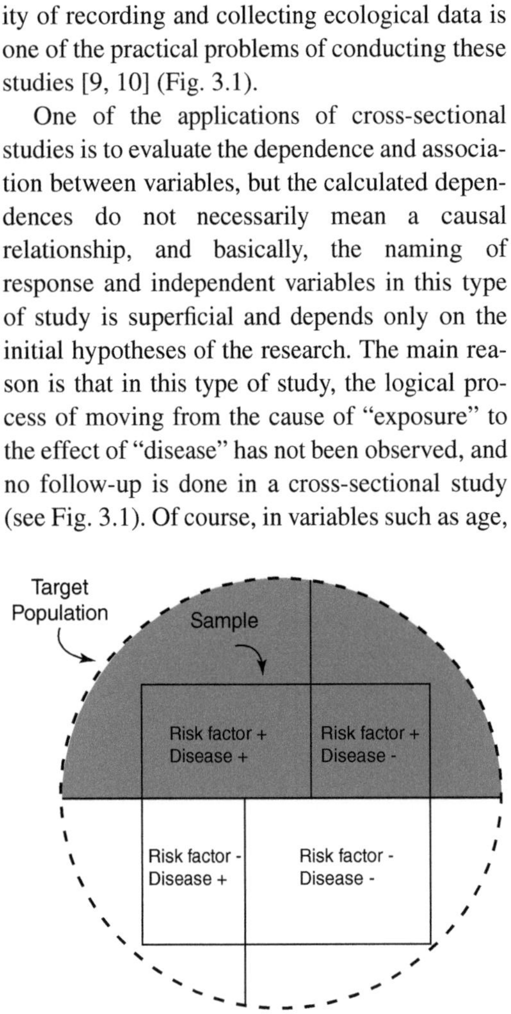

Fig. 3.1 In cross-sectional studies, researchers first take a sample from the community and then measure disease-related variables and risk factors

Advantages and disadvantages of cross-sectional studies:

- One of the most important advantages of cross-sectional studies compared to cohort and intervention studies is that we do not need to wait for the final event to occur. This makes the study quick and inexpensive.
- There is no problem with missing items in the follow-up.
- Cross-sectional studies are usually the starting point of analytical studies (to determine exposed and nonexposed groups, as well as healthy and sick people) in the research process. A cross-sectional study is a study in which we can calculate the prevalence of a disease or risk factor.
- One of the weaknesses of cross-sectional studies is the challenges and difficulties in stating a causal relationship between what the researcher calls the disabled and the risk factor.
- When the outcome under study is rare, a cross-sectional study is not practical, especially when the goal is a sampling from the normal population (e.g., in a cross-sectional study to determine the prevalence of stomach cancer in people aged 45–59, about 10,000 samples are needed to find one case of cancer).

3.3 Observational Studies

Observational studies include two general groups: case-control studies and cohort studies. Each of these studies is examined in this section.

3.3.1 Case-Control Studies

To investigate the causes of the disease, in most cases, cohort and cross-sectional studies based on sampling from the population of healthy people are expensive, and it is necessary to examine thousands of samples to determine the risk factors (e.g., in the case of a rare disease such as stomach cancer). Sometimes, clear risk factors can be demonstrated by a group of patients suffering from a certain type of disease (e.g., injecting drugs and AIDS). In this case, we have used our previous information about the prevalence of the risk factor in the base population. But in most cases, it is necessary to specify a reference group so that the size of the risk factor in people with the disease (cases) is comparable to the size of the risk factor in normal people (controls). Figure 3.2 shows how this study plan works.

Designing case-control studies is very challenging due to the possibility of encountering different cases, but there are many examples of well-designed case-control studies that have produced important results. In case-control studies, we are not able to estimate the incidence or prevalence of the disease, because the ratio of diseased and healthy people in the study is determined by the researchers and not by random sampling from the population. What is obtained from a case-control study is an estimate in the form of an odds ratio.

Advantages and disadvantages of case-control studies: The most important advantages of case-control studies are as follows:

- Case-control studies are cheaper and faster than follow-up studies. Because no time is spent waiting for the disease to develop. This issue is very favorable in the study of diseases that take a long time to appear.
- Many risk factors can be checked simultaneously in this study. This issue causes the examination of many hypotheses in a case-control study.
- These studies are a relatively suitable method for investigating risk factors in rare diseases.
- Case-control studies require a much smaller sample size than similar cohort studies. For example, in comparison with similar cohort studies, when the total sample size is small, the evaluation of confounding variables and the interaction of risk factors are done with a higher statistical power.
- Due to the nonobservance of time sequence in case-control studies, we are not able to accu-

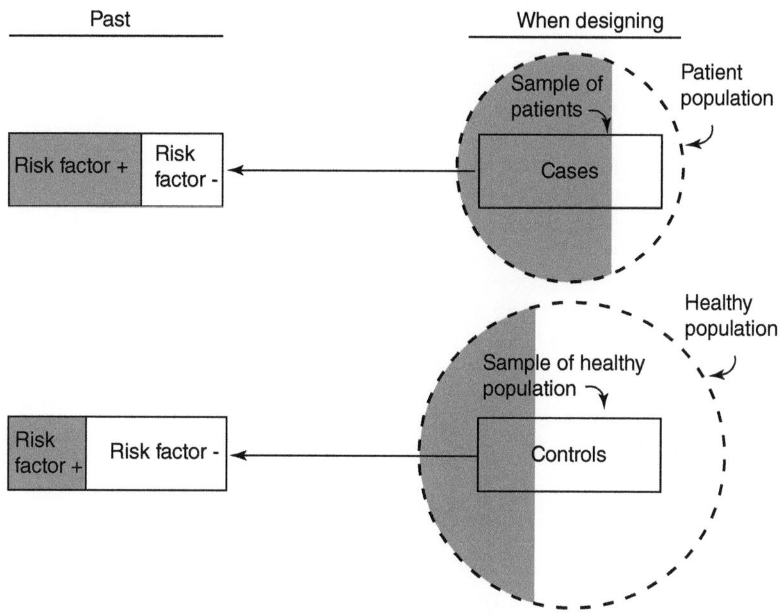

Fig. 3.2 In case-control studies, researchers first take a sample from the population of patients (cases) and then a sample from the population of people at risk but healthy (controls) and measure the risk factors of the disease

rately evaluate causal relationships in these studies.

- In case-control studies, we are not able to estimate the risk, and only in certain cases, an approximation of the relative risk can be calculated (with these, the odds ratio is an indicator whose calculation has enough credibility and scientific appeal).
- In case-control studies, the sources of potential bias are very wide. In most cases, the source of corruption is the way controls are selected.

3.3.2 Selection of Cases in Case-Control Studies

Sampling in case-control studies begins with the collection of cases. It is very important to know which group of patients represents which part of the patients under study. Ideally, case sampling includes a random sample of all people suffering from the disease in question. With this idea, the first question that arises is to know who has the desired disease and who does not have this disease. In cross-sectional and cohort studies, researchers regularly examine the presence of disease in all subjects. But in a case-control study, the cases are selected from a community in which the presence of the disease has already been diagnosed and reported. This sample is not a suitable and unbiased and completely random representative of all affected patients, because undiagnosed, misdiagnosed, unreported and referred, and deceased cases were excluded from the selection. For this reason, the selection of subjects under study in case-control studies is of double importance. Figure 3.3, which is known as the disease iceberg, shows this issue [11–13].

Before selecting cases, a precise definition of the disease under investigation should be provided. If the definitions are not clear, there is a risk of misclassification. If the definition of cases includes a wide range, the case-control study will be ineffective. For example, mental illness is a general word that includes different diseases. There are two main sources for selecting case group people:

1. Hospital
2. Population

The specific advantage of hospital cases is the simple access to people and ease of conducting the study in terms of logistics, but the main problem of this source is the selection bias in using this method. Selecting cases from the community minimizes the possibility of selection bias. In this method, the need for accurate recording and reporting systems about the disease under study is very vital. Another point in choosing a group of items is the method of selecting the group of items (new items or existing items). Figure 3.4a, b shows how to select items in each of these two modes. Figure 3.4a is related to the selection of available items. In this study, only cases 2, 6, 7,

Fig. 3.3 It is possible that the case-control study is not a suitable representative of the patient population

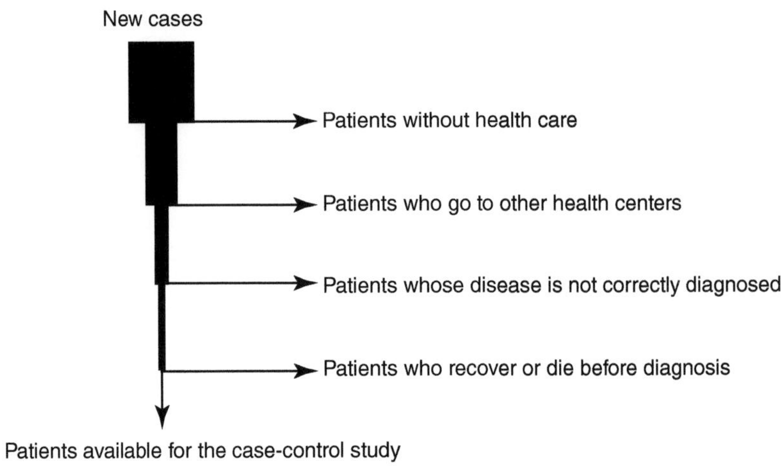

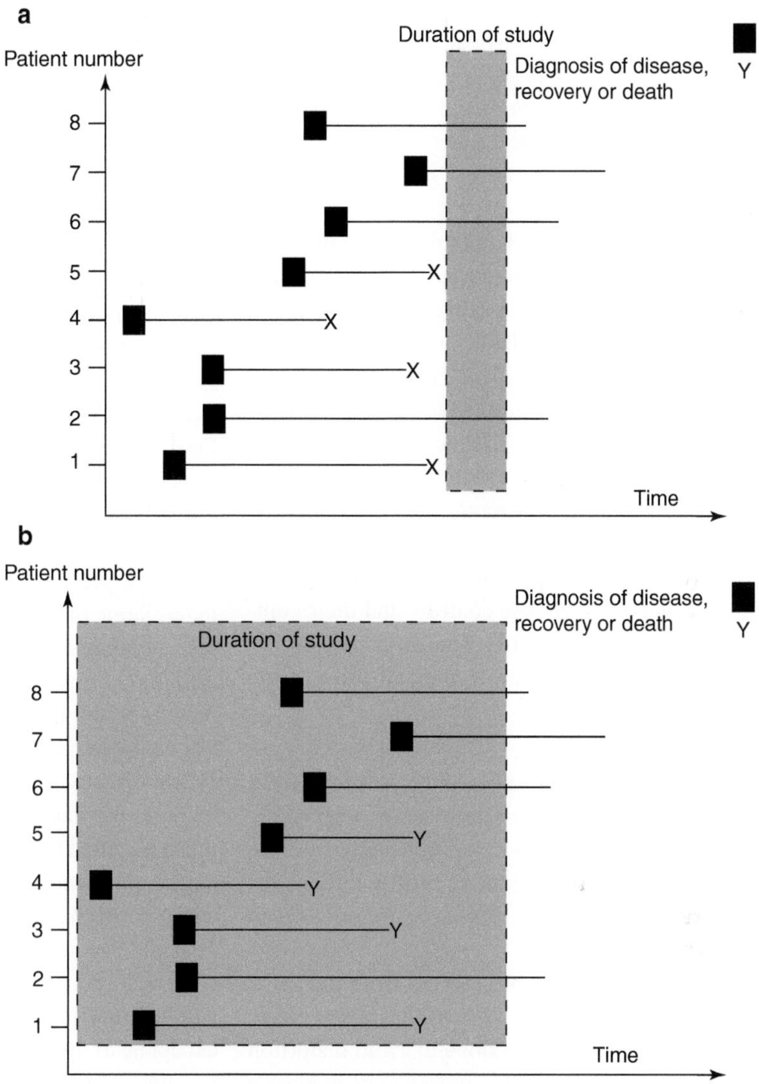

Fig. 3.4 Methods of selecting cases in a case-control study. (**a**) The method of selecting cases in the case-control study. In this method, only patient numbers 2, 6, 7, and 8 are included in the study. (**b**) The method of selecting new items. In this method, all patients whose disease was diagnosed during the study period are examined in the study

and 8 who are sick and alive at the time of the study are examined.

Figure 3.4b is related to the selection of new items. In this study, all cases diagnosed during the study (regardless of how long after the diagnosis, they are sick or alive) are examined. The important point in choosing new cases is that since the purpose of the study is to investigate the factors that cause the disease, there is no need for follow-up.

Entry and Exit Criteria Sometimes only groups of diseases are considered in the study that have or lack certain characteristics. For example, removing groups that have one or more co-morbidities or exceptional cases in which the risk factors are extremely higher than other people is very effective in increasing the internal validity of the study. In some circumstances, it may be necessary to limit the collection of items to a certain period and a certain place. For this reason, in many studies, cases are collected from a limited source (in terms of time and place). On the other hand, for some studies, it is necessary to remove many items from the collection, because there was a small chance of encountering risk factors for them.

Sources Cases are usually patients diagnosed in the medical system. Hospital records, operating room records, and pathology reports are common sources in this field. Sometimes, a combination of these sources is used to select items.

Selection of Controls (Control Group) in Case-Control Studies In practice, the resources of patients who make up the cases are limited. For this reason, choosing them for the study is relatively simple. The difficult part of decision-making in any case-control study is the selection of appropriate controls. The selection conditions of the control group, except for the criteria related to the diagnosis of the disease, must be under the selection conditions of the case group. The most important and controversial topic in case-control studies is how to choose controls and their comparability with cases [14]. The following principles should be observed in the selection of the control group:

- The control group should be selected from people who are free of the disease under study. Usually, the control group consists of people who, although they are currently without the disease under study, expect to be infected in the future.
- This group should be selected from the same base society from which the items were selected. This issue is done to avoid distortion of exposure effects, the presence of unknown or unmeasured risk factors, and potential confounding factors. The criteria for entering and exiting the study (except for the disease under study) should be similar in the two groups.
- The control group should potentially have the chance of contracting the disease. For example, women whose uterus has been removed should not be selected as evidence in a study related to endometrial cancer.
- The control group should be selected from the same place as the people of the target group. In other words, when the source of a selection of cases is the population, the controls must also be selected from the population, and when the source of a selection of the cases is the hospital, the controls must also be selected from the hospital. The following strategies are common in the selection of controls.
- Hospital control group.
- Matching.
- Sampling-based on healthy people in the community.

Using multiple control groups, now we discuss the mentioned sources for the selection of case-control study controls.

3.3.2.1 Hospital Controls

One of the available methods to eliminate the selection bias in these studies is to use a control group who were hospitalized in the same hospital or clinic. Many influential factors make patients choose a particular clinic or hospital for treatment. Some of these factors include financial status, residential area, ethnicity, and religious affiliation similar to the cases. This neutralizes the effect of influencing factors to a large extent. For example, in a case-control study on the association between smoking and heart attack in women, the case subjects can be selected from those admitted to the Cardiac Care Unit (CCU) of the hospital and the control subjects from those admitted to the surgical, orthopedic, and wards. And the medical services of the same medical centers are accepted and include musculoskeletal and internal patients and all kinds of diseases except heart diseases. There are several important practical and scientific advantages to using a hospital control group. First, it is easy to identify these people, and they are available easily and in sufficient numbers, so the study expenses and the practical work to be done are minimized. Second, because these people are in the hospital, they tend to know more about the history of exposure or past events than healthy people. In this way, the similarity between the two groups for reporting information reduces the recall bias. Thirdly, the use of hospitalized patients who are being treated for other reasons means that there were similarities between this group and the cases under study that made them refer to a specific clinic or hospital. Fourth, the hospital control group, like the case group, shows a greater desire to cooperate than healthy people, so the stress caused by nonresponse and noncooperation is reduced. The most important drawback of using a hospital control group is that, according to the definition, these people are sick and therefore different from normal people. Therefore, the condition of these patients may not be a suitable representative to investigate the prevalence of risk factors in the population from which the case group was taken. Studies conducted on hospital and nonhospital control groups have proven that, for example, hospitalized patients smoked more, used more birth control pills, or consumed more alcohol in western countries than nonhospitalized people. For this reason, if a case-control study is conducted using hospital controls on the use of coffee and bladder cancer, it may lead to a significant relationship between these two variables, and if another control group was used, this result was not obtained. The question of which category or categories of patients should be included in the hospital control group is an important issue. An issue that should be considered is that the type of disease for which the control group was hospitalized may be related to the studied risk factors. Therefore, in practice, patients who have a positive or negative correlation with the desired risk factors should be excluded from the control group. For example, smoking is an important risk factor for many respiratory diseases such as bronchitis and pneumonia. Placing such patients in the comparison group of a case-control study about smoking and lung cancer causes a high proportion of smokers to be included in the control group; as a result, this group is not a suitable representative of healthy people in society. A suitable strategy in selecting a hospital control group is to select patients from different departments of the hospital who do not have diagnostic similarities with the studied disease or are not related to the risk factors of the studied disease.

3.3.2.2 Matching

Matching is one of the simple and effective methods to make the group of cases and controls comparable. In this method, the important factors related to the disease, which the researcher does not want to investigate the effect on the disease, are matched. For example, many factors and diseases are related to age and sex. For this reason, comparing two groups while they are not comparable in terms of age and gender does not seem very logical. One of the ways to avoid this problem is to match controls and cases in terms of age and sex. In addition, many risk factors that are difficult to measure (such as environmental, genetic, and hormonal factors) that are related to age, sex, and family history are adjusted by matching in the study. Assimilation is done in two ways: individual and group assimilation. In individual assimilation, a similar control (in terms of desired variables) is selected for each person in the study group. In group assimilation, the people of the control group are selected in such a way that the ratio of certain variables among them is similar to the ratio of those variables in the people of the case group. For this example, if 30% of the people in the case group are workers, 30% of the people in the control group are also selected from the workers. Usually, in this method, all the people of the selected group and the people of the control group should be selected according to them.

3.3.2.3 Sampling Based on Healthy People in the Society

Selection of the control group from the normal population is done in various ways. When conducting studies that require sampling from specific target areas, researchers often resort to methods such as selecting random phone numbers or identifying individuals through census maps. However, when it comes to selecting healthy individuals from the general population, certain challenges arise. Determining and examining controls from the general population is usually more expensive and time-consuming than hospital controls. The list of people in the community is not always available, and due to their busy schedules and due to the situation of their departure times, it is usually difficult to contact and establish a relationship with them. In addition, the quality of information between the two groups of cases and controls may be different, because those who live in normal society may not remember the risk factors as much as those who have the disease. Also, people who have not had any health problems recently have less motivation to participate in the study. Therefore, the number of people who refuse to participate in the program in the community control group is almost always more than in the case group and the hospital control group. Another source of control selection includes special groups such as friends, relatives, companions, or neighbors of the cases. These groups have some advantages over the control group of society because they are healthy and have a greater desire to cooperate than the normal population. The advantage of this method is that some main confounding factors related to race, economic, social, and environmental status are controlled.

3.3.2.4 Using Multiple Control Groups

Sometimes the use of a control group has certain shortcomings that can be compensated by using another group. For example, in a case-control study about the relationship between coffee consumption and pancreatic cancer, patients should be compared with a group of controls who were hospitalized for other reasons. While using a hospital control group is appropriate due to its low cost and easy access, the important thing is that hospital controls are different from healthy people in society in terms of coffee consumption. To correct this situation, another control group that includes normal people in society should be selected. The comparison of the observed correlation between coffee consumption and pancreatic cancer in each of the control groups proves the information about the real effect of this factor and also the inadequacy of using a hospital control group to study such a hypothesis. After determining the source and number of control groups, it is necessary to decide on the ratio of controls to cases. The best ratio of control to the patient is one to one, but when the sample size of patients is limited or the cost of obtaining information in the case group is high, the ratio of control to the patient can change to some extent. But usually, it is not recommended that this ratio be more than 4 to 1. After defining the characteristics and sources of selection of case and control groups, information about the disease and exposure should be obtained. Another important point is the accuracy and correctness of comparison and comparability of information sources. The necessary information about the condition of the disease can be obtained from several sources, such as reviewing death certificates; registering cases in monitoring programs, doctors' office files, hospital admission, and discharge files; and operating room offices and the pathology department. Exposure information can be obtained from study subjects including questioning and information included in medical records. The approaches used to obtain information in both control and case groups should be similar as possible. For example, the location and conditions of the interview should be the same in both groups, and in situations where there is a possibility of blinding the questioner or the summarizer of medical records about the condition of the cases and controls, this issue must be observed. After all, the people who are responsible for collecting information should be kept as ignorant as possible about the hypotheses of the study. This work is very necessary to minimize the observer's distortion [14].

3.3.3 Cohort Studies

Cohort studies are a type of epidemiological studies in which subjects are followed over time. There are two main goals in conducting cohort studies:

- Description: To describe the occurrence of specific events over time.
- Analysis: To evaluate association and dependence between response and independent variables. In general, cohort studies are generally divided into two types: prospective and retrospective (and combined).

3.3.4 Prospective Cohort Studies

In prospective cohort studies, researchers select or define the desired sample and then measure characteristics such as lifestyle, activity pattern, place of residence, employment, and any other

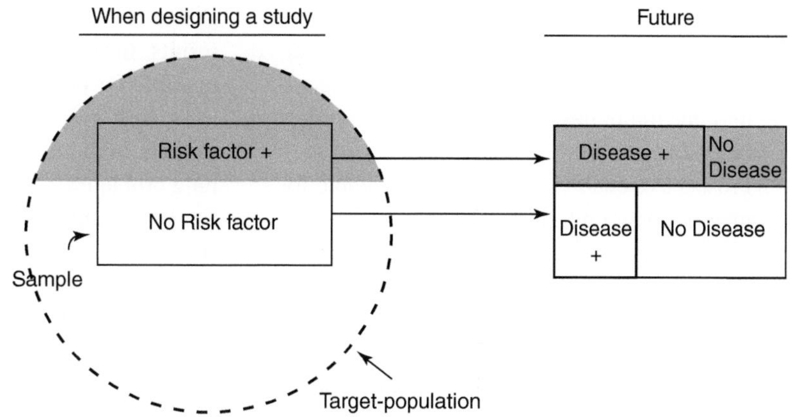

Fig. 3.5 In prospective cohort studies, researchers take a sample from the community and measure the variables related to prognosis and risk factors, and during the follow-up of this population, the incidence of the disease is measured

variable that is likely to predict the incidence of the desired event. These members are continuously examined in the follow-up phase, and their important characteristics are measured again, and the occurrence or nonoccurrence of the desired event in them is investigated. Figure 3.5 shows how to conduct this study.

A cohort study in its simplest form includes the selection of two groups of people in the society (base population), which are one group of exposed people. Exposure is a special characteristic that makes members with this characteristic be among the high-risk groups for suffering from the desired event (e.g., smoking in case of lung cancer), and the other group is people who have no exposure. Two groups are followed for a certain period. This follow-up can continue until the death of the last person in each group, and the occurrence of the desired event in the two groups is compared. For example, in a study conducted on the dangers of exposure to coal, miners working in coal mines and other heavy industry workers can form two target groups (base population). These two groups are followed for a certain period (e.g., 10 years) to compare the incidence of bronchitis between these two groups.

The nonexposed group (workers working in heavy industries) is included in the study to be examined as a control group for the comparison of disease cases related to the exposure factor (coal). Ideally, only those who are initially free of the desired disease or outcome are allowed to enter the study. Therefore, in the previous example, only people without bronchitis symptoms should be considered as the base population.

A prospective cohort study is a powerful strategy for describing the occurrence and examining the possible causes of an event in various conditions because the potential factors causing the disease are measured before the consequences occur. The correct time sequence strengthens the theory that the measured factors are the cause of the result. The prospective study offers researchers the opportunity to fully and accurately measure all important factors. This issue is very important in some variables, such as the daily diet, whose measurement is very important due to the taste of the answers and the error of forgetting. The measurement of some variables, after the onset of the disease, due to errors and distortions caused by knowledge of the patient or biological intervention, becomes invalid and careless. This problem disappears in prospective cohort studies.

3.3.5 Advantages and Disadvantages of Cohort Studies

- Prospective cohort studies are usually very expensive and time-consuming. The main reason is planning to follow a large group of people over a long period.
- These studies are not suitable for examining long-term diseases. Because the study period will be unacceptably long. For example, if

healthy young smokers and nonsmokers are followed until the development of lung cancer, we need at least a 20-year follow-up program until the tumor develops and reaches the stage of diagnosis.

- Prospective cohort studies are not suitable for investigating rare diseases, because in this case, we need a very large base population with a very long follow-up, both of which can be unacceptable. For example, when the incidence of a disease is five cases per 100,000 people per year and we want to study about 100 cases to investigate a significant relationship between exposure and disease, we should follow an initial cohort population of 200,000 people for 10 years. The study of an initial cohort population of 400,000 people with 5 years of follow-up has a similar result. The effect of the study is an important factor that may affect some changeable characteristics in the subjects under study. For example, it is possible that the studied members, after being studied and continuously monitored, may consciously change their lifestyle, diet, and daily activity level, or eliminate the exposure factor. It is assumed that they quit smoking or do not expose themselves to direct sunlight. This issue strongly affects the accuracy of the inferences about exposure and nonexposure groups.
- The exposure factor, especially in studies that have a long follow-up time, may be removed or reduced, added, or intensified without being related to the research effect. For example, a smoker may quit smoking or increase the number of threads consumed per day. In addition to creating a problem in measuring the amount and duration of exposure, this issue also complicates the analysis of the results.
- The withdrawal of people from the study is a factor that can affect the results. Withdrawal from the study can be done for reasons not related to the disease, in which case special statistical methods should be used in their adjustment, or it can be related to the disease and occur regularly, which causes error in the results, for example, exposure With coal, it is possible for people with bronchitis to migrate to an area with hot weather, or for smokers to migrate from the city to the countryside due to lung problems.
- The main study is designed only for one exposure factor and one event or disease. When different risk factors and different events are considered, more complex methods are needed.

3.3.6 The Retrospective (Historical) Cohort Study

The historical cohort study design is similar to the prospective cohort study. A group of people in society are followed over time, and the potential risk factor variables are measured in them, and it is ensured that they have a disease or injury. The only difference is the history of events (measurement of basic risk factors, follow-up, and confirmation of disease occurrence), which is entirely in the past. This type of study can only be done if appropriate and high-quality data are available. It is possible that these people were followed up in a cohort study for another purpose. Figure 3.6 shows the model of how to conduct this study.

Cohort studies are historical in determining risk factors and predictors. These studies are faster and more economical compared to the prospective cohort study. Because the historical cohort study was done in the past and the researcher did not have a role in the initial measurements, follow-ups, and diagnosis of the disease, the quality of the data may not be suitable. Usually, the available data does not include much of the information needed to evaluate the research questions. In the historical studies of missing data, the measurement of variables with a method other than that intended by researchers and the incompleteness of information forms are serious research problems.

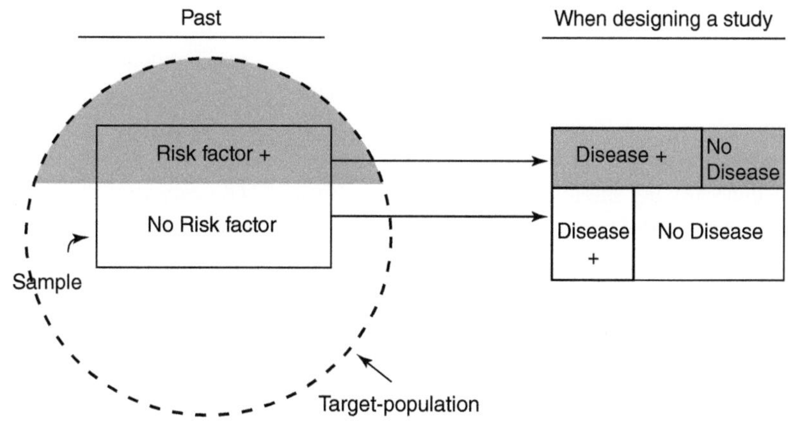

Fig. 3.6 In retrospective cohort studies, the researcher reconstructs the cohort population that existed in the past and collects information about the risk factors and prognosis of the disease that were measured in the past. Then it measures the incidence of the disease

3.3.7 Selection of the Exposed Population

The people who are selected to be considered as the exposed population in a cohort study may be from various sources. The selection of a specific group depends on many scientific and operational considerations, some of which are the frequency of exposure under study, the need to have complete and accurate information about the exposure, the possibility of reaching the people under study, the traceability of the people under study, and the nature of the questions asked in research, which are evaluated [14].

If the exposure is relatively common (such as smoking or exposure to direct sunlight), a sufficient number of exposed people can be identified among the target population. But in rare exposures such as exposures related to a specific profession, environmental factors, and special climatic conditions, choosing a special population is more effective. Special risk groups can include people from a certain profession such as rubber factory workers, uranium miners, shipbuilders, and patients who are undergoing radiation therapy due to cancer, or who have had repeated fluoroscopy examinations to diagnose tuberculosis. People who live near a harmful environment, such as a nuclear test site or a toxic waste storage site, people whose daily diet is different from normal people or have a special lifestyle, and people who have faced a special exposure in a special event (the dropping of the atomic bomb in Hiroshima or industrial accidents in large factories) are examples of this. The advantage of selecting the population with a specific exposure is that it is possible to follow the exposed people in a reasonable time and sufficient numbers.

The use of these cohorts can identify the cause of the disease in the special conditions under investigation. In addition, cohorts can be an efficient tool to identify risk factors that exist in the reference population. Therefore, to evaluate the relationship between physical activity and coronary artery disease, some cohort studies were conducted among groups with special exposure such as bus drivers and porters in London. With the information obtained from these studies, considering their obvious advantages, in terms of the small sample size and the ability to reveal the exposure and proper follow-up of the participants to determine the desired outcome, the results of the study to evaluate the role of physical activity in the etiology of coronary artery disease have been generalized to the general population [15].

In addition, by using a cohort with specific exposure, it is possible to evaluate rare outcomes. Even if an outcome is very rare in the general population, it may be common enough in a group with a specific exposure that it is possible to collect a sufficient number of cases. For example, the annual incidence of mesothelioma in the general population is close to 8.24 per million. Therefore, in a cohort study that includes 20,000 people, it is impossible to identify every case of this disease within 5 years of follow-up. But because the incidence of mesothelioma is relatively common among those who deal with fireproof cotton, a cohort study of 20,000 workers who work with this material might produce enough cases to look for exposure relationships. Illness is enough. Thus, although the cohort study is generally not suitable for the evaluation of rare diseases if the desired outcome is not rare in the exposure group, a cohort design with appropriate efficiency can be used.

The first requirement for the validity of the cohort study is the ability to obtain complete and accurate information about the participants, especially in terms of proving the data related to the desired exposure and outcome; for this reason, cohort studies are often conducted among groups that have been specifically selected. Different groups that are targeted for cohort studies can include workers in a factory, people in a union, pensioners, students of a particular university, or participants in medical care programs. Each of these groups has specific advantages for the researcher, which range from the availability of annual records to periodic follow-up mechanisms and the provision of complete medical and occupational reports. The reason for choosing these groups is not high levels of exposure, but the possibility of better follow-up and study leads to these choices.

In this way, the selection of a special group as a cohort population is related to the hypothesis under investigation and the special aspects of the study plan. For example, to evaluate the possible relationship between exposure to halal and the risk of cancer, a cohort study can be designed on some people working in factories that use halal, and reports about their occupational exposure are available. Such a study was conducted on plastic, linoleum, and rubber workers at six major rubber factories in the United States. In this study, the consequences related to industrial exposure and cancer risk were investigated [14].

For this type of research on important risk factors in relatively chronic and common diseases to be effective, the best choice for the study population is a general cohort that can be examine and prove the initial exposure of these people to risk factors and can then be periodically reexamined to determine the next consequences in them. A classic design of this type of study is the study of heart diseases in the city of Framingham, United States. In this study, a prospective cohort with a population of nearly 5100 residents over 30 years of age in Massachusetts was examined. The city of Framingham was not chosen as a study site because its population had specific characteristics related to exposure or outcome that would allow for further investigation, but because it allowed the researchers to identify and follow the participants for several years in this city, it was chosen. The population of this city was stable, and its industries were known. A major and large hospital in this city covered a very large part of the population, and the lists that make it easy to follow the participants were available annually and timely. These are the cases in the successful implementation of a prospective cohort study with the general population that allows the evaluation of the effects of a wide range of factors that are considered risk factors for many diseases. In this study, it was possible to investigate coronary artery disease, rheumatic heart disease, heart failure, angina, and some eye diseases [16, 17].

3.3.8 Selection of the Comparison Group (Nonexposed Population)

After determining the sources and selecting exposed subjects, the next important step is to select a suitable comparison group of nonexposed subjects. Choosing a comparison group in a cohort study is as difficult and important as choosing a control group in a case-control study. The main principle underlying this decision is that the comparison groups should be similar to the exposure groups as much as possible in terms of all the factors that can be related to the disease (except for the exposure factor under investigation) so that if there is no correlation between the exposure and disease, indices are similar in both populations. Another important point is to ensure that the information obtained from the nonexposed group is sufficient for comparison with the exposed population.

In cohort studies in which a general cohort is given and then its members are classified according to different categories of exposure, a comparison group within the cohort can be used. That is, experience with a specific exposure in a subgroup of members of the same classification group is compared with the experience of another subgroup of members of the same group who were without exposure or had exposure of different intensity. For example, in a cohort study of English physicians conducted in 1950 by Dahl and Hale, the incidence of lung cancer among those who had never smoked was compared with the incidence of this disease among all smokers and those who smoked in different amounts. The researchers found that the death rates from lung cancer among smokers have increased compared to nonsmokers, and also a significant and continuous increase in the incidence of lung cancer is observed with the increase in the number of cigarettes smoked [18]. Similarly, in the Framingham study, the baseline level of blood cholesterol, systolic, and diastolic blood pressure was determined, and the participants were divided according to exposure percentiles. In the continuation of the study, the rates of coronary artery disease in each of the levels were calculated and compared. It is important to pay attention to this point that when several risk factors are considered at the same time, the nonexposed group should include people who do not have any of the evaluated risk factors [19].

It is usually very difficult to identify that part of the cohort that can be safely assumed to be without exposure and to be used for comparison in cohort studies that are designed to investigate a specific exposure group such as labor groups or special climatic conditions. In this case, external comparison groups are used. One of the external comparison groups is the general population of the region where the cohort lives. The rate of disease observed in the study group is compared with the estimated rate of disease in the general population during the follow-up of the cohort. For example, to evaluate the potential risks related to working in a rubber factory, the damping observed in the rubber factory workers was compared with the damping of the general population of that area, which was adjusted in terms of age, sex, and other potentially important risk factors [20].

Of course, the comparison with population rates is only possible for outcomes that have population-related rates available. Examples include cancer incidence, cancer remission, or similar situations where outcome data can be obtained. Apart from this, the use of the general population as a reliable indicator of the experience of the unexposed group is based on the assumption that only a small part of that population is exposed in practice and through any type of risk factor source under investigation. Depending on the scope of that part of the general population that has exposure, the real correlation between exposure and disease is underestimated.

The major drawback of using the general population as a comparison group is that the individuals within the general population may not be directly comparable to those within the target group. This discrepancy arises because, firstly, people who are employed tend to be on average healthier than those who are not. Since the general population includes people who cannot work due to illness, and this group includes working people, the rates of illness and death in the general population are almost always higher than the rates of illness and death among those subject to labor law. This phenomenon is called the healthy worker effect.

The reference population and the cohort population may be similar in terms of some factors such as demographic and geographic characteristics, but they are completely different in terms of other disease risk factors (including smoking, diet, and consumption of alcoholic beverages). Because this information is not available for the general population, the observed differences may be due to the failure to control confounding factors.

Another way to use disease rates in the general population as a comparison group is to compare the experience with a specific exposure of a cohort with a cohort similar in terms of demographic characteristics but without exposure. In studies related to occupational exposures, such a group includes workers of different types of jobs who work in different locations of an industrial center. For example, the disease rates in the unexposed group of administrative workers of a factory can be compared with the disease rates of the production workers group in the same factory. One of the studies conducted is a cohort study that investigates the exposure of pilots who flew chemical bombs during the Vietnam War. These pilots are compared with a group of Air Force personnel working in the air transport sector in the same region of Vietnam during the same timeframe [21]. Also, to evaluate the risk of long-term exposure to low amounts of ionizing radiation in radiologists, these people were compared with internal medicine specialists [22]. Because internal medicine specialists are similar to radiologists in terms of demographic characteristics, attention to health, and use of medical care, this comparison seems very justified. In a study about exposure to fireproof and its relationship with lung cancer, a group of workers exposed to fireproof cotton who worked in the spinning industry was compared with normal cotton spinning workers. These two groups have similar job duties, and they have common socioeconomic characteristics, but from the occupational point of view, the second group is not exposed to fireproof cotton [23]. The advantage of using the same group in comparison with the use of the general group is that it is possible to choose a group that is more compatible and similar to the exposed group. Furthermore, information about potential confounding factors can be obtained about the studied subjects and residual differences can be controlled during the analysis.

In many cohort studies, especially when no group seems to be sufficiently similar to the exposed individuals, there is no assurance of the validity of the comparison. In these cases, it is beneficial to have several comparison groups. In such conditions, if a similar correlation is obtained from different groups, the result of the study is more justified. For example, in the fireproof cotton study described earlier, in addition to comparing fireproof cotton workers with regular cotton mill workers, damping rates were also compared with the white male population of the United States. Workers working in refractory cotton spinning departments had higher rates of mortality from all causes, lung cancer, other respiratory diseases, and hypertension compared to ordinary cotton spinning workers and the general population. In this way, the damping rate of fireproof cotton workers was not only higher than the general population but also significantly higher than the group of men who had similar work but fireproof cotton was not in their work environment. The compatibility of the results of these two comparisons strengthened the theory that the workers of fireproof cotton factories are at risk of developing diseases related to their jobs. Also, in evaluating the adverse consequences related to the use of oral contraceptive pills (OCP), it is very important to choose a proportional comparison group. For comparison, a group should be selected that uses some kind of contraception other than oral pills. Women who do not use any method of preventing pregnancy may be different from those who use any type of contraception in terms of the ability to get pregnant, the desire to get pregnant, and the nature of sexual behavior. On the other hand, women who use various forms of birth control methods are probably different from women who use oral pills in terms of socioeconomic status and other factors affecting health and lifestyle. Therefore, no type of comparison group may be superior. The first cohort study in Iran evaluated the outcome of permanent hypothyroidism and predictive factors of thyroid dysfunction and showed that a large proportion of women with moderate and severe PPTD, especially at the age of 30 years and older, have recurrent hypothyroidism [24].

3.3.9 Data Sources

When designing any type of cohort study, the main focus is on the availability of accurate and complete information that allows the classification of all members of the cohort (in terms of exposure to the researched risk factors or the occurrence of any desired outcome) to be provided. Information about exposure can be obtained from several sources, including records collected independently of the study (such as medical or employment records), information obtained from the study itself (through questionnaires or questionnaires), data obtained from the medical examination or other tests performed for the participants, and direct measurements at the place of residence or work of the group members. Information about outcomes can also be collected from pre-existing records such as death certificates or medical records, questionnaires, or physical examinations. Each of these data sources has its advantages and disadvantages, which should be considered when designing or interpreting the study.

3.4 Types of Interventional Studies

In the type of cohort study, exposed groups are compared with nonexposed groups, but the exposure factor in clinical trial studies is often an intervention, but in cohort (observational) studies, the factor under investigation is usually the factor that people face. Understanding the difference between these two designs is very important in terms of interpreting the results. In cohort (observational) studies, unlike experimental observations (randomized clinical trials), the subjects' exposures are not assigned randomly and by the researchers' will. For this reason, when a relationship between exposure and disease is obtained in a nonrandomized study, this relationship may be due to the nonrandom (targeted) selection of study subjects.

Experiments or interventions provide the most definitive evidence to investigate a causal relationship. Medical studies are no exception to this. Interventional studies differ according to the presence or absence of comparison groups (parallel or simultaneous), conducting studies on patients or healthy people, and random assignment of subjects.

3.4.1 Experimental Studies

In experimental studies, subjects under study receive the desired intervention only when the researcher assigns these interventions to each member based on a precise protocol and possibly using random assignment methods. In these studies, the prescription of each of the interventions for the people under study is not based on the need or choice of the people under study or special environmental conditions, but based on the research protocol, and the researchers allocate the interventions to the people under study. For instance, in a scenario where a doctor administers treatment for headaches, it is common for them to prescribe a brand-name drug to financially capable patients in order to establish trust. Conversely, for economically disadvantaged patients, the doctor may opt to prescribe the same drug but with a generic name to reduce treatment expenses. In this case, it is important to note that this particular study does not qualify as experimental due to the fact that the prescription of medicine to patients is contingent upon individual preferences and subjective judgment. To conduct an experimental study, the doctor must prescribe the drug to the patients based on a written protocol to neutralize any potential changes caused by other factors. The allocation of treatments in experimental studies is to avoid the effect of changes in other factors on the comparisons as much as possible. If personal judgments, the clinical conditions of the patients, and the taste of the study administrators influence the assignment of the intervention, it is still possible to compare the methods with each other by designing a semi-experimental or nonexperimental study.

There are many ethical considerations in the design and implementation of experimental studies. The reason is that the purpose of the study determines the way of assignments and the clinical needs of the patients are not considered. Experimental studies are ethically applicable only when they are considered useful for patients. In particular, there must be acceptable scientific reasons to show that two or more of the existing treatments proposed in the study protocol are the best available treatments. Consequently, it is essential for each of the proposed treatments or interventions to demonstrate a minimum level of efficacy in terms of treatment or prevention. These inherent limitations, such as those encountered in toxicology studies, often render them nonexperimental in nature. Considering all these issues, the fully informed consent of the subjects under study is the main license to conduct experimental studies.

Despite these limitations, many studies of this type are designed and implemented in various medical fields. Most of these studies are classified as clinical trials. Clinical trials are studies designed to compare different treatments in patients. Experimental studies that are designed with the aim of primary prevention are called field trials or community interventions.

3.4.2 Clinical Trial (Study or Research)

A clinical trial is a study in which patients are the members under investigation. The main goal of any clinical trial is to evaluate a new treatment for a disease or to find suitable methods to prevent the complications of a disease such as death or physical disability. A comprehensive definition of clinical trials can be as follows.

A clinical trial is a human research conducted to discover or confirm the clinical, pharmacological, or other pharmacodynamic effects of an investigational product or to identify any adverse reactions. The product is done to prove its safety or effectiveness.

The goal of researchers in clinical trials is to test treatment methods (under the title of intervention) on people under study and observe their effects. The most important strength of trials compared to observational studies is the ability to make causal inferences. The act of randomly assigning the intervention can eliminate the effect of confounding variables and blinding eliminates the possible effects of bias in judgment.

However, in general, clinical trials are expensive and time-consuming and sometimes can be risky for the people under study, and usually, clinical studies answer only one very specific research question. For this reason, clinical research is used only in cases where research goals and questions have reached a certain level of development [25].

Now, we examine the different steps for designing an experimental study.

3.4.3 Selection of Patients

In every clinical trial, we need a precise definition of eligible patients to enter the study. The main goal is to make sure that the patients who enter the trial are representative of the class of patients that the trial findings will be applied to in the future. In addition, it is desirable to focus the treatment with the new drug on those patients who are likely to benefit the most from the drug. At the same time, the entry of patients should not be limited, and the trial should not be so small that the findings lose their generalizability. The main aspects that need attention are as follows:

- Source of patient choice.
- The condition of the disease under study.
- Specific criteria for patient discharge.

The issue of choosing the source of patients should be considered with special care. For example, in the study of depression, if we go to hospitalized patients, we will find an unusual group. These patients include mostly chronic and severe cases. While the antidepressants under study are usually used by a larger group of depressed patients under the care of doctors.

3.4.4 Determining the Entry and Exit Criteria

In determining the entry and exit criteria of any clinical trial, the overall amount of the intended outcome, the approximate amount of effectiveness of the active intervention, the generalizability of the findings, easy access to the studied subjects, possible side effects, and the possibility of follow-up of the sample should be taken into consideration.

If the intended outcome, such as breast cancer, is rare, it is usually necessary to select the subjects under study only from high-risk subjects so that the sample size and follow-up period are acceptable; on the other hand, limiting the entry criteria to high-risk people reduces the ability to generalize the results and also makes it difficult to access the sample members.

Researchers should have reliable estimates of the overall outcome under study. These results may be obtained from current statistics, longitudinal studies, or outcome measures in the nonintervention group (control group).

Limiting the study of high-risk people can reduce the sample members. If the risk factors have a predetermined outcome, the inclusion criteria can be based on having a minimum estimate of risk exposure. For example, in a clinical study on the effect of tamoxifen in preventing breast cancer, a combination of risk factors for this cancer was used as one of the criteria for entering the study. This study showed that the benefit of tamoxifen is seen only in elderly women with a previous heart attack and a low risk of recurrence [26]. Another way to increase the access to the sample members of the outcome rate is to limit the study to the study of affected people. For example, in a study that investigated increasing the amount of estrogen and progesterone hormones in reducing the incidence of coronary artery disease (CHD), 2763 women who had previously suffered from this condition were used. These methods are more practical and less expensive than a similar study with women who did not suffer from CHD complications (which requires a sample size of over 25,000 people).

Limiting the entry criteria to high-risk groups has two major limitations. First, the results obtained from the study on high-risk groups may not be generalizable to low-risk groups. For example, in the study of estrogen and progesterone, which only investigated women with CHD complications, there is no guarantee for the effectiveness of this method in women without CHD complications. In addition, collecting documents and sufficient information about high-risk groups, such as the history of CHD, may require the collection of data, information, or multiple measurements, which makes the study complicated, time-consuming, and expensive.

In determining the exclusion criteria of a clinical study, a decision should be made in such a way as to prevent the unnecessary exclusion of patients from the study as much as possible because the unnecessary removal of patients from the study reduces the generalizability of the study and complicates and costs the collection of samples. The main reasons for excluding patients from the study are given in Table 3.1.

3.4.5 Measurement of Basic Variables

In general, in every clinical trial, information related to four categories of variables should be collected: variables related to the identification of study subjects such as name and family name, contact phone number, birth certificate number, and home address; demographic variables such as age and gender; confounding variables; response variable; and different levels of intervention.

Measurements performed on patients should be accurate and repeatable and should not depend on the person responsible for the measurement or the observer. Unfortunately, many evaluations are

Table 3.1 Reasons for excluding people under study in clinical trials

Reason
The active treatment carried out has an unexpected destructive side effect
Unexpected danger due to receiving a placebo threatens the subjects of the study
Active treatment is not effective because the subject:
– Basically, it is not exposed to the risk of infection
– He/she is suffering from a special disease that removes the effectiveness of the treatment under study
– Takes drugs that interfere with the active treatment
– Does not follow active or passive treatment continuously and accurately
Incomplete follow-up
The basic problems of the patient to participate or continue cooperation in the study

quantitative, and experienced observers are needed. For example, mental illness is evaluated based on clinical diagnosis. The main issue is that the collected information is structured. For example, in the case of depression, it is not appropriate to reach a general and scattered statement about the patient's condition. Instead, specific depression diagnosis methods (e.g., the Hamilton scale) have been developed, which use structured interviews to record information. In difficult cases for clinical evaluation, it is very useful to form a composite group of two or three observers whose main task is to agree on a common opinion (after initial independent evaluation and then consultation with each other). This issue is very appropriate and practical for evaluations that do not require the presence of the patient, for example, CT scan interpretation.

In some diseases, it is not possible to evaluate the effects of treatment unless we ask the patient's opinion. For example, pain relief in the trial of antirheumatic drugs is an example of this issue.

3.4.6 Evaluation of the Patient's Response

After the start of the trial, the therapeutic progress of each patient needs an objective, accurate, and stable evaluation to evaluate the relative merits of the treatments. Therefore, the methods of evaluating and recording the progress of the patients need a precise definition in the study proposal. In fact, for patient evaluation in a clinical trial, normal case notes are inappropriate, because they are usually written very vague, irregularly, unstable, and subjective. The patients present in the trial are evaluated for the following reasons:

1. Baseline assessment before starting treatment.
2. The main criteria of the patient's response.
3. Secondary criteria such as side effects.
4. Other aspects of patient monitoring In each of these four stages, careful planning is necessary for collecting information and recording data in forms or designing new forms.

At the same time, one should first decide which aspects to measure or observe.

3.4.7 Main Patient Response Criteria

Clinical trials may require extensive observations for each patient, which may make data interpretation difficult. Therefore, before the trial begins, solutions should be provided regarding the relative importance of various measurements. If a certain scale is used to examine the patient's response and compare the treatments, useful work has been done.

3.4.8 Sub-Criteria and Side Effects

After the main criterion of patient evaluation is clearly defined, there are other major aspects that researchers tend to investigate. For example, in drug trials, it is important to evaluate the safety and efficacy of the drug. Therefore, there is a need to compare treatments to determine their side effects. If the side effects are known, this is clear (e.g., decreased heart rate due to beta-blocker use, differential decrease in white blood cells due to drugs with a toxic effect on the cell). But it is more difficult to record side effects in the case of a relatively new drug. In such a situation, we should put a lot of emphasis on the patient's evaluation of side effects. A conventional method is to prepare a checklist of all symptoms and diseases at certain intervals and ask the patient. For example, Table 3.2 can be useful in a trial of antidepressants.

Note that this list should be expressed in words that patients can understand. Another method is that the patient is asked to explain any adverse event he experienced. For each patient, the events are entered on a special form and kept for the next classification [25, 27].

Table 3.2 An example of the list of side effects for evaluating a new drug

Paresthesia	Nausea	Headache
Shivering	Vomit	Tiredness
Hyperhidrosis	Indigestion	Insomnia
Edema	Xerostomia	Getting confused
Convulsions	Skin dryness	Diarrhea
Aggression	Arthralgia or joint pain	Constipation

3.4.9 Randomization

The next step in clinical studies is the random assignment of different treatment groups to patients. In the simplest design, one group receives active treatment, and the other group receives a placebo. The random assignment of patients to each of the treatments is the basis of performing statistical tests on the data.

3.4.10 Methods of Randomizing Treatments

3.4.10.1 Simple Random Method

In any randomized trial with two treatments (A and B), the simplest method is to use the table of random numbers. Below is an example of tables displaying random numbers ranging from 0 to 9. To randomly assign two treatments to patients, it should be done in this order.

We choose an optional point from the table of random numbers and extract the required number of numbers listed in the table. For example, it is possible to obtain the following sequence.

9 0 9 6 2 3 7 0 0 0 9 3 and so on

We consider numbers 0–4 for treatment A and numbers 5–9 for treatment B. In this case, a list with the following random order will be created:

A B A A A B A A B B A B and so on.

It is very easy to generalize this rule to more treatments, and for example, in the case of three treatments A, B, and C, we act as follows:

Figures 3.1, 3.2 and 3.3 for treatment A
Figures 3.4, 3.5 and 3.6 for treatment B
Figures 3.8, 3.9 and 3.10 for treatment C

And we ignore the number 0. In this case, if the sequence

1 9 0 8 2 6 6 5 9 8 3 2 6 4 6 1 1 etc.

Extracted from the table of random numbers, the random assignments of the three treatments are as follows:

A A B B B A A C C B B B A C - C A and so on.

The advantage of this method is its simplicity and the unpredictability of the subsequent treatment, but one of the problems of this method is the unequal number of people in each treatment group. This is not an obvious difference when out of 20 patients under investigation, eight patients received treatment A, and 12 patients received treatment B, but when four patients receive treatment A and 16 patients received treatment B, the power of the study is reduced to a large extent. To avoid this problem, more efficient methods such as randomization with placement, random replacement blocks, and classified randomization, which include the slant coin method and classified randomization, have been invented.

3.4.10.2 Blinding

If possible, double blinding of the subjects is a very suitable way to increase the reliability of the study. In two-way blinding, the patients and the research team are unaware of which of the study subjects received which treatment. After the study is completed and the results are collected, the codes for each patient are available to the research team. Usually, in studies where one of the groups does not receive treatment, blinding is done by prescribing placebos similar to the main drug.

3.4.11 Standard Report of Clinical Trials

In clinical trial studies, in addition to scientific and principled design, other important points are important. These steps are how to guide and report the results of studies. Unfortunately, the details of the implementation steps, how to deal with unforeseen regular errors, and the points that are included in the study to improve the quality of the study and increase the reliability and repeatability of the study are not reported or are stated very briefly. During the last decade, many efforts have been made to standardize the quality of reports in clinical trial studies, which resulted in the CONSORT guidelines in 1996 AD and its updated version in 2001 [28, 29]. Very useful information about this on the website http://www.consort-statement.org (Accessed date 7/29/2022).

Figure 3.7 shows the general structure of the examined items, and Table 3.3 shows a checklist of the important items examined in the CONSORT guidelines. Although the CONSORT guidelines are generally prepared for the analysis of designs with two parallel groups, it is also possible to use it in more complex cases such as factorial, cluster, or multicenter and crossover designs. New versions of CONSORT guidelines for reporting such studies are being prepared and regulated.

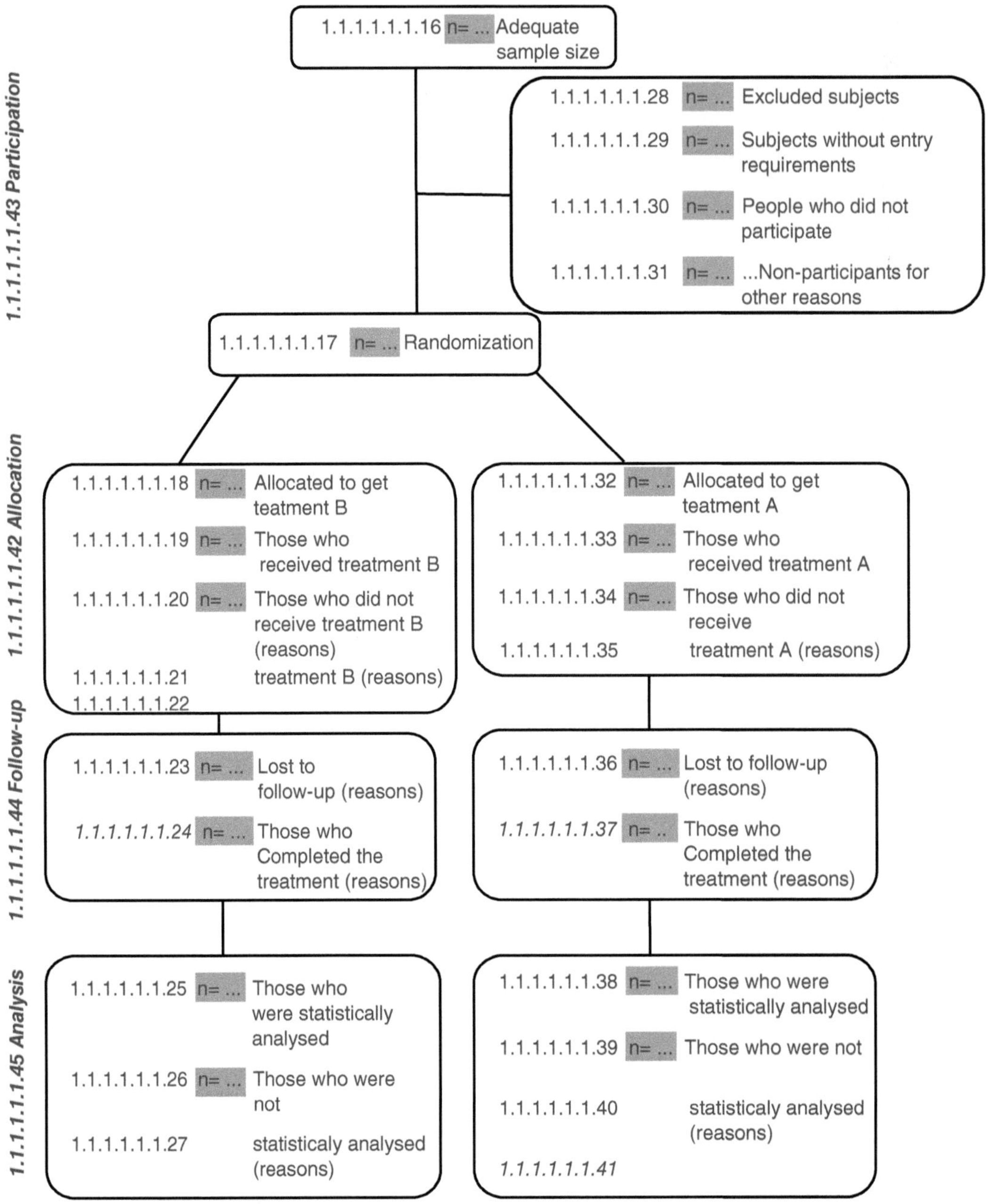

Fig. 3.7 Completing the patient acceptance process according to the CONSORT guidelines for reporting randomized clinical trials

Table 3.3 CONSORT guideline checklist for reporting randomized clinical trials

Contents	Items must be fully explained
Title and abstract	
	1\. How to allocate treatments to study subjects (e.g., random allocation or replacement blocks method)
Introduction	
General issues	2. Literature review and problem statement
Methods	
Participants in the study	3. Patient selection criteria, time and place of data collection
Intervention (treatment)	4. Details of the interventions applied in each group, how and the exact time of admission
Objectives	5- specific objectives and hypotheses related to the study
Outcomes	6. Definition of primary and secondary outcomes, time, and method of measuring variables. Methods used to ensure the quality of measurements
Sample size	7. Sample size calculation and, if necessary, the number of periodical analyzes when conducting the study and rules for completing the study earlier
Randomization	
Generating a sequence of random numbers	8. The methods used to generate the sequence of random numbers and the details of the existing restrictions (e.g., blocking or classification of data)
Concealment of the random sequence of treatment allocation	9. Determining the methods used to keep the random sequence of assignments secret after the start of the study
Execution	10. Mention the people who generated the sequence of random numbers and the people who were responsible for assigning patients to each of the treatments.
Blindness	11. Implementation or non-implementation of the blinding method, people who were blind to the type of treatment used and how to evaluate the degree of success in the implementation of blinding
Statistical methods	12. The methods used to compare groups in terms of desired outcomes. Performing side analyses such as modeling, how to adjust confounders, and analysis in subgroups
Results/findings	
Number of participants	13. Participants at each stage (preferably shown in a diagram). In particular, the number of samples required for study in each treatment group, samples that were randomly allocated, those who received treatments, who were lost during the follow-up, and who were analyzed should be mentioned. Cases of deviation from the study protocol must be reported with the reason
Reception	14. The admission time of each patient in the study and the details of the follow-ups
Universal findings	15. Demographic and clinical characteristics of the subjects under study
The number of patients analyzed	16. The number of people and participants in each study group that have been analyzed should be mentioned in exact numbers (e.g., 10.20, not 50%)
Estimating effects and outcomes	17. For each of the primary and secondary outcomes, the effect size of the treatment used along with its accuracy (e.g., 95% confidence interval) should be mentioned
Sub-analyses	18. Sub-analyzes that can include multivariate, subgroup, or classified analyses
Adverse outcomes	19. All important adverse effects or side effects in each treatment group should be listed
Discussion	
Interpretation of the results	20. According to the test of study hypotheses, potential sources of biases and risks arise from the inconsistency of the analysis results with the previous findings
Generalizability of the results	21. Examining the degree of generalization (external validity) of the findings
General conclusion	22. Interpretation and final inference from the results according to the previous studies

Source: Retrieved from CONSORT Statement https://www.consort-statement.org

3.4.12 Types of Clinical Trial Studies

A detailed review of all types of clinical studies is beyond the scope of this book, and only general categories are presented in this section. For further see references [25, 27–31].

3.4.12.1 Trial with Independent Simultaneous Controls

For accurate examination and direct supervision of the experiment, it is necessary to have two groups:

The first group receives the new treatment (experimental group), and the other group has prescribed a placebo or standard treatment (control group). The control group and the experimental group should be identical in all aspects, except for the intended treatment method, and the difference between the responses in the two groups should be caused only by the applied treatment method (and not by any other factor). The best way to ensure that the treatment of the two groups is the same is to plan at the same time and at the same time in both groups. This type of design is called a study with parallel controls. Figure 3.8 shows an overview of this study.

3.4.12.2 Parallel Design

Most randomized clinical trials have a parallel design. In these studies, each group of participants is exposed to one of the study interventions (Fig. 3.9).

3.4.12.3 Factorial Study

When researchers want to investigate the combination or separation of two or more interventions with different levels (more than two drug levels) along with the control group, one of the efficient and very suitable options is to use the factorial design.

The easiest way to learn factorial study is to study it through the simplest form of factorial design, that is, a study with two interventions (A and B) at two levels and four treatment groups. In this study, n number of patients are studied in each treatment group. One of the groups does not receive any of treatments A and B, the next group receives both treatments A and B, and the next two groups receive only treatment A and the other only treatment B. Groups that do not receive one or both treatments are likely to receive a placebo. This study is called a 2 × 2 factorial design. Despite its simplicity, this design has most of the characteristics of a factorial experiment. Using this study, enough information is provided to investigate the effects of treatments A and B alone and the simultaneous effect of treatments A and B. A simple overview of this study is shown in Table 3.4.

It is possible to generalize the 2 × 2 factorial study to more complex designs.

One of the most famous factorial studies with the order of 2 × 2 is the study of physicians' health. In this study, approximately 22,000 doctors from the United States were investigated to

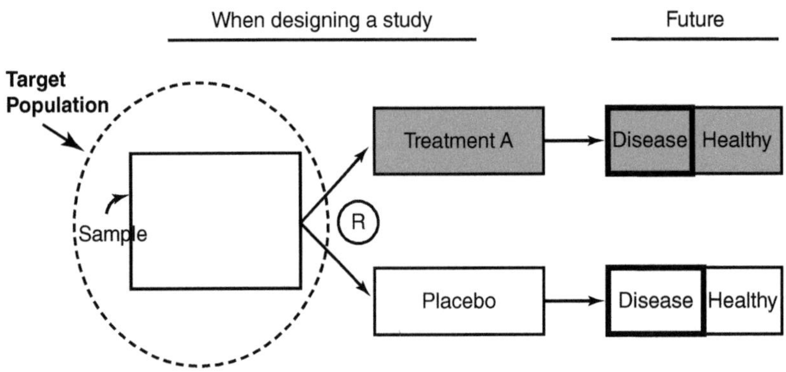

Fig. 3.8 In a randomized trial, the researcher collects a sample from the community and measures background variables. Then the participants in the trial will receive one of the interventions by chance. During the follow-up of these people, variables related to disease outcomes are collected and analyzed (R stands for randomization)

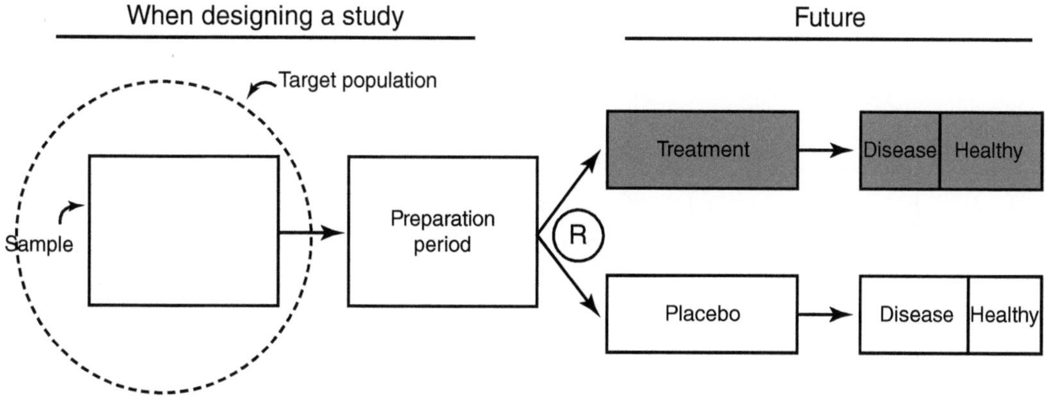

Fig. 3.9 Sometimes, in conducting randomized clinical studies, a preparation period is prescribed to investigate the possible side effects of each intervention (or the administration of a placebo)

investigate the effects of 1-aspirin in reducing mortality from cardiovascular diseases and 2-beta-carotene in reducing the incidence of cancer. Each doctor was placed in one of the following four groups:

1. He takes aspirin and beta-carotene.
2. He does not use aspirin and beta-carotene.
3. He takes aspirin, but instead of beta-carotene, he uses a placebo.
4. He uses beta-carotene, but instead of aspirin, he uses a placebo.

Table 3.5 shows the random assignment of doctors in these four groups [32].

The most important limitation in conducting these studies is the possibility of interaction between the treatments and the intended outcome. It is possible to design factorial studies despite mutual effects, but these studies are complex and require a large sample size, their implementation is difficult, and their interpretation is not easy. The best cases for using factorial design are when we want to examine two relatively separate research questions. Randomization of matched pairs is one of the most appropriate strategies to balance basic confounders, such as age and sex. In this type of study, one of the two treatments is randomly assigned to each of the matched couples. One of the interesting applications of this study is the use of paired body parts as matched pairs. For example, in a study on diabetic retinopathy patients, each of the patients, one eye was treated with laser, and the other eye remained untreated (control group). Figure 3.10 shows a simple example of factorial design.

Table 3.4 Four treatment groups with equal sample size in each group (balanced design) in a 2 × 2 factorial study

	Treatment B		
Treatment A	Not received	Received	Total
Not received	n	n	$2n$
Received	n	n	$2n$
Total	$2n$	$2n$	$4n$

Table 3.5 Factorial design to study the effect of aspirin and beta-carotene

	Beta-carotene		
Aspirin	Not received	Received	Total
Not received	5517	5520	11,037
Received	5520	5514	11,034
Total	11,037	11,034	22,071

3.4.12.4 Crossover Design

By making small changes in the sequential study design, a combination of simultaneous and sequential evidence can be obtained. In this plan, two groups of patients are used: one group to receive the experimental treatment and the second group to receive standard drug or placebo treatment.

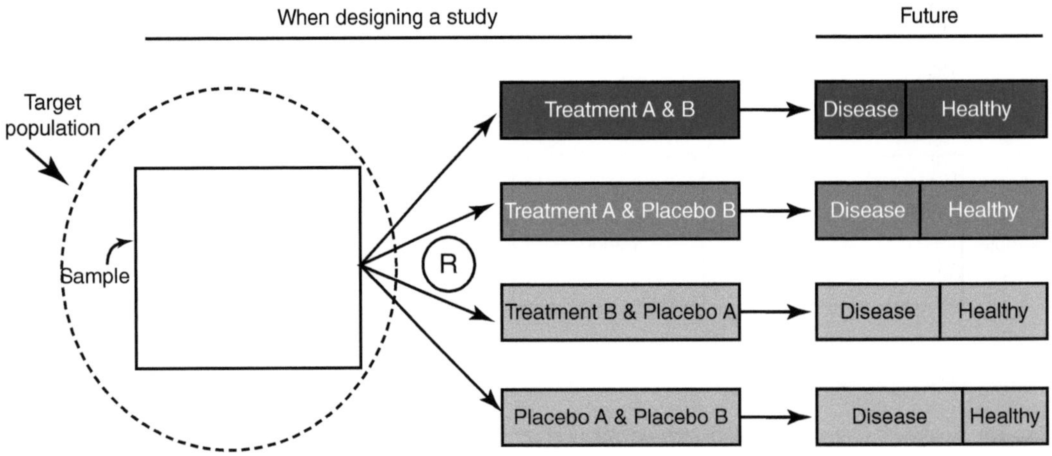

Fig. 3.10 In factorial studies, researchers select a sample from the community and measure background variables. Then, two effective interventions and similar placebos are randomly assigned to four groups. During the follow-up after prescribing the drugs, the desired outcomes are measured

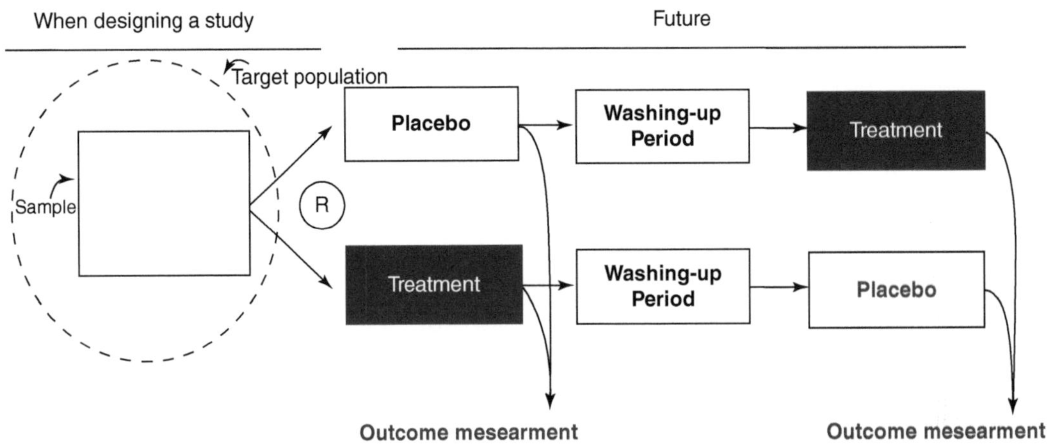

Fig. 3.11 In cross-sectional studies, researchers take a sample from the community and measure background variables. Then, they randomly assign one of the desired interventions (drug, placebo) to the subjects, and after applying the intervention, they measure the related consequences. After a washing period, the allocation of interventions is reversed, and the above steps are repeated

In these studies, at the beginning of the study, half of the participants are randomly assigned to the control group and the rest to the active treatment group. In the second phase of the study, which is usually followed by a washout period, the two groups are switched. This method (which turns into a Latin square design when there are several treatments) practically allows analysis between groups and within groups. Figure 3.11 shows how to do this design.

In this study, because each member is used as a control in the next stage, by removing some potentially confounding variables, the statistical power will be higher than in parallel designs. However, performing the design for each patient requires at least two steps, and the complexity of the analysis and interpretation of the results due to the possibility of a transfer effect is one of the disadvantages of these studies. The transfer effect occurs due to the remaining effects of the primary treatment from the first period and its effect on the desired outcome on the evaluations related to the second stage of treatment. For example, the effect of blood pressure treatment using diuretic treatments probably remains for months, which makes the observed blood pressure level remain affected by diuretic treatments in the evaluation of a new treatment that starts immediately after this treatment.

In general, in crossover trials, only short-term responses during the treatment and at the end of the treatment period are considered. Any long-term transfer effect caused by the first treatment is undesirable in the next period and distorts the results. If there is a possibility of a transfer effect, there should be an appropriately timed washout period after each treatment period. At the same time, in many cases, due to ethical aspects, it is not possible to stop the treatment period. To design cross-sectional studies, the following characteristics regarding intervention and disease must be present:

- Interventions are usually used in chronic diseases that do not have quick treatment.
- The effects of the intervention should have a quick onset and a short duration. The condition of the disease must be stable.

In some ways, this study includes the advantages of parallel and sequential designs.

Sometimes the crossover design can be extended to more than two treatments and consecutive courses for each patient. The studies that are in the first stages of testing for the development of drugs are mostly of this category due to the short time interval between treatments and implementation on healthy volunteers. For example, we can refer to the study of the short-term effects of polluting gases on the lung function of volunteers. In this study, for each pollutant (e.g., sulfur dioxide), there were four levels: none, low, medium, and high, which each volunteer received in random order on four consecutive days [23]. This study had a Latin square design in blocks of four, which used random assignments with numbers 1–4 for the sequence of prescription values. Different doses of pollutant were previously randomly marked with letters A, B, C, or D. Thus, the following table was designed to complete the study.

		Study days			
		1	2	3	4
The sequence of treatments	1	A	B	C	D
	2	B	D	A	C
	3	C	A	D	B
	4	D	C	B	A

3.4.13 Evaluation of Trial Progress

In many clinical trials, patients are studied one by one, and their responses to treatment are observed gradually. For the following reasons, researchers are obliged to evaluate the progress of the experiment:

- Ensuring compliance with the study protocol.
- Evaluation of adverse effects, especially side effects and severe toxic reactions of new treatments.
- Data processing and quick attention to any errors, inconsistencies, or missing items in information forms.
- General information about how the trial is progressing.
- Interim comparisons while the trial is still ongoing to ethically prevent patients from receiving ineffective treatments.
- Evaluation of short-term responses to treatments.

In inter-period comparisons, only a certain number of variables should be considered, because, otherwise, it becomes difficult to interpret multiple comparisons. It is recommended that only one treatment comparison be investigated and a formal stop order defined for it. Other comparisons can be used informally for any important characteristic. The decision to stop or change a trial is not a purely statistical act. In this case, other issues such as effect size, a significant amount of differences, practical aspects of treatment (such as ease, acceptability, and cost), and new ideas should also be considered. If there are interim analyses in the study, the precise definition of the stopping rule in trials requires special statistical methods. In these methods, the significance levels of the tests are adjusted based on multiple comparisons, which is necessary. This type of analysis is known as group sequential analysis.

3.4.14 Sample Size in Clinical Trials

In designing clinical trials, researchers are always faced with the question, "How many patients are needed to conduct the trial?" To achieve the goals of the clinical trial, statistical methods are used with appropriate power to determine a sufficient number of patients. Appendix C shows more details.

At the same time, it is very important to note that these methods are only used as guidelines. Practical issues such as access to patients, resources, and ethical requirements of research should also be considered.

Usually, when statistical methods are used to determine the sample size, researchers are surprised by the large and unexpected number of patients needed in the study. In such cases, it is possible to decide to forget the statistical principles and conduct the experiment in any possible way. Unfortunately, this method often leads to small trials that have little scientific merit. The logical method is to start working with statistical methods to determine the sample size and then examine the financial resources, the number of available patients, and other resources. The next step is to evaluate the rate of patients participating in the trial. Usually, this work is done by estimating the number of qualified patients in a year. After estimating the size of patients needed in the trial and the rate of patients entering, the time required for entering patients can be estimated. It should also be remembered that an additional period of follow-up may be included.

Often, individual patient resources, whether from hospitals, private practices, or research centers alone, are insufficient to conduct clinical trials of an appropriate size; therefore, at the time of designing clinical trials, determining whether it is possible to conduct a study in only one center is of particular importance. If there is a need to conduct multicenter trials, the reasons, advantages, and disadvantages should be carefully investigated.

Some advantages and disadvantages of multicenter trial studies are as follows:

- The main advantage of multicenter trials is the faster entry of patients. For this reason, the sample size in the experiment can be considered larger, or the final results can be obtained in a shorter time.
- Conducting a trial in several centers increases the resources of patients and also the diversity of the treatment group; for this reason, the generalization of the results in these studies is done with more confidence.
- Planning and administration of multicenter trials are more complicated than normal trials.
- Implementation of multicenter trials is very expensive in terms of manpower and resources.
- Ensuring that all centers will follow the study protocol is very important.
- Quality control of measurements, clinical observations, and data recording is very necessary for these studies; for this purpose, it is necessary to provide adequate training and explanations to the research group.
- Data collection and data processing in multicenter trials require an experienced and organized group.
- In general, the more centers there are in a clinical trial, the more the problems and complexity of the trial increase.
- Statistical analysis of data from multicenter trials requires special methods.

3.4.15 Design with Consecutive Controls (Semi-Experimental Study)

An interventional study has a sequential design, where each participant receives all or some of the study's interventions in consecutive periods. Which participant receives which intervention is randomly determined. In the successive design of each of the participants, they are their controls. In medicine, it becomes necessary to use this plan when, due to the dangerous side effects of the drug or the possibility of a very serious effect of the treatment in dangerous diseases, from the ethical point of view, the least number of patients should be studied in the research. Figure 3.12 shows how this study was done.

3.4.16 Trial with External Controls

Another way to control experiments is to use controls outside the scope of the study. It is possible that, in this method, the results of other research are used as a comparison. Sometimes, control subjects, called historical controls, are patients that the researcher has already treated in another way.

Historical evidence is often used in cancer research. During studies with historical controls, the researcher should also pay attention to the changes in other factors (treatment time of control subjects), because the resulting difference may be caused by changes in these factors and not in the treatment itself.

3.4.17 Studies without Controls

In this category of studies, there is an intervention, but there is no control. In a more precise definition, we do not call this class of studies experiments or experiments. When evaluating a diagnostic method, studies without controls are often used.

The main weakness of such studies is that, unfortunately, researchers consider their method the best. The history of medicine is full of examples where the used drug was abandoned after conducting a controlled clinical trial. The most important problem in uncontrolled studies is that, unfortunately, unproven treatment methods have become common, and this issue makes conducting controlled studies difficult. Has done.

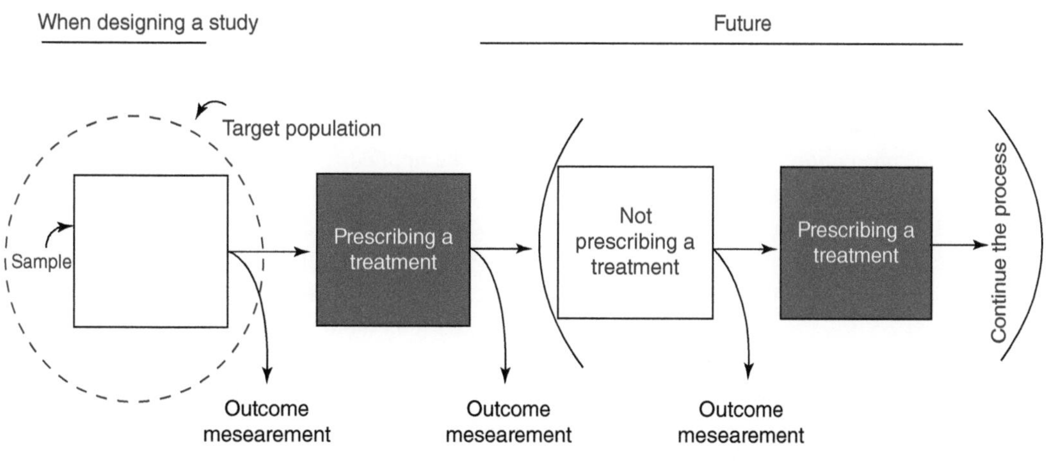

Fig. 3.12 In studies with consecutive controls, researchers select a sample from the community and measure background variables and then prescribe a type of intervention to all group members and measure variables related to the desired disease or outcome during follow-up. Sometimes the type of intervention is changed and the above steps are repeated

3.4.18 Nonrandomized Trial

The selection of patients for treatment methods is not always random. Studies whose patients are not randomly selected are called nonrandomized trials. Many researchers have been exposed to many types of errors, so their results are highly questionable. Studies with nonrandomized control subjects are much weaker in terms of validity than experimental studies. Because there is no way to prevent distortions caused by the nonrandom assignment of patients.

3.4.19 Field Trials

Field trials are different from clinical trials in that, in these studies, the trial is focused on healthy people. In clinical trials, the possibility of short-term complications of the disease is very high. However, the possibility of short-term side effects in field trials is very rare. For this reason, these studies are usually very extensive and require a large sample size. On the other hand, since healthy people are considered in these studies, it is not logical to expect these people to refer to special centers such as hospitals or clinics, and for examination and access to the people under study, it is often necessary to go to the people's place of residence, work, or study, and special centers should be provided to guide the study and encourage the people under the study to refer to it. All these issues make this kind of study expensive. For this reason, these studies are performed only in the prevention of very common or extremely dangerous diseases. For example, several field trials have been designed and implemented regarding the consumption of large amounts of vitamin C and the prevention of colds [23–34].

Polio disease is also a rare but very dangerous disease that caused the largest experimental study on humans due to the importance of its complications. In this trial, the polio vaccine or placebo was injected into hundreds of thousands of school children [35].

In these studies, like clinical trials, the way of assigning the studied methods should be in such a way that the groups under study are comparable. Random assignment can be an ideal option. But the practical problems of using this procedure in studies with a very large sample size may cause researchers to withdraw from this method. For example, injecting an iodized oil solution into students in mountainous and hyperendemic areas and comparing it with a suitable control group in reducing the degree of goiter and increasing the concentration of thyroid hormones and its effect on the progress of growth and psychomotor ability is a suitable example of this type of trials [36].

3.4.20 Community Interventions and Cluster Randomized Trials

Trials based on community interventions are a special type of field study that covers the entire society. For example, adding fluoride to the drinking water of a city to investigate the possibility of preventing tooth decay in comparison with another urban community that only uses ordinary water is a trial based on community intervention.

A clear example in this regard is the preventive program of the national committee to combat iodine deficiency in the production, distribution, and promotion of the consumption of iodized salt throughout the country [37].

Sometimes, interventions defined for study are used in smaller groups than the whole community. For example, interventions related to diet may be applied to family members. Some environmental interventions may be tested and evaluated on residents of a residential unit or employees of an office. New sports equipment may be studied in a sports team. The groups on which the desired intervention is tested can include different army units, schools, villages of a city, or any other similar group that has the same members (in terms of the important exposures of the influencer and the studied intervention). Intervening in such groups is much easier and more practical than extensive field studies and community interventions. Such studies in which the investigated interventions are attributed to some groups instead of individuals are called cluster-randomized studies.

3.5 Studies Based on Existing Data

Many of the research questions can be checked with the appropriate speed and efficiency using the data that has already been collected. In general, there are three main methods for using available data in research: secondary data analysis, sub-studies, and regular review.

The fast and cost-effectiveness of these methods is the most important advantage of using them in research. Sometimes, investigating a research question conventionally may require a lot of financial resources and a very long time. But by using the available data, it is possible to reach the objectives of the study quickly and cheaply. For example, an intervention study with several risk factors and a different intervention with the abbreviation MRFIT was designed to investigate the effective factors in the prevalence of cardiovascular diseases. During the study, the information related to the pattern of smoking in the subjects under study was examined and recorded. After completing the study, one of the researchers realized that it was possible to investigate the effects of involuntary exposure to cigarette smoke and the prevalence of cardiovascular diseases. The results of this study showed that the prevalence of heart diseases in nonsmoking men with a smoking wife is twice that of married men with a nonsmoking wife. A result that was much more interesting and new than the main goals and findings of the study [38].

However, studies based on available data have limitations. Choosing the right sources for data collection is one of the complex parts of these studies [39]. Apart from this, the method of measuring and recording information in these data is out of the researchers' control. Data quality is very important and subject to various factors such as missing and erroneous data. According to their characteristics, the categories of data can be in the form of master, reference, transactional, historical, and metadata. For example, it is possible to collect a dichotomous variable for having or not having high blood pressure. It is also possible that the data quality is not suitable, and there are many missing or wrongly recorded cases [40]. There is also the possibility of not recording and collecting important intervening factors, main consequences, and final results of the subjects under study. All these limitations can be summed up in the statement that, in research based on existing data, researchers have no control over how data is collected.

3.5.1 Secondary Data Analysis

In data reanalysis, information is available in both individual and macro forms. Individual data are data that contain the information of each person separately. These data can be obtained from previous studies, medical records, hospital records, death certificates, and many other sources. In such data, the existence of a relationship between the desired characteristics and the sample is investigated using the information obtained from the files and documents. The next steps of the research are exactly similar to the process where the researchers collect measurements and information directly from the study members. One of the important sources of information collection for members under study is the data collected from previous studies. In many studies, more data is collected than researchers can analyze. The second type includes a large set of national and regional data that are generally available and not exclusive to a particular group. For example, referring to the Iranian Statistics Center makes it possible to access these data faster. When individual data is not available, big data is sometimes useful. In big data, only information related to large groups of society (a city or a province) are available (e.g., death rates due to colon cancer in all provinces of the country). With such data, relationships between population groups are investigated by comparing the information on a risk factor (such as meat consumption per capita) and the size of the desired event (colon cancer).

Analysis of available data is possible in two ways:

- The researcher may be interested in investigating a specific research question and try to find a set of data that can answer that question. This method is the usual method of clinical research.
- The researcher examines and analyzes the available data and then examines the questions that can be answered by this data set. The problem with this method is finding meaningful relationships among a lot of information.

The different stages of finding a data bank suitable for the research question are as follows:

- Finding a research question and reviewing related scientific texts.
- Preparing a list of response and confounding variables.
- Finding appropriate data banks that contain the required information.
- Choosing the best data set that is compatible with the research objectives.
- Setting research hypotheses and specifying appropriate statistical methods to analyze the results.
- Data analysis.

The different stages of designing research questions, according to the available data, are as follows:

- Choosing the right data bank.
- Familiarity with collected variables and how to measure them.
- Determining the variables or subgroups of information that seem appropriate to answer the research questions.
- Reviewing sources and consulting with other researchers about the importance and new aspects of the research question.
- Setting up the research hypotheses and specifying the statistical methods of analyzing the results.
- Data analysis method.

3.5.2 Auxiliary Studies

Designing the study by the method of data reanalysis requires answering the research question for which the relevant information is available. In the secondary study, the researcher can measure and record a limited number of new variables in addition to what was predicted in the research. Secondary studies have many benefits in secondary data analysis. At the same time, compared to these studies, they have fewer limitations. Sub-studies can be added to any type of study (e.g., cross-sectional studies and case-control studies), but large prospective cohort studies and randomized trials are well suited for such study designs. Measurements in a sub-study designed for randomized trials are usually useful and informative when they are planned before the trial begins, but it is very difficult to collect this information for people who were not members of the research group from the beginning. When the variables are measured at the beginning, their measurement during or at the end of the trial can provide useful information to the researcher. In most prospective cohort studies, the researcher periodically adds new measurements. This issue is an ideal situation for designing sub-studies.

The possibility of designing sub-studies should be continuously followed, especially by novice researchers who have limited time and resources. For example, a researcher who is interested in investigating the effects of weight loss on arthritis pain may start by defining interventions such as diet, exercise, habit change, and the use of drugs effective in weight loss. In this study, intervening variables may be determined by consulting weight loss experts or reviewing articles. The next step is to classify the different degrees of arthritis in patients and also to define how to measure the response variables, that is, the amount of pain and weight change (as a sub-measure). After this stage, the researcher should be looking for a study that provides a good opportunity for secondary measurements. Attracting the opinion of the main researchers is the most important stage of this type of research. Most researchers tend to add some sub-criteria and measurements in the main study, of course, if they state an important question and do not hinder the implementation and guidance of the main study. For example, most researchers welcome the addition of a questionnaire or a series of interesting, low-cost, and quick measurements, while they have little desire to include time-consuming, expensive, dangerous, and unpleasant or unethical measurements such as endoscopy. In general, the inclusion of a second study in the research process requires the permission of the main researcher or the study committee.

The disadvantages of secondary studies are few, but in some cases, there are practical problems to obtain official permission to conduct the study to train those who perform the measurement, or to obtain consent from each participant. It is possible that the executive of the second study is not aware of the objectives and the way of conducting the main study, and as a result, it is difficult to obtain all the information.

3.5.3 Systematic Review and Meta-Analysis

In a regular review, attention is paid to the review, evaluation, and criticism of completed studies that seek to answer a research question. The purpose of this study is the general and final summary of a specific research question. In comparison with other methods of reviewing sources, regular review is a standard and well-known method for defining all studies related to the research question, stating the results in justified studies and, if possible, calculating the summary estimates obtained from all the results. Statistical methods of systematic review (calculation of effect and variance estimates, statistical tests for homogeneity, and statistical studies of publication bias) are called meta-analysis. Regular review is a good opportunity for a novice researcher. Although regular review requires a lot of precision and effort, it does not require a financial burden or additional resources. To conduct a regular review, the researcher must be completely familiar with the literature on the research topic and the history of the research question. Systematic reviews are planned based on a comparative and unbiased search of completed studies. The regular review proposal should have suitable entry and exit criteria for the study, and these criteria should be specified before starting work. Inclusion and exclusion criteria in meta-analysis studies are usually things such as the time frame of conducting and publishing the study, the population under study, the desired disease or conditions, the intervention of the study, the need to blind the study, the randomization of the tests, the acceptable control groups, the number of missing data in the follow-up, and the minimum follow-up period. They specify what is acceptable. When these criteria are determined, the study is reviewed by two or more researchers. In general, regular reviews include the following information.

- Summary of the important indicators of each study, which often includes the sample size of the studies, response rate, follow-up period, demographic indicators of the study, and statistical methods used.
- Reviewing the specific results of each study, which includes risk estimates and confidence intervals. Please refer to references No. 52 and 53 for more information about meta-analysis or meta-analysis studies.

References

1. Merrill RM. Introduction to epidemiology. Burlington, MA: Jones & Bartlett Learning; 2021.
2. Kohn G. Principles of epidemiology. Independently Published; 2020.
3. Goldsmith JR. Environmental epidemiology: epidemiology investigation of community environmental health problems. United Kingdom: CRC Press; 2021.
4. Gómez-Ochoa SA, Rojas LZ, Echeverría LE, Muka T, Franco OH. Global, regional, and national trends of Chagas disease from 1990 to 2019: comprehensive analysis of the global burden of disease study. Glob Heart. 2022;17(1):59. https://doi.org/10.5334/gh.1150. PMID: 36051318; PMCID: PMC9414802
5. Leavy P. Research design: quantitative, qualitative, mixed methods, arts-based, and community-based participatory research approaches. Guilford Publications; 2022.
6. Doyle YG, Furey A, Flowers J. Sick individuals and sick populations: 20 years later. J Epidemiol

Community Health. 2006;60(5):396–8. https://doi.org/10.1136/jech.2005.042770. PMID: 16614328; PMCID: PMC2563964

7. Southwood TRE, Henderson PA. Ecological methods. Germany: Wiley; 2016.
8. Ainy E, Soori H, Ganjali M, Baghfalaki T. Deriving fatal and non-fatal road traffic injury cost by willingness to pay method using Bayesian analysis. Quarterly. J Transp Eng. 2017;8(4):657–69.
9. Ehsani-Moghaddam B, Martin K, Queenan JA. Data quality in healthcare: a report of practical experience with the Canadian Primary Care Sentinel Surveillance Network data. Health Inf Manag. 2021;50(1-2):88–92. https://doi.org/10.1177/1833358319887743. Epub 2019 Dec 5
10. Sarafidis M, Tarousi M, Anastasiou A, Pitoglou S, Lampoukas E, Spetsarias A, Matsopoulos G, Koutsouris D. Data quality challenges in a learning health system. Stud Health Technol Inform. 2020;270:143–7. https://doi.org/10.3233/SHTI200139.
11. Khankeh HR, Vojdani R, Saber M, Imanieh M. How do cancer patients refuse treatment? A grounded theory study. BMC Palliat Care. 2023;22(1):10. https://doi.org/10.1186/s12904-023-01132-5. PMID: 36750817; PMCID: PMC9903566
12. Deakin University. Quantitative study designs. Accessed February 20, 2023.
13. Mansori K, Soori H, Farnaghi F, Khodakarim S, Mansouri Hanis S, Khodadost M. A case-control study on risk factors for unintentional childhood poisoning in Tehran. Med J Islam Repub Iran. 2016;30:355. PMID: 27453885; PMCID: PMC4934449
14. Amini Niks S, Shujaei Tehrani H, Klishadi R, et al. Epidemiology in medicine by Charlie H. and Boring J., Cardiovascular Research Center, Isfahan University of Medical Sciences, Isfahan 2006.
15. Regmi M, Siccardi MA. Coronary artery disease prevention. [Updated 2022 Aug 8]. In: StatPearls. Treasure Island (FL): StatPearls Publishing; 2022.
16. Brown JC, Gerhardt TE, Kwon E. Risk factors for coronary artery disease. 2022 Jun 5. In: StatPearls. Treasure Island (FL): StatPearls Publishing; 2022.
17. Menard S. Handbook of longitudinal research: design, measurement, and analysis. Netherlands: Elsevier Science; 2007.
18. Doll R, Hill AB. Mortality in relation to smoking. The 25-year observation of British doctors. Br Med J. 2009;1964:1.
19. DeCarli C, Pase M, Beiser A, Kojis D, Satizabal C, Himali J, Aparicio H, Flether E, Maillard P, Seshadri S. Secular trends in head size and cerebral volumes in the Framingham Heart Study for birth years 1902-1985. Res Sq [Preprint]. 2023 Jan 30:rs.3.rs-2524684. doi: https://doi.org/10.21203/rs.3.rs-2524684/v1. PMID: 36778357; PMCID: PMC9915799.
20. Azari MR, Hosseini V, Jafari MJ, Soori H, Asadi P, Mousavion SM. Evaluation of occupational exposure of shoe makers to benzene and toluene compounds in shoe manufacturing workshops in East Tehran. Tanaffos. 2012;11(4):43–9. PMID: 25191437; PMCID: PMC4153221
21. Hall DE. The 44th Medical Brigade in the Great War: Vietnam, 1966-Activation, Deployment, and Initial Operations. Med J (Ft Sam Houst Tex). 2022 Oct-Dec;(Per 22-10/11/12):5-24.
22. Gregorich SL, Sutherland-Smith J, Sato AF, May-Trifiletti JA, Miller KJ. Survey of veterinary specialists regarding their knowledge of radiation safety and the availability of radiation safety training. J Am Vet Med Assoc. 2018;252(9):1133–40. https://doi.org/10.2460/javma.252.9.1133.
23. Bridgman S. Community health risk assessment after a fire with asbestos containing fallout. J Epidemiol Community Health. 2001;55(12):921–7. https://doi.org/10.1136/jech.55.12.921. PMID: 11707487; PMCID: PMC1731804
24. Azizi F. Age as a predictor of recurrent hypothyroidism in patients with post-partum thyroid dysfunction. J Endocrinol Investig. 2004;27(11):996–1002. https://doi.org/10.1007/BF03345300.
25. Tai BC, Machin D, Fayers PM. Randomised clinical trials: design, practice and reporting. United Kingdom: Wiley; 2021.
26. Chlebowski RT, Haque R, Hedlin H, Col N, Paskett E, Manson JE, et al. Benefit/risk for adjuvant breast cancer therapy with tamoxifen or aromatase inhibitor use by age, and race/ethnicity. Breast Cancer Res Treat. 2015;154(3):609–16. https://doi.org/10.1007/s10549-015-3647.1. Epub 2015 Nov 24
27. Butcher NJ, Monsour A, Mew EJ, Chan AW, Moher D, Mayo-Wilson E, et al. Guidelines for reporting outcomes in trial reports: the CONSORT-outcomes 2022 extension. JAMA. 2022;328(22):2252–64. https://doi.org/10.1001/jama.2022.21022.
28. Moher D, Schulz KF, Altman D. The CONSORT statement: revised recommendations for improving the quality of reports of parallel-group randomized trials. JAMA. 2001;285:1987.91.
29. Friedman LM, Furberg C, Demets DL. Fundamentals of clinical trials. New York: Springer; 1998.
30. Smith PG, Marrow R. Field trials of health interventions in developing countries. London: Mac Milan; 1996.
31. Donner A, Klar N. Design and analysis of cluster randomization trials in health research. London: Arnold; 2000.
32. Data from the steering committee of the physician's health study research group: final report on the aspirin component of the ongoing physician's health study. N Engl J Med. 1989;1:129–35.
33. Dykes MHM, Meier P. Ascorbic acid and the common cold: evaluation of its efficacy and toxicity. JAMA. 1975;231:1073–9.
34. Karlowski TR, Chalmers TC, Frenkel LD, et al. Ascorbic acid for the common cold: a prophylactic and therapeutic trial. JAMA. 1975;231:1038–42.
35. Franci ST, Napier JA, Voigh BS, et al. Evaluation of the 1954 field trial of poliomyelitis vaccine:

final report. Ann Arbor, MI: Poliomyelitis Vaccine Evaluation Center, University of Michigan; 1957.
36. Mirmiran P, Nazarabadi M, et al. The effects of iodized oil solution injection in students suffering from disorders caused by iodine deficiency, a three-year study. Research in medicine, year two, April and June 2006, 54–64.
37. Azizi F, Sheikhul Islam R. National program to combat iodine deficiency. Medicine and Cultivation, numbers 19 and 20, summer 2005, 18–22.
38. Svendsen KM, Kuller LH, Martin MJ, et al. Effects of passive smoking in the multiple risk factor intervention trial (MRFIT). Am J Epidemiol. 2007;126:783–95.
39. Haghdoost A. Structured review and meta-analysis, concepts, applications, and calculations. Tehran: Taimurzadeh Publications, Spring; 2016.
40. Mahanti R. Data quality: dimensions, measurement, strategy, management, and governance. United States: ASQ Quality Press; 2019.

4 Precision, Validity, and Repeatability of Measurements and Diagnostic Tests

Shallow men believe in luck; strong men believe in cause and effect. Cause and effect, means and ends, seed and fruit, cannot be severed; for the effect already blooms in the cause, the end preexists in the means, the fruit in the seed.

—Ralph Waldo Emerson (1803–1882)

4.1 Types of Measurement Errors

Sources of measurement error process may be due to the following reasons.

4.1.1 Mistake

Mistakes occur due to carelessness and human error. The mistake can be caused by incorrect use of the tool, registration error, or calculation error. The nature of the mistake is undetectable. When the error is minimized, the obtained measurements are more correct. Mistake and error are often used interchangeably but have differences in contexts. A mistake is an action or decision that is incorrect, or misguided due to a lack of knowledge or misunderstanding. A wrong outcome is achieved despite a correct intention. Mistakes are often made by humans and are considered a natural part of the learning process. Mistakes are related to human behavior, judgment, and decision-making, while errors are often related to technical and mechanical functions.

4.1.2 Error

An error is an action, calculation, or measurement that is wrong or inaccurate due to improper techniques, a faulty system, or a technical malfunction. Errors are not usually intentional but can have serious consequences if not identified and controlled.

4.1.3 Random Errors

Random errors occur due to the nature of the measurement, the instability of the environment, the limitations of the measurement tool, and the lack of assumptions. In such errors, positive and negative values cancel each other out in the long run.

H. Soori, *Errors in Medical Science Investigations*, https://doi.org/10.1007/978-981-99-8521-0_4

4.1.4 Sampling Error

Sampling errors occur due to estimates obtained from sampling. If sampling is done with probability-based methods, positive and negative errors will tend to cancel each other out. The measurement of the sampling error is estimated by the population variance and the sample measurement.

4.1.5 Bias

Any bias and regular measurement error cause bias in the results. The errors caused by the network do not cancel each other out in the long run. Systematic errors originate from defects in tools and equipment, technical problems, or researcher bias.

When the sum of the errors that happened is small, we consider the measurements or estimates to be correct; however, there is no specific definition regarding the classification of errors into different categories in terms of their measurement. In general, the error has two components: systematic error and random error. This chapter is dedicated how to evaluate, estimate, and control these errors in measurements and diagnostic tests in medical studies.

4.2 Scientific Reports of Measures

One of the misleading mistakes in writing scientific texts is reporting measurements as absolute numbers. Because no measurement is error-free, therefore, every measurement report should include the range in which we expect the actual value of the measurement to be. For example, when we are measuring with a 30 cm wooden ruler, due to the change in the temperature of the environment, there may be a length change of 3 mm in the length of the ruler. Therefore, when we see the length of an object as 300 mm, the actual measurement is between 297 and 303 mm. In this example, if the length measurement report of one side with a wooden ruler is between 297.303 mm and the other length measurement report with a metal ruler is reported as values between 285 and 315 mm, the area of a square whose one side is 297.303 mm and the other side is 285–315 should be reported as 84,645–95,445 square millimeters.

4.2.1 Validity and Precision in Clinical Studies

Every applied study usually includes the process of measuring some parameters and collecting information related to them. Measurement error is one of the important factors that researchers should take care of and effort in controlling. Unfortunately, there is no standard word to express these concepts in scientific texts. The terms validity and accuracy are equivalent, and the words precision, repeatability, compatibility, and reliability are equivalent to each other.

One of the best ways to describe these concepts is in Fig. 4.1. This figure shows the results of shooting by four different people at four similar targets. The shots of person "A" are gathered around the center of the target and close to each other. By observing this phenomenon, it can be argued that the gun's aim is set correctly, so the bullets hit where they were aimed. And also the shooter "A" was a skilled person who aimed with high precision. This information indicates high precision and reliability in targeting. Shooter "B" did not shoot in a close cluster. However, on average, his shots tend to hit the center of the target. It may be assumed that the gun's aim was properly adjusted, but the shooter did not have much skill, which caused the scattering of shots. These results indicate low precision and high reliability in targeting. On the other hand, person "C" is a skilled shooter because his shots are close together, but there is no precision focus on the target, which is probably related to the non-adjustment of the gun's aiming device. This state indicates the high precision and low validity of markings, but person "D" was not a skilled shooter, nor was his gun's aiming device well adjusted. Because his shots hit the target board

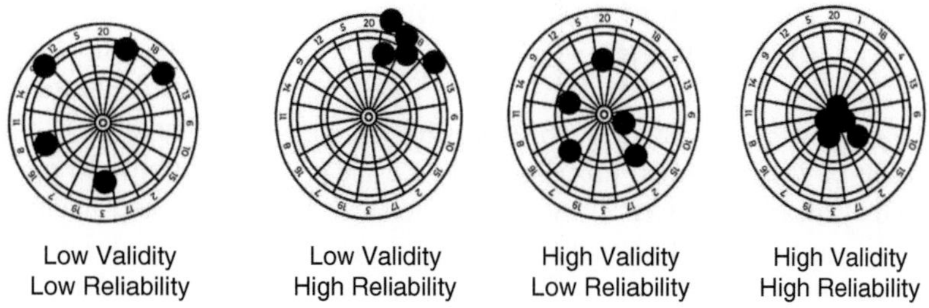

Fig. 4.1 Showing the validity and precision of pointing to the target

unintegrated and far from the center of the dartboard, this issue can indicate low precision and reliability in shooting; wrong marks can be related to factors such as the intensity and direction of the wind, the performance of the weapon's aiming system, or the intensity and precision of the shooter's vision. These factors can cause a systematic error in a certain direction and turn the arrows away from the middle spot of the dartboard.

Bias is the result of a systematic error, which, in such a case, the precision recording of measurements regularly and continuously tends to value higher (or lower) than the real value. The word error is used in this context only when the true value of the measurement is known, and generally, the word changes are used instead. Precision in measurements is related to the number of random changes from a fixed point (regardless of the validity of the measured value). A loose measurement is sometimes more than a fixed size and sometimes less. If we define the error as the difference between the observed value and the true value, then the mean of the random errors becomes zero. It can be considered that the errors have a normal distribution and are independent of each other.

4.2.2 Precision

Precision measurements are repeatable; in this case, almost the same results are recorded in each test or measurement. Using a precision scale to measure weight will record precision measurements. If using the interview method to measure the quality of life is a process that undergoes much wider changes, as a result, the repeatability of this method is less. Precision is one of the important factors in the statistical power of any study.

The precision of measurement is affected by random errors (chance). The more and more effective the random errors are, the less the precision will be.

In general, three factors of measurement tool, observer, and intrinsic changes of the studied members are involved in creating random changes.

Intrinsic changes of the studied organs: These changes are caused by momentary biological changes in people. Temperament and physical fitness, which are constantly undergoing transformation and change, are considered as such.

Observer changes are related to changes in measurement that are caused by the fluctuations of the observer, such as the words used in interviews or the level of skill of the operator in using the devices.

Changes in measuring instruments that are related to changes caused by measuring instruments due to factors such as temperature change, altitude, and consumption.

Therefore, the instrument measurement process is unreliable if:

The researcher measured the characteristics of a person in different conditions and obtained different results (observer changes).

Different researchers with the same measurement tool obtain different results about each member of the study (measurement tool changes).

The person under study (the respondent or the quantity to be measured) should give different answers to a test, questionnaire, or measuring instrument in different conditions (intrinsic changes of people under study).

4.2.3 Evaluation of the Precision of the Results

Evaluation of precision is only possible as a result of repeated tests. Precision can be evaluated by measuring the consistency and agreement of the results obtained from the repetition of measurements. To achieve this goal, an experimental study may be designed by keeping all conditions constant and changing one of the three sources of change mentioned above. In this case, the following four situations can be checked.

- Evaluation of the Repeatability of Each Observer's Results.
- Each observer (user) measures a certain parameter at certain times on a set of samples (within-observer reproducibility).
- Evaluation of the Repeatability of the Results of Several Observers.
- A group of observers (operators) measures a specific parameter a certain number of times on a set of samples (between-observer reproducibility).
- Evaluation of the Repeatability of the Measurement Tool.
- In this case, the observer uses a measuring tool to measure the desired parameter at certain times in a series of samples (within-instrument reproducibility).
- Evaluating the Repeatability of Different Measurement Tools.
- The process of measuring a certain parameter in a set of samples is repeated a certain number of times with different measuring tools (between-instrument reproducibility).

4.2.4 Different Strategies to Increase the Validity

There are five methods to reduce random errors and increase measurement validity, which are as follows:

1. Standardization of measurement methods: The protocol of each study should include scientific and precise definitions of the parameters of the study. For example, there should be specific instructions for taking measurements. These definitions should include written instructions how to prepare the environmental conditions, the members to be studied, how to record and maintain the results of measurements and interviews, how to set up the devices, and so on. Such instructions are necessary for conducting extensive and complex studies, and it is recommended to provide these instructions in studies with smaller dimensions. Even in cases where there is only one parameter to measure, providing brief instructions for each measuring device helps to make the results uniform.
2. Training and confirmation of observer skills: Training improves and uniformity of measurement methods. The importance of this issue is much greater when there is a need to use several observers.
3. Improvement of measurement tools: The use of accurate mechanical or electronic devices usually reduces changes. Also, when using interviews and questionnaires, the use of written forms and standard methods reduces unknown and confusing points and increases the transparency of the obtained information.
4. Use of automatic devices: Those changes caused by observer error in measurement can be prevented by using automatic devices or questionnaires that are completed by the people under study. The use of this method will reduce changes only when the automatic tools have higher validity than human measurements.
5. Repetition: The effect of random errors regardless of their source can be reduced by repeating the measurement and using the average of observations instead of single measurements. Using this method increases validity. The only limitations of this method are possible costs and practical problems in repeating measurements.

In the measurement process, researchers must agree on how to use each of these five methods to ensure the validity of the measurements. Decision-making in this field depends on the

Table 4.1 Different strategies to increase precision

Strategy to reduce random error	Source of random error	Examples of random error	Examples of how to avoid
1. Standardizing measurement methods in the research process	Observer/rater	Changes in the size of blood pressure result from the recording of blood pressure at different times after the subsidence (sometimes faster and sometimes slower than 2 mmHg/s)	The deflation time of the cuff should be determined exactly at the 2 mmHg/s point
	Subjects	The change in the size of the blood pressure occurs from the change in the resting time of each person before the measurement	Providing conditions where each person can rest for 5 min in a quiet room before blood pressure measurement
2. Training and confirmation of the observer	Observer/rater	Change in the size of blood pressure originates from the different methods of each observer	All users should be taught the same technique
3. Improvement of measuring devices	Measuring instrument or observer	Change in blood pressure measurement resulting from the preference for rounding to specific digits (rounding to 0 or 5 when recording)	Using the table of random numbers to round the last digit seen
4. Automating measuring devices	Observer/rater	Changes in blood pressure measurements due to individual errors in reading or recording measurements	Using digital sphygmomanometers to record the results
5. Repetition of measurement	Observer, subject, measurement tool	All sources of random error	Using the average blood pressure obtained from two or more measurements

importance of the desired variable, potential factors effective in the occurrence of random errors in the study, and the cost and feasibility of each strategy.

In general, standardization and training methods are always used, and a repetition strategy is an option that guarantees high validity if possible.

Table 4.1 lists various strategies to reduce random error and increase validity in the blood pressure measurement process that can be used in a study to treat high blood pressure.

4.3 Validity

Validity refers to the degree to which a measure or test accurately measures what it is intended to measure. There are several types of validity such as the following:

- *Internal validity:* Internal validity refers to the extent to which a study can establish a cause-and-effect relationship between variables.
- *External validity:* External validity refers to the extent to which the findings of a study can be generalized to other populations, settings, or conditions.
- *Construct validity:* Construct validity refers to the extent to which a study accurately measures the construct or concept it claims to measure. A study with high construct validity measures what it is intended to measure.
- *Content validity:* Content validity refers to the extent to which a study covers all aspects of the construct being measured. A study with high content validity is one that covers all aspects of the construct being measured.
- *Face validity:* Face validity refers to the extent to which a study appears to measure what it is intended to measure. A study with high face

validity appears to measure what it is intended to measure.

- *Criterion validity:* Criterion validity refers to the extent to which the results of a study are consistent with those obtained from other measures of the same construct or with a known criterion. A study with high criterion validity is one where the results obtained from the study are consistent with other measures of the same construct or a known criterion.

Every research needs accurate, repeatable, and reliable data, but these features do not guarantee the quality of the data or the fundamental relevance of the data to the research objectives. For example, children with visual or hearing impairments may score low on a standardized intelligence test.

Ensuring the validity of measures is important in research where accurate measurements are necessary for decision-making and analysis.

Certainly, inappropriate materials and methods cannot lead to fair results. For example, if goiter disease is measured by touching the throat of the subjects under study, the measurement results will not be valid.

Validity is a function of systematic errors. The higher the systematic error, the weaker the validity of the results. The three main factors of systematic error are as follows:

- Observer bias: Any conscious or unconscious distortion in the provision or reporting of observations by the researcher, such as the use of directed questions, biased judgment, etc.
- Subject bias: Distortion of measurements made by the subjects under study. For example, women who have been diagnosed with breast cancer and know that excessive consumption of fat is one of the risk factors associated with this cancer may exaggerate the amount of fat consumed in their youthful diet during the interview.
- Instrument bias: This error can be caused by the structural causes of the instrument to be measured. For example, a scale that has not been controlled and adjusted may consistently show the weight of the people under study to be less or more than the actual weight.

Table 4.2 Validity and precision in measuring a feature

	Precision	Validity
Definition	A criterion that determines how variable an attribute is in repeated measurements	A criterion that determines how accurate the measurements of a parameter are
The most important evaluation method	Comparison of repeated measures	Comparison with a standard method
Worth checking out	Increasing the statistical power in the detection of effects	Increasing the accuracy of the results
Threatening factors	Random error caused by an observer, subject, measuring instruments	Systematic error caused by: Observer people under study measuring instruments

We emphasize once again that precision and validity are not necessarily related to each other. They are both important concepts in measuring. Precision refers to the level of exactness in a measurement. Validity refers to the degree to which a measure accurately measures what it is intended to measure. Ideally, both precision and validity are important for measures. Table 4.2 shows the differences between validity and precision.

4.3.1 Evaluation of Validity of Results

The most important method to evaluate the validity of the measurements is to compare the results with the measurements obtained from a reference standard method, and we are sure of the accuracy of the results. In measurements that have a continuous scale, the average difference between the investigated method and the reference standard method can be calculated. In the sizes that are categorized, comparison with the reference standard method is possible by calculating the sensitivity and specificity. When there is no standard reference method, researchers usually assume the correctness of common methods to evaluate the accuracy of a new technique.

4.3.2 Different Strategies to Increase the Validity of the Results

The main ways to increase the validity of the results include the first four strategies listed in increasing validity, along with the other three methods described here:

1. Standardizing measurement methods.
2. Training and confirmation of observer skills.
3. Improving measurement tools.
4. Using automatic devices.
5. Inconspicuous measurements: Sometimes it is possible to measure some characteristics without the knowledge of the studied members. This situation can cause the elimination of some potential sources of torque. For example, when studying the feeding pattern of elementary school children, instead of asking the children directly, the number of chocolate wrappers in the trash can be counted at the end of each day.
6. Blinding: This strategy does not increase the overall accuracy of the measurements, but it can eliminate the bias, preferably in the way of evaluating the subjects under study. In a double-blind study, the person under study and the treating team do not know the content of the drugs used (or even the placebo). In observational studies, it is also possible to use this procedure for people who are responsible for measuring the desired outcome.
7. Adjustment of measuring devices: The validity of the results of many measuring instruments, especially mechanical and electrical devices, always remains at the desired level in case of periodic adjustment.

Adhering to the two strategies of standardization and training is inevitable. Whenever it is possible to perform the blinding procedure, its implementation is mandatory, and periodic adjustment of devices that potentially lose their sensitivity over time is also essential.

Table 4.3 lists various strategies to reduce systematic errors and increase accuracy in the blood pressure measurement process that can be used in a study to treat hypertension.

4.3.3 Internal Validity and External Validity

The appropriateness of the methods and the level of trust in each research is determined by evaluating its internal and external validity. Internal validity is the degree of correctness of the inferences that can be made regarding the causal relationship in the study. In other words, the internal validity of research is high when we can be sure that the observed effect is completely related to the applied intervention and not other disturbing (confounding) variables.

External validity is related to the ability to generalize research findings to the target population under normal conditions. High internal validity requires creating artificial and unnatural conditions (laboratory) or being limited to specific cases in the research. This issue may cause the inability of the researcher to generalize the research findings in normal conditions.

When evaluating the validity of a measurement tool, it can be important to pay attention to the following points.

- Face validity: Measurements should be related and similar to what it is claimed to measure. Of course, this is not a guarantee that the method is scientific.
- Content validity: The measured characteristics should be an appropriate representative of the target population. For example, when we intend to examine the amount of daily physical activity in patients, the sample members cannot be the only patients who can walk. Another example is measuring the quality of life. Measuring such quality should include

Table 4.3 Different strategies to reduce systematic error to increase validity

Strategy to reduce systematic error	Source of systematic error	Examples of systematic error	Examples of strategies adopted to avoid errors
1. Standardizing measurement methods in the research process	Observer/ rater	One of the users regularly recorded the degree to which the sound stopped while measuring the diastolic blood pressure	Operational definition of diastolic blood pressure so that the degree of the sphygmomanometer is recorded at the moment of hearing the sound of the pulse
2. Training and confirmation of observer skills	Observer/ rater	Excessive recording of blood pressure due to not following the measurement instructions in the research plan	Training the user and verifying the correctness of the work using a two-hand pressure gauge
3. Improving measurement accuracy	Subject	Excessive recording of diastolic blood pressure, because the members participating in the plan climb the stairs of the clinic	Considering a private room for people participating in the project so that they can rest for 5 minutes
	Measuring tool	Excessive recording of blood pressure due to the use of standard cuffs in people with very large arms	Using a larger cuff in obese people
4. Automating the measurement tool	Observer/ rater	The conscious or unconscious tendency of the observer to record blood pressure lower than the actual value in the new treatment group	Using a digital sphygmomanometer that records the results automatically
	Subject	Blood pressure increased due to the respondent's anxiety in dealing with the medical staff	Using a digital sphygmomanometer so that the people under study can measure blood pressure by themselves
5. Imperceptible measurement	Subject	Tendency to exaggerate the use of blood pressure medication	Measuring the amount of drug consumed in urine
6. Blinding	Observer/ rater	Conscious or unconscious tendency to under-record blood pressure in the new treatment group	Using a double-blind procedure in which users and people under study are unaware of the type of drug used
	Subject	The tendency of the subjects under study to exaggerate the side effects of the new drug	Using a double-blind procedure in which users and subjects under study are unaware of the type of drug used
7. Adjusting and calibrating the measurement tool	Measuring tool	Measuring more than the actual value of blood pressure due to the non-adjustment of the blood pressure device	Continuous control and calibration of blood pressure measuring device

questions about social, health, emotional, and mental functions.

- Structural validity: The measuring instrument must be consistent with existing theoretical assumptions and scientific theories. For example, if we believe that a new drug is more effective than a standard drug due to changes in a series of characteristics, the measurement tool used should be able to measure this difference.
- Experimental validity: The results obtained from the measurement process should be consistent with the results obtained by similar measurement methods.

4.3.4 Choosing Appropriate Methods for Measuring Research Variables

Medical tests, such as those used to screen risk factors, diagnose a disease, or predict the course of a disease, are very important subjects of medical research. These tests, which are usually expensive, play an essential role in treatment and prevention. For this reason, we need criteria for the proper selection of each of these methods. Table 4.4 shows the important questions that determine the usefulness of each medical test, along with suitable study designs to answer these questions and statistical indicators related to each.

Important points for designing studies whose purpose is to compare medical tests are reviewed in this section. The first point in the design of these studies is to examine the test results for a wide range of people, including healthy people to people with severe diseases. Since most of these studies are descriptive (in the early stages), the way of selecting sample members has a great impact on the results. For this reason, if the sample people (healthy or sick) are different from the target population in important features, the results will be distorted. For example, the patient members in the sample can be selected from among the patients with acute conditions that are easier to diagnose and the control group (without disease) in the sample to be selected from among the healthier people in society. In this case, probably many diagnostic tests have ideal results. Misleading results appear when the issue of diagnosis between two diseases with similar symptoms is raised, or the diagnosis between a healthy person and a person who has mild initial symptoms when the disease appears. For this reason, the subjects under study in such designs should be selected from the entire spectrum of the disease to determine the capabilities of the test from a clinical point of view.

The next point is to pay attention to the sources of changes, the ability to generalize the results, and the sampling design in the study. In some research questions, the main source of changes is the people under study (patients). For example, white blood cells increase in babies who have a bacterial infection in their blood. The diagnosis of this matter probably does not depend much on the person who takes the blood sample or the laboratory that measures the number of blood cells. Instead, in many tests, the results depend a lot on the person who performs the tests or the people who interpret the results. For example, the sensitivity, specificity, and validity of the interpretation of mammography results are highly

Table 4.4 How to evaluate medical tests

Question	Prospective study design	Statistical indicators to express the results
How repeatable are the results obtained?	Studies that evaluate intra- or inter-observer variations or intra- or inter-device variations	Agreement ratio, kappa coefficient, coefficient of variation, mean and standard deviation of differences
How valid are the tests?	Cross-sectional, case-control, or cohort studies in which test results are compared with standard reference methods	Sensitivity, specificity, positive and negative predictive value, ROC curve, and accuracy ratio
To what extent do the performed tests affect clinical decisions?	Evaluating the accuracy of differential diagnoses with the help of tests	The ratio of anomalies, the ratio of discordant results, the ratio of changed clinical results with the help of the test, and the cost of each case of anomaly or a change in each clinical decision
Does the test improve clinical outcomes or does it only have side effects?	Randomized trials, cohort studies, or case-control studies where the intervening variable, performing or not performing the intended test, and the response variable include mortality, morbidity, and cost related to the disease or new test	Risk ratio, odds ratio, hazard ratio, number of people who need treatment, ratio, and rate of side effects

dependent on the quality of the equipment used and the skill of the pathologist. Repeating the experiment by several experts or interpreting the results of the laboratory by several experts increases the generalizability of the results of studies that require skill and experience. When the credit or cost is different from one institution to another, to reach generalizable results, it is necessary to examine a sample of these institutions in the research.

Another important issue in the design of these studies is to pay attention to the subjects' blindness. Researchers should do their best to keep other clinical and paraclinical results related to the diagnosis of the disease hidden while performing the test and interpreting its results. For example, when the purpose of the study is to evaluate the results of sonography in the diagnosis of appendicitis, the people who interpret the results should not be aware of the previous records of the patient and the results of clinical examinations. In the same way, the people who are responsible for making the final decision about the presence or absence of appendicitis in patients (a completely valid final diagnosis with which the sonography results are compared) should not be aware of the results of the sonography test. Blinding removes biases, subjective backgrounds, and additional information that can influence decisions about test results.

4.4 Designing Studies that Examine the Repeatability of Tests

4.4.1 Designing Studies that Examine the Reliability of Tests

Sometimes the test results are variable based on where or when the tests were performed or who performed them. The change in the results determines the repeatability of the tests when the results of a sample are repeated by a user or laboratory at different times. For example, if a radiologist interprets the chest X-ray images twice at different times, what proportion of the images have similar interpretations on both occasions? Or if the same photos are presented to two radiologists for interpretation, what proportion of the interpretations are similar?

When the repeatability between observers or a single observer is weak, diagnostic tests are ineffective on this basis. Tests that are designed to evaluate repeatability do not need a standard reference test to determine the validity of the results. This means that two observers (or all observers) can agree on a wrong interpretation, in this case, the results are repeatable. For this reason, the reproducibility of the results guarantees the validity, but it has nothing to do with the validity of the results.

Cross-sectional studies are used to compare the results of tests between two or more observers or to compare the results of one observer in different situations.

4.4.1.1 Analysis

In the previous section, it was explained how to design studies that examine the repeatability of tests. In this part, some statistical indicators are examined to show the difference between the results of these studies.

4.4.1.2 Nominal Variables

The simplest criterion for agreeing with observers is the ratio of agreeable results to all comparisons. This ratio is called the agreement rate. However, when there are more than two categories, the interpretation of the agreement rate becomes complicated. A more appropriate criterion for agreeing is the Kappa coefficient. This criterion expresses the net agreement rate, which is adjusted to observe the agreements caused by accident. The Kappa coefficient changes from −1 as a complete disagreement to +1 as a complete agreement. Kappa equal to zero indicates the existence of completely random agreements [1].

This standard is shown with Greek letters. If Aobs represents the ratio of agreement between two observers and Aexp, the ratio of agreements resulting from chance, the coefficient is calculated as follows:

Table 4.5 Interpretation of the results of pathology photos by two pathologists

	Physician 2		
Physician 1	Abnormal	Normal	Total
Abnormal	20	15	35
Normal	10	55	65
Total	30	70	100

$$K = \frac{A_{obs} - A_{\exp}}{1 - A_{\exp}}$$

A Kappa coefficient greater than 0.75 indicates a very high agreement. A Kappa coefficient between 0.75 and 0.45 indicates moderate agreement, and a Kappa coefficient less than 0.45 indicates weak agreement. Table 4.5 shows a summary of the mammography results of 100 people (normal or abnormal) interpreted by different pathologists.

The kappa coefficient to summarize the results related to the agreement between two pathologists is calculated as follows:

$$A\left[\frac{\frac{30\times 35}{100}+\frac{70\times 65}{100}}{100}\right]_{\exp}$$

$$A_{obs} = \frac{20+55}{100} = 0.75$$

$$K = \frac{0.75-0.56}{1-0.56} = \frac{0.19}{0.44} = 0.43$$

4.4.1.3 Continuous Variables

The criteria expressing changes between observers in continuous variables depend to a large extent on the design of the study. Some studies are designed only to evaluate the degree of agreement between two devices or two methods (e.g., temperatures obtained from two different thermometers). The best way to describe this type of data is to report the average size difference of each sample. Reporting the number of times this difference is greater than the clinically sensitive value can also be useful. For example, when a difference of 0.5 °C in the temperature measured by two thermometers is clinically important, it is important to report the average of the observed differences and the times when this difference is greater than 0.5 °C. Other studies are designed to assess variation between multiple groups of observers, methods, laboratories, or devices. In these cases, the results are generally reported by calculating and announcing the coefficient of change (the coefficient of variation is calculated by dividing the standard deviation of the sample by the mean). If the results are normally distributed, 95% of the observations fall within a distance between two standard deviations from the mean (mean ± 2SDmean).

Another standard criterion is the calculation and reporting of the intraclass correlation coefficient (ICC). This coefficient is calculated as follows:

$$\text{ICC} = \frac{\sigma_u^2}{\sigma_u^2 + \sigma_e^2}$$

In this regard, it is the variance of the actual measurements within each group and the variance of the measurement errors. The smaller the measurement error is, the smaller the increase in measurement error changes, and the ICC value is closer to 1. When all the measurements have been done correctly and as a result ICC = 1. In this case, all observed changes are due to variance between measurements. The scope of this criterion is between zero and one, where ICC = 1 indicates complete agreement and repeatability. For example, in a part of a case-control study to investigate the existence of a relationship between asthma and antioxidant consumption in the diet (the information was collected by completing a questionnaire by the patients), two measurements were made to determine the amount of selenium consumption 3 months apart. Figure 4.2 shows the results for 94 patients aged 15–50 years. As can be seen, although there is a clear correlation between the first and second measurements, there is a fundamental difference between the answers in the first and second questionnaires. The mean and standard deviation of the logarithm of selenium consumption in the first measurement was 3.826.0401 and 3.768.0372 in the second measurement. It seems that there is a significant decrease in the mean observed for the second measurement compared to the first measurement

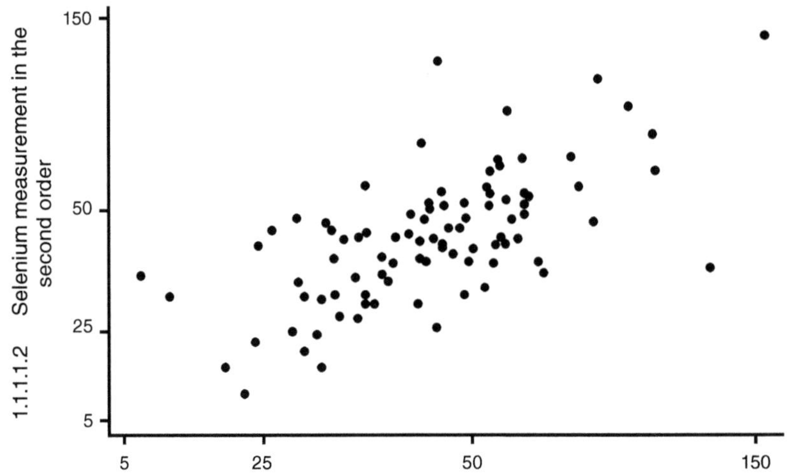

Fig. 4.2 Distribution of selenium intake in 94 patients

(mean difference 0.058 with significant value $P = 0.083$) [2]. Estimates of variance components to calculate ICC equal to:

$$\text{Variance of measurement errors}, \sigma_e^2 = 0.0535$$

$$\text{Variance within each group, } \sigma_\mu^2 = 0.0955$$

$$\text{Total Variance, } \sigma_\mu^2 + \sigma_e^2 = 0.1491$$

and as a result:

$$\text{ICC} = \frac{\sigma_\mu^2}{\sigma_e^2 + \sigma_\mu^2} = \frac{0.995}{0.1491} = 0.6410$$

Therefore, in this example, 64.1% of the total variance is related to the changes within the groups, and therefore, it seems appropriate to use the diet assessment questionnaire only once.

4.5 Studies that Examine the Accuracy of Tests

The studies that are reviewed in this section are related to the issue of "to what extent does the proposed test lead to correct results?" pays. To get the answer to this question, there needs to be a method by which the correct result of the tests is determined. There is such a standard method for some diseases. For example, the result of a tissue biopsy usually determines the presence or absence of disease. (However, histological tests are not ideal because sampling errors, improper tissue preparation, or wrong diagnosis may distort the results of this test.) There is a standard contract method for some other diseases. For example, 50% blockage of at least one of the main coronary arteries, which is determined by angiography, is considered as a criterion for diagnosing coronary artery blockage disease. But in many diseases, such as rheumatic diseases, for the diagnosis of the disease, the examined person must have a minimum of clinical symptoms, syndromes, or unusual paraclinical cases to be considered as a patient. In these conditions, it is natural that the validity of symptoms, syndromes, or diagnostic tests, which are part of the disease diagnosis criteria, cannot be evaluated.

4.5.1 Design

Studies that investigate the accuracy of diagnostic tests can be cross-sectional or case-control. And the studies that evaluate the accuracy of the tests predicting the disease state are usually of the cohort type. In case-control studies, patients and healthy people are sampled separately, and the test results are compared in two groups. Unfortunately, it is very difficult to consider a wide range of people under study in the sample (including clinically healthy people and patients). In sampling for such studies, patients and healthy people should not be selected from the extreme parts of the spectrum, that is, completely healthy people and patients with clear symptoms of the disease that are easily recognizable. Healthy people should also include a group that has symptoms and syndromes similar to patients. For this reason, case-control studies in evaluating the validity of diagnostic tests should be limited to rare diseases for which there is no other sampling design or which are associated with difficulties.

The design of cross-sectional studies in the evaluation of accuracy usually gives more reliable results that are easier to interpret.

To evaluate the accuracy of the tests that predict the course of the disease, there is a need to design cohort studies (prospective or retrospective). In prospective cohort studies, the desired test is performed when the members enter the study. These members are followed up to observe the progress of the disease in the future. In special circumstances, it is also possible to use retrospective cohort studies. For example, the accuracy of the "viral load" test in AIDS patients can be evaluated by a cohort of these patients who have already been followed up and whose blood samples are available. When the desired disease is rare or the test is very expensive, a nested case-control study design is relatively efficient. Usually, we expect the results of nominal tests to be in the form of positive or negative answer. But ranked or continuous answers are also possible. Whenever possible, ranked or continuous answers are preferred because they contain more information. In the case that the response variable is dichotomous (positive/negative), it is easily possible to evaluate it using a standard test.

4.5.2 Analysis

In determining the accuracy of the test or diagnostic method, two points should be considered:

First, what is the effectiveness of the method in diagnosing the desired situation? (What percentage of patients who have a positive test result are infected with the disease?) This point is called test sensitivity. If the sensitivity of the test is high, the false-negative rate is low. In other words, the test result is not falsely negative in a large number of patients with this disease. Sensitivity can be defined in different ways: the probability of a positive test result for patients suffering from the disease in question, the proportion of patients with the disease with a positive test result, or the true positive rate.

The next point is that the accuracy of a test is the amount of correct identification of those people who are not suffering from the disease in question. This part of the accuracy of the test is called the characteristic (specificity) of the test. If the specificity of a test is high, the false-positive rate of the test is low. The characteristic of an experiment can be defined in the following ways. The possibility is a negative test result in people who do not have the desired disease. The proportion of people who do not have the desired disease and the test result is negative in them or the actual negative amount.

To determine the sensitivity and specificity, it is done in the following order:

A group of patients who are surely suffering from the desired disease (or condition) is selected. Another group that we are sure is not suffering from the desired disease is also selected. We experiment with two groups. Then we get the percentage (or percentage) of patients with the desired disease who have a positive test result. In addition to sensitivity and specificity, it is very important to know the probability that the examined members are sick, if the test result is positive, or if they are healthy if the test result is negative. These quantities can be shown by indicators of positive test predictive value and negative test predictive value. The method of completing the agreement table for these tests is shown in Table 4.6.

Table 4.6 How to set up the 2 × 2 table in diagnostic tests

	Disease	
Result	D^+	D^-
T^+	TP	FP
T^-	FN	TN

4.6 Evaluation of the Diagnostic Test

To evaluate the diagnostic test, the indicators of sensitivity, specificity, the positive and negative predictive value of the test, and the percentage of false positives and false negatives are important. Table 4.7 shows how to calculate these indicators.

Table 4.8 shows how to calculate these indicators in a study about the ability of parents to remember vaccine injections. Comparison with health files has shown [3].

The sensitivity and specificity of a test indicate the correctness of that test, but when it comes to making decisions based on the positive and negative results of a test, sensitivity and specificity are not very useful. The positive predictive value shows the probability of the presence of the disease if the test result is positive, and the negative predictive value shows the probability of the absence of the disease if the test result is negative. These two possibilities measure the validity and usefulness of any diagnostic practice test. Another point about these indicators is to pay attention to the prevalence of the desired disease in society and its relationship with these indicators. Sensitivity and specificity are indicators that the prevalence of the disease does not affect their value. But the predictive value of the tests depends on the severity of the disease prevalence in the studied community. To understand these relationships, pay attention to the hypothetical example below. In this example, a hypothetical population of 100,000 people has been considered in a test with 90% sensitivity and 80% specificity with different prevalences of the disease under investigation.

A: Prevalence equal to 0.001.

$$\text{Positive predictive value} = \frac{90}{90+19980} = 0.0045$$

$$\text{Negative predictive value} = \frac{79920}{79920+10} = 0.9998$$

	Reality		
Result	Disease	Healthy	Total
Positive	90	19,980	20,070
Negative	10	79,920	79,930
Total	100	99,900	100,000

Table 4.7 Evaluation indices of diagnostic tests

Indicator	Calculation method
Sensitivity	$\frac{TP}{TP+FP}\times 100$
Specificity	$\frac{TN}{TN+FN}\times 100$
Positive predictive value (PPV)	$\frac{TP}{TP+FN}\times 100$
Negative predictive value (NPV)	$\frac{TN}{FP+TN}\times 100$
False-positive percentage	$\frac{FP}{TP+FP}\times 100$
False-negative percentage	$\frac{FN}{FN+TN}\times 100$

Table 4.8 Calculation of indicators in a study about the ability of parents to remember vaccine injections

	The information on the injection of the BCG vaccine obtained from the health record (standard reference of the test)				
Parents report the injection of the BCG vaccine based on memory.		**Yes**	**No**	**Total**	
	Yes	55	5	60	Sensitivity $\frac{55}{70}\times 100 = \%78.6$
	No	15	25	40	Specificity $\frac{25}{30}\times 100 = \%83.3$
	Total	70	30	100	
		Negative predictive value $\frac{25}{40}\times 100 = \%62.5$	Positive predictive value $\frac{55}{60}\times 100 = \%91.7$		

B: Prevalence equal to 0.01.

	Reality		
Result	Disease	Disease	Total
Positive	900	19,800	20,700
Negative	100	79,200	79,300
Total	1000	99,000	100,000

$$\text{Positive predictive value} = \frac{900}{900 + 19800} = 0.0434$$

$$\text{Negative predictive value} = \frac{79200}{79200 + 100} = 0.9987$$

C: Prevalence equal to 0.1.

	Reality		
Result	Disease	Healthy	Total
Positive	9000	18,000	27,000
Negative	1000	72,000	73,000
Total	10,000	90,000	100,000

$$\frac{9000}{9000 + 18000}, \text{ Positive predictive value} = 0.3333$$

$$\frac{72000}{72000 + 1000}, \text{ Negative predictive value} = 0.9863$$

D: Prevalence equal to 0.5.

$$\frac{45000}{45000 + 10000}, \text{ Positive predictive value} = 0.8181$$

$$\frac{40000}{40000 + 5000}, \text{ Negative predictive value} = 0.8888$$

	Reality		
Result	Disease	Healthy	Total
Positive	45,000	10,000	55,000
Negative	5000	40,000	45,000
Total	50,000	50,000	100,000

E: Prevalence equal to 0.9.

	Reality		
Result	Disease	Disease	Total
Positive	81,000	2000	83,000
Negative	9000	8000	17,000
Total	90,000	10,000	100,000

$$\frac{81000}{81000 + 2000}, \text{ Positive predictive value} = 0.9759$$

$$\frac{8000}{9000 + 8000}, \text{ Negative predictive value} = 0.4705$$

F: Prevalence equal to 0.99.

	Reality		
Result	Disease	Disease	Total
Positive	89,100	200	89,300
Negative	9900	800	10,700
Total	99,000	1000	100,000

$$\frac{89100}{89100 + 200}, \text{ Positive predictive value} = 0.9978$$

$$\frac{800}{9900 + 800}, \text{ Negative predictive value} = 0.0748$$

G: Prevalence equal to 0.999.

	Reality		
Result	Disease	Disease	Total
Positive	89,910	20	89,930
Negative	9990	80	10,070
Total	99,900	100	100,000

$$\frac{89910}{89910 + 20}, \text{Positive predictive value} = 0.9998$$

$$\frac{80}{9990 + 80}, \text{ Negative predictive value} = 0.0079$$

Figs. 4.3a, b show the relationship between positive and negative predictive value and disease prevalence in this hypothetical example.

4.6.1 ROC[1] Curves

The previous methods for evaluating diagnostic tests are used when the result of the diagnostic method is positive or negative. Nevertheless, in many experiments, quantities are measured on a continuous scale. When the values of the test results are determined continuously, the sensitivity and specificity levels depend on the place where the point of differentiation between positive and negative diagnosis is set. This situation can be shown by using two normal distribution curves related to testing result values (one distribution curve for people with the disease and the other distribution curve for people without the desired disease). In Figs. 4.4b, two hypothetical

[1] Receiver Operating Characteristic (ROC)

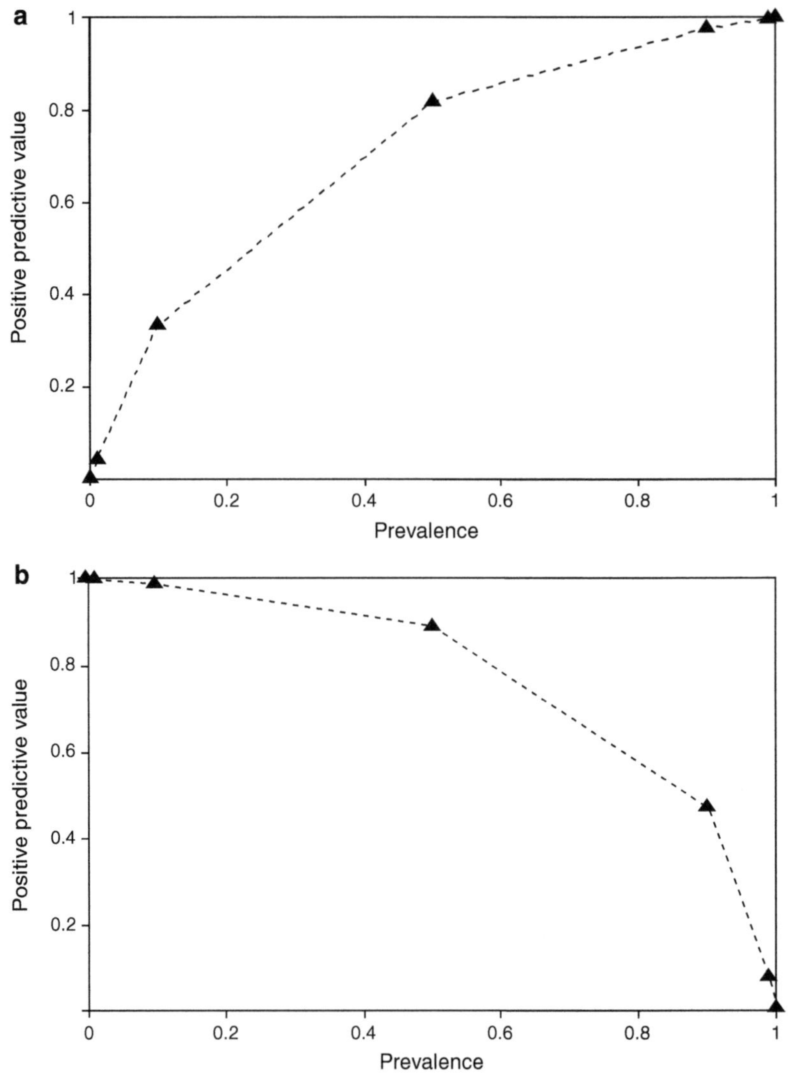

Fig. 4.3 (**a**) Prevalence relationship and positive predictive value for 90% sensitivity and 80% specificity in a hypothetical population of 100,000 people. (**b**) Prevalence relationship and negative predictive value for 90% sensitivity and 80% specificity in a hypothetical population of 100,000 people

distribution curves are shown in the case where the average value of the subject (e.g., cholesterol concentration in the blood) is 75 for people with the disease and 45 for people without the disease.

If we consider the decision differentiation point as 60, as seen in Fig. 4.4, about 10% of people without disease are considered "abnormal" in terms of the test, because their test results are higher than 60. In the same way, about 10% of people with the disease are considered "normal" in terms of the test, because the value of their test result is less than 60. In other words, in this test, the sensitivity is 90%, and the specificity is 90%.

Let's assume that medicine is willing to use a test with higher sensitivity. In other words, the doctor prefers to have more false positives than people who have the disease. In Fig. 4.4b, this state, that is, increasing sensitivity, is shown by reducing the point of differentiation between the normal and abnormal values from 60 to 55. The sensitivity of the test increased, but the specificity of the test decreased.

There is a more effective method to show the relationship between the specificity and the sensitivity of experiments whose results are continuous. In the field of communication, ROC curves have been created to show the ratio of signal to disturbing noise. To understand the application of

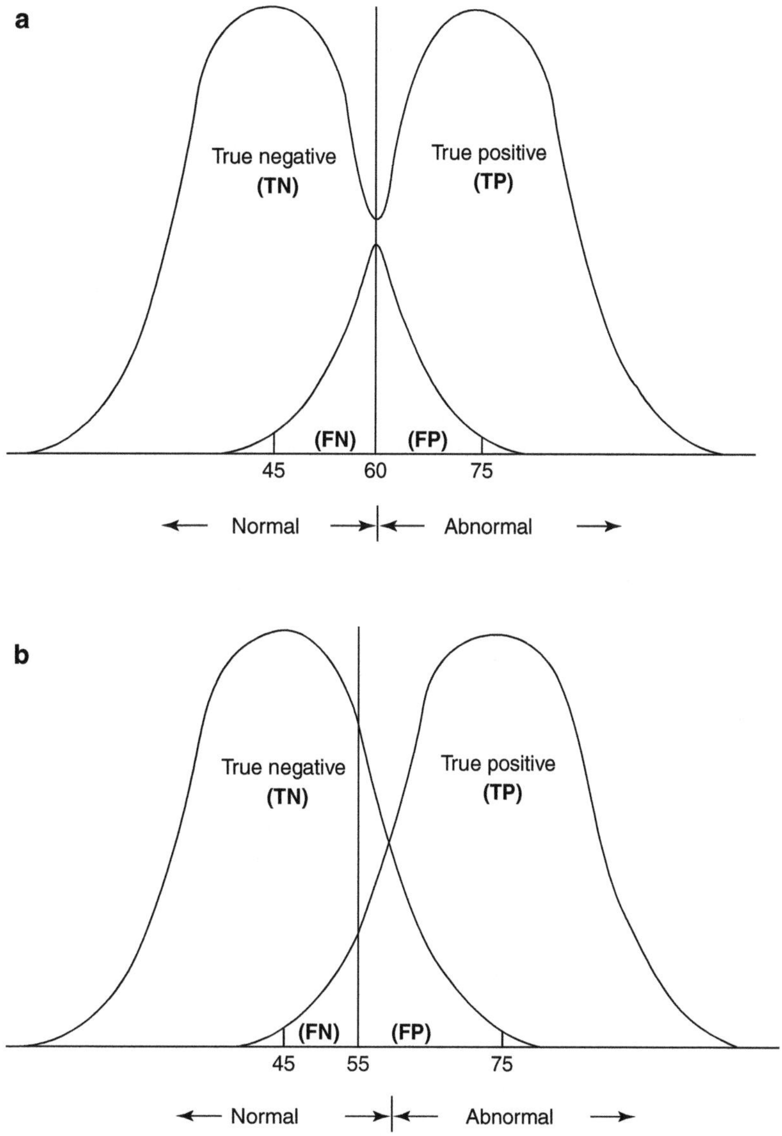

Fig. 4.4 (**a**) Figure of two hypothetical distributions for the decision line equal to the differentiation point of 60. (**b**) Figure of two hypothetical distributions er decision line equal to 55 differentiation point

this curve, in a diagnostic method, we consider a true-positive result as a "correct signal" and a false-positive result as "interference." ROC curve is a graph obtained from the ratio of sensitivity (true positive rate) to false-positive rate. The dashed line in the middle of Fig. 4.5 corresponds to a test that is randomly positive or negative. The closer the ROC curve is to the upper left corner of the figure, the more accurate it is, because the true positive rate becomes one and the false positive rate becomes zero. The more precisely the positive test criteria are defined, the point related to sensitivity and specificity (point A) on the curve moves down and to the left (i.e., less sensitivity and more specificity) [3].

If fewer criteria are required for the test result to be positive, the point related to sensitivity and specificity (point b) on the curve will move up and to the right (i.e., more sensitivity and less specificity).

ROC curves are useful graphical methods for comparing two diagnostic methods. For example, both radionuclide scans (RN) and computerized tomography scans (CT) are used to detect brain

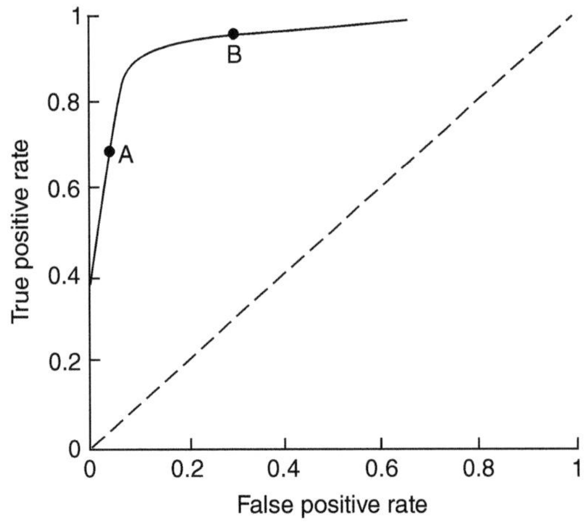

Fig. 4.5 ROC curve

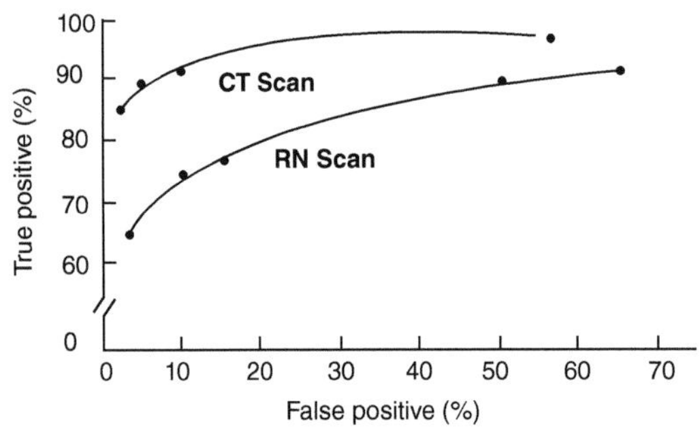

Fig. 4.6 Showing two ROC curves for evaluating two diagnostic methods

tumors. ROC curves have been used to compare these two methods. Figure 4.6 shows the ROC curves of these two methods [4].

By performing a statistical test, it is possible to determine whether the two ROC curves have a significant difference or not. In this method, the area under each ROC curve is determined and compared using the modified Wilcoxon rank sum method.

4.6.2 4-5-5 Correctness Ratios

Although the information of a diagnostic test can be expressed by sensitivity and specificity in dichotomous variables and by ROC curves in continuous variables, there is a better method. The correctness ratio for a positive and negative test allows the researcher to summarize all the information available in a test. For each of the positive or negative tests, the correctness ratio is stated below.

$$\text{Likelihood ratio} = \frac{\text{Probability}\left(\text{Test result / Disease}\right)}{\text{Probability}\left(\text{Test result / Healthy}\right)}$$

In the case of nominal variables, the correctness ratio of the positive test is equal:

$$\text{Likelihood ratio of positive test} = \frac{\text{Sensitivity}}{1-\text{Specificity}}$$

And the correctness ratio of the negative test is equal:

$$\text{Likelihood ratio of negative test} = \frac{1-\text{Sensitivity}}{\text{Specificity}}$$

The reason for using the validity ratio is that when a test is not completely valid, being informed about the result of this test will not determine whether a person is sick or not. The probability of these events can be predicted by using probability ratios. The higher the validity ratio, the more the ability of the test to correctly diagnose the disease. Validity ratios above 100 are ideal. The smaller the validity ratio is (closer to zero), the greater the ability of the test to correctly diagnose healthy people. When the correctness ratio is equal to one, it indicates that no new information is obtained from the test. For example, Table 4.9 shows the results of the study to investigate the possibility of predicting bacterial meningitis or the appearance of bacteria in the blood by the number of white blood cells in infants with fever [5].

As can be seen, the number of white blood cells less than 5000 or more than 20,000 is more common among babies with meningitis or with bacteria in the blood. The correctness ratio shows this issue very simply. For example, 8% of babies whose white blood cell count is less than 5000 have the disease, while only 4% do not have the disease. Therefore, the correctness ratio is equal.

Table 4.9 The relationship between bacterial meningitis or the presence of bacteria in the blood and the number of white blood cells in newborns

White blood cell count	Meningitis or bacteria in the blood		
No. white blood cell	Yes	No	Likelihood-ratio
>5000	5 (8%)	96 (4%)	2.0
5000–9999	18 (29%)	856 (39%)	0.7
10,000–14,999	12 (8%)	790 (36%)	0.3
15,000–19,999	17 (27%)	2 (13%)	2.1
≤20,000	15 (24%)	151 (7%)	3.4
Total (%)	63 (100%)	2177 (100%)	

4.6.3 Evaluation of Diagnostic Methods in Continuous Data

In this section, appropriate analysis methods for studies that compare different diagnostic methods for measuring the same parameter are reviewed. The most famous method for analyzing these studies is using the Bland and Altman method [6, 7].

The data shown in Fig. 4.7 is dedicated to the British Women's Heart Health Study. A total of 1236 women participating in this study were asked to report their weight, and then their weight was measured in the study. This scatter figure describes these two sizes. These two measures have a high correlation. For example, the Pearson correlation coefficient between these two measures is equal to 0.982. However, the high correlation does not indicate the existence of a good agreement between the two quantities. Because, for example, if one variable is always twice the other variable, their correlation coefficient is exactly equal to one. Apart from this issue, the correlation coefficient is a quantity dependent on the extent of the data. The wider the range of data, the higher the correlation, and the closer the data are, the lower the correlation.

The theoretical line in Fig. 4.7 defines the region where the two measurements have exactly equal values. If all the points are on this line, the two measurements have a complete agreement. As it is clear from the figure, the majority of observations are below this line. This shows that the weight reported by the study subjects is usually lower than its real value [8].

Bland and Altman [9] suggested that the degree of the agreement should be checked by drawing a graph of the difference between each pair of sizes (on the vertical axis) against the average of each pair (on the horizontal axis). This figure, which is usually known as the Bland and Altman figure, is shown in Fig. 4.8. If one of the measurements is correct, the average of the observed difference determines the presence of distortion in the new measurement. In this example, the average reported weight is 68.88 kilograms, and the average measured weight is 69.85 kilograms. The average difference between these two measurements is −0.93 kg (with a 95% confidence interval, −0.80 to −1.07 kg). Accordingly, there is a clear trend in reporting less weight, the average of which is 0.93 kilograms. Figure 4.8 shows the mean along with the 95% confidence interval of the agreement between the two measurements.

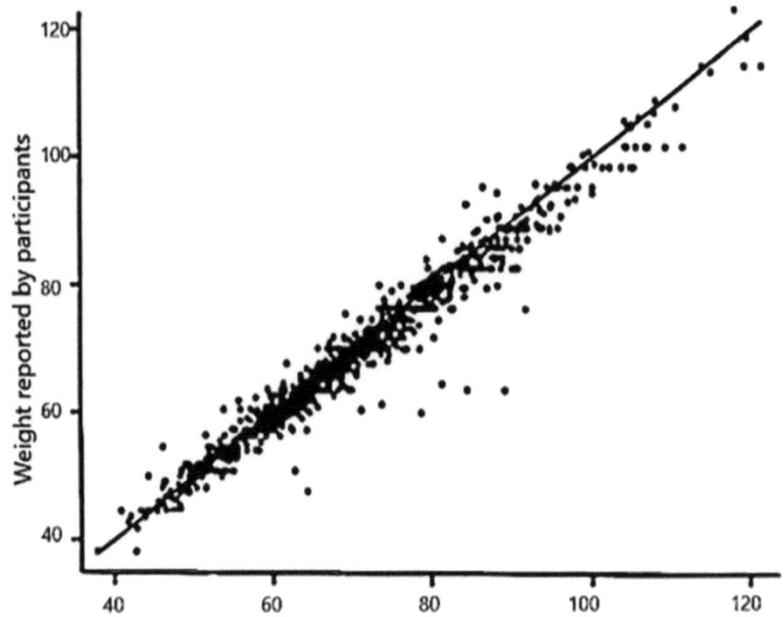

Fig. 4.7 Scatterplot of weight reported by the study subjects against measurements taken in 1236 women participating in the Women's Heart Study in Britain

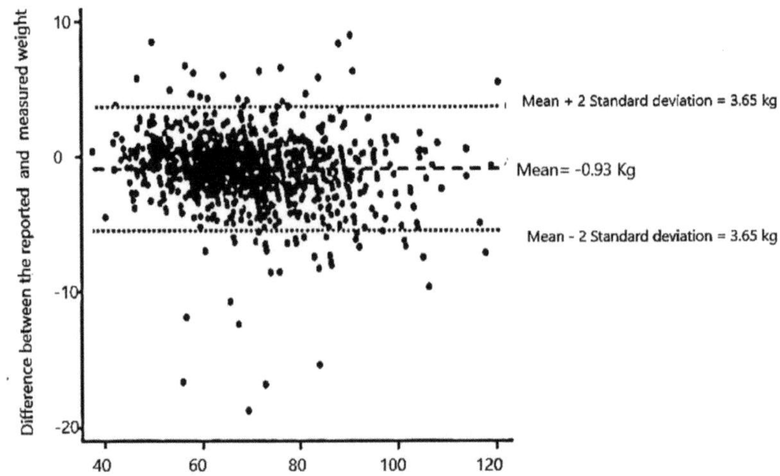

Fig. 4.8 Bland and Altman figure of the difference between reported weight (vertical axis) and mean reported weight and measured weight (horizontal axis) in 1236 women participating in the Women's Heart Study in Britain

4.7 The Effect of Measurement Error in the Analysis of the Results

The issues and problems that occur due to the existence of errors in the measurement of the outcome under study with variables related to exposure are shown in Table 4.10.

4.7.1 Weakening of the Effects in the Regression Model

Due to the existence of errors in the classification of consequences, the estimated effects for measuring the effect of exposure tend toward the zero hypothesis (ineffectiveness of exposure). In this way, the size of the correlation between the expo-

Table 4.10 Problems caused by measurement or classification errors

	Type of error		
		Misclassification (nominal variables)	Measurement error (continues variable)
Variable	Outcome	Attenuation of the effects in the regression model	Regression around the mean
	Exposure	Attenuation of effects in the regression model of potential problems to control confounders	

sure and the outcome is estimated to be less than the actual size.

In exposures that are of a continuous type, this strain is related to the intraclass correlation coefficient (ICC). In the linear regression model, this relationship is as follows.

$$\text{ICC} \times \text{true effect} = \text{estimated effect}$$

This relationship is approximately maintained in Cox and logistic regression models when the true effect size and error variance are not too large.

In serial exposure, the estimated effect size can be corrected by performing repeated measurements in all or some individuals. However, the methods of calculating the real effect size are much more complicated than in the previous case. The main reason is the correlation of errors with the real values of measurements [10, 11].

4.7.2 Regression Around the Mean

The phenomenon of regression around the mean was reported for the first time by Galton. When mixing bean pollen, he realized that the product made from two long beans is shorter than both beans and vice versa.

The same phenomenon occurs in the repeated measurement of a quantity despite the measurement error. Large values in the first measurement become smaller in subsequent measurements, and small values in the first measurement become larger in subsequent measurements. There is a negative correlation between the first size and other sizes.

Figure 4.9 shows the relationship between two diastolic blood pressures in a six-month interval in 50 volunteers [8], and Fig. 4.10 shows the distribution of the difference between two observations (vertical axis) against the initial size observed (horizontal axis). As it is clear from the figures, the initial measure of high blood pressure tends to decrease in the second measurement (6 months later) and vice versa. If there is no relationship between the actual reduction of two sizes and the actual size of the first order, the regression coefficient related to the observed correlation (β_{obs}) between the difference between the two sizes and the size of the first order is calculated as follows.

$$\beta_{obs} = ICC - 1$$

The greater the variance of the measurement error, the smaller the ICC and the larger the observed regression coefficient.

One of the common methods to reduce the effect of regression around the mean is to use the mean of measurements. Figure 4.11 shows the scatter figure of the difference between two blood pressure measurements against the average of the two measurements. As can be seen, the effect of regression around the mean has been adjusted to a large extent [12, 13].

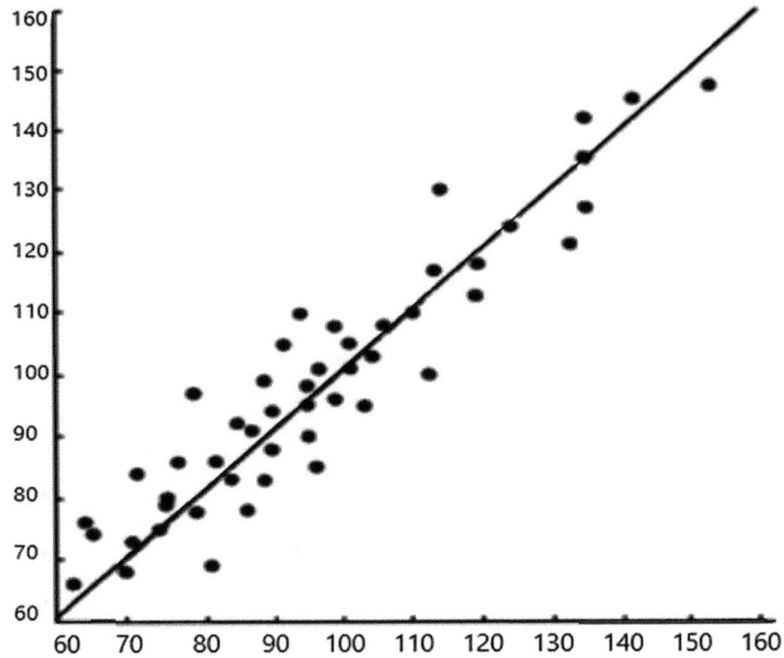

Fig. 4.9 The relationship between two measures of diastolic blood pressure measured in 6 months

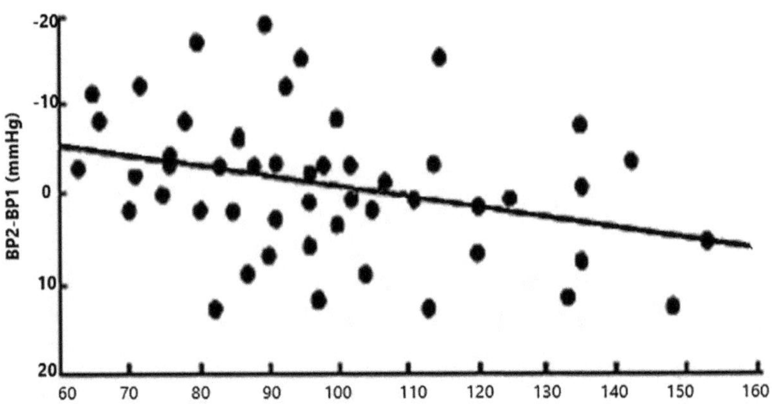

Fig. 4.10 Diastolic blood pressure changes against initial values. Correlation coefficient along with the direct regression line fitted to the data

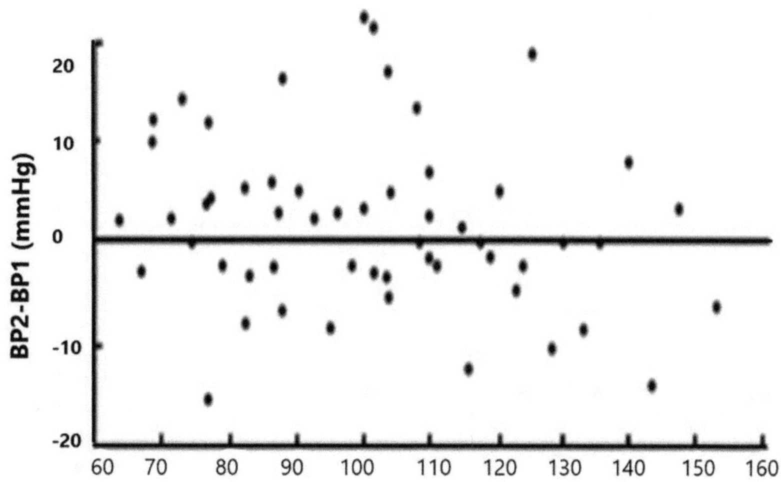

Fig. 4.11 Diastolic blood pressure changes against the average of primary and secondary values. Correlation coefficient along with the direct regression line fitted to the data

4.8 Studies that Investigate the Effect of a Test in Diagnosing a Disease

A test may be valid, but if the disease is rare, the test will be positive only in very few cases. This issue is equivalent to the fact that this test is not necessary for prescription in many cases. Other tests may often have positive results but do not affect clinical decisions. Because no new informants add to the treatment information compared to what is obtained from the patient's history, clinical examinations, or other tests [13–15].

In this part, the design of studies that evaluate the usefulness of tests in disease diagnosis and their effects on clinical decisions are discussed.

4.8.1 Design

The studies that investigate the usefulness of the test in the diagnosis of the disease answer such questions.

- When this test is prescribed for a specific situation, how many percent of abnormal cases are determined?
- Can the test results be predicted using other available information about the disease?
- What happens to patients who have anomalies? Do they benefit from the test results?
- These studies examine the proportion of positive results among patients who have specific symptoms. It is usually logical to assume:
- The probability of seeing positive results (presence of complications or consequences) is higher for patients for whom this test is prescribed than for other people.
- People whose test results are negative do not benefit from the test (because the treatment process does not change them).

With these assumptions, if the amount of positive results of a test is low, it can be argued that the application of this test is not useful in this particular case. To evaluate the direct effect of test results on clinical decisions, before and after comparison studies are designed. In these studies, the types of treatments and operations prescribed by the medical team before and after the test results are determined are usually compared [15–17].

For instance, in a study examining the impact of sonography on clinical decisions regarding acute abdominal pain in children, a research team assessed the initial clinical diagnosis and prescribed treatments for 94 children before undergoing sonography. Subsequently, they compared these findings with the results obtained from the sonography. The study revealed that in 46% of the cases, the additional information provided by sonography had an influence on the clinical diagnosis and subsequent treatment decisions [16].

Changing clinical decisions alone does not guarantee the usefulness of the test for patients. This issue is confirmed only when there are useful and effective treatments for the diagnoses obtained from the test. In the example above, there is a very high probability that patients will benefit from the new test. For example, changing clinical decisions from "discharge from the hospital" to "surgery" in children with appendicitis, or changing the decision from "surgery" to "under investigation" in the hospital in children with vague abdominal pains are the results that can be obtained using sonography.

4.8.2 Analysis

Statistical analysis and reporting of the results of these studies are usually simple. Often, the proportion of positive tests and tests that cause a change in management or (potentially) improved outcomes are calculated and reported along with the corresponding confidence intervals. Studies that examine the feasibility, costs, and risks of the test are one of the most important parts of clinical studies. These studies examine the applicability and practicality of diagnostic tests and are usually descriptive. The sampling design is very important in these studies [18] because the results often differ from one institution to another and also among patients.

References

1. Duwarahan J, Nawarathna LS. An improved measurement error model for Analyzing Unreplicated method comparison data under asymmetric heavy-tailed distributions. J Probab Stat. 2022;2022:3453912. https://doi.org/10.1155/2022/3453912.
2. Patel BD, Welch AA, Bingham SA, Luben RN, Day NE, Khaw KT, et al. Dietary antioxidants and asthma in adults. Thorax. 2006;61(5):388–93. https://doi.org/10.1136/thx.2004.024935. PMID: 16467075; PMCID: PMC2111195
3. Petrie A, Sabin C. Medical statistics at a glance. 4th ed. Hoboken: John Wiley and Sons Ltd; 2020.
4. Lu CM, Nicoll D, McPhee SJ. Guide to diagnostic tests. 7th ed. United Kingdom: McGraw-Hill Education; 2017.
5. Pantell RH, Newman TB, Bernzweig J, et al. Management and outcomes of care of fever in early infancy. JAMA. 2004;291(10):1203–12. https://doi.org/10.1001/jama.291.10.1203.
6. Suen YN, Cerin E. Measurement error. In: Michalos AC, editor. Encyclopedia of quality of life and well-being research. Dordrecht: Springer; 2014. p. 3816–21. https://doi.org/10.1007/978-94-007.0753-5_1758.
7. Mansournia MA, Waters R, Nazemipour M, Bland M, Altman D. Bland-Altman methods for comparing methods of measurement and response to criticisms. Glob Epidemiol. 2021;3:100045.
8. Kirkwood BR, Sterne JA. Essential medical statistics. Germany: Wiley; 2010.
9. Carstensen B. Comparing methods of measurement: extending the LoA by regression. Stat Med. 2010;29(3):401–10. https://doi.org/10.1002/sim.3769.
10. Berglund L. Regression dilution bias: tools for correction methods and sample size calculation. Ups J Med Sci. 2012;117(3):279–83. https://doi.org/10.3109/03009734.2012.668143. Epub 2012 Mar 8. PMID: 22401135; PMCID: PMC3410287
11. Weisberg S. Applied linear regression. 4th ed. Hoboken: Wiley; 2014.
12. Keogh RH, Shaw PA, Gustafson P, Carroll RJ, Deffner V, Dodd KW, et al. STRATOS guidance document on measurement error and misclassification of variables in observational epidemiology: part 1-basic theory and simple methods of adjustment. Stat Med. 2020;39(16):2197–231. https://doi.org/10.1002/sim.8532. Epub 2020 Apr 3. PMID: 32246539; PMCID: PMC7450672
13. Wu Z, Frangakis CE, Louis TA, Scharfstein DO. Estimation of treatment effects in matched-pair cluster randomized trials by calibrating covariate imbalance between clusters. Biometrics. 2014;70(4):1014–22. https://doi.org/10.1111/biom.12214. Epub 2014 Aug 27. PMID: 25163648; PMCID: PMC4284983
14. Lee MJ. Basics of treatment effect analysis. In: Micro-econometrics for policy, program and treatment effects. Advanced Texts in Econometrics. Oxford: Oxford Academic; 2005. 21–78. https://doi.org/10.1093/0199267693.003.0002.
15. Abdolrazaghnejad A, Rajabpour-Sanati A, Rastegari-Najafabadi H, Ziaei M, Pakniyat A. The role of ultrasonography in patients referring to the emergency department with acute abdominal pain. Front Emerg Med. 2019;3(4):e43.
16. Haynes RB, Straus SE, Glasziou P, Richardson WS. Evidence-based medicine: how to practice and teach EBM. United Kingdom: Elsevier/Churchill Livingstone; 2005.
17. Carrico CW, Fenton LZ, Taylor GA, et al. Impact of sonography on the diagnosis and treatment of acute lower abdominal pain in children and young adults. Am J Roentgenol. 1999;172(2):513–6. https://doi.org/10.2214/ajr.172.2.9930816.
18. Soori H, AnsariFar A, Mubasheri F, Mahmoudlou A, Noorafkan Z, Bakhtiari M. An overview on causation in epidemiology. Iran J Epidemiol. 2012;7(4):73–80.

Problems Related to Etiology in Medical Sciences

5

One of the first things taught in introductory statistics textbooks is that correlation is not causation. It is also one of the first things forgotten.

—Thomas Sowell (born June 30, 1930)

5.1 Introduction

Making causal inferences from the relationships observed in studies is one of the most important issues in clinical research. This chapter is dedicated to the investigation of etiology problems in medical studies. First, we will introduce the methods of avoiding artificial relationships, and then we will investigate real noncausal relationships. In the following, the role of chance and confusion in creating noncausal relationships is investigated.

5.2 Spurious Association

The relationship between an independent variable and an outcome variable is seen in a study, but this relationship is not true either due to chance or bias in society. For example, observational studies have shown an increased risk of road traffic injuries (RTIs) among women who drive slowly. However, a randomized trial found no effect on the risk of RTIs, suggesting that the association observed in the cross-sectional study was spurious.

A spurious association is a statistical relationship that is found between two variables but that is not causally related. In other words, the association between the two variables is due to a third variable that influences both of them.

For example, a spurious association may occur when there is a correlation between ice cream sales and crime rates. If one were to look at the data, one may be tempted to conclude that more ice cream causes more crime or vice versa. However, the spurious association comes from a third variable; the real cause behind both correlations is summer weather. In this case, summer weather leads to more ice cream sales and also higher crime rates, but it is not an actual causal relationship between ice cream consumption and crime.

Spurious associations can be particularly problematic in research, as they can lead to incorrect conclusions and a waste of resources. To avoid spurious associations, researchers must carefully consider potential confounding variables and attempt to control or adjust for them in their analyses. They may also conduct experiments to establish cause-and-effect relationships between variables.

H. Soori, *Errors in Medical Science Investigations*, https://doi.org/10.1007/978-981-99-8521-0_5

The spurious correlation is not a new concept and was first proposed and defined by Carl Pearson (March 27, 1857 to April 27, 1936), an English mathematician and biostatistician, in 1897. He explained how to obtain a significant value for a correlation coefficient. The variables are not correlated. He called this phenomenon a spurious correlation.

A spurious association or spurious correlation is sometimes a mathematical relationship in which two or more events or variables are related, but due to chance or the presence of a specific invisible third factor (such as a common response variable, confounding factor, moderator variable, or latent variable), this relationship is not causal.

Knowing the causes of diseases is necessary not only for prevention but also for diagnosing and applying correct treatments. If we make a mistake in determining the causal relationship or make a mistake in inferring from raw and descriptive findings, we may be misled both in the diagnosis of the disease and in choosing the appropriate treatment methods and the appropriate choice of preventive interventions. Fallacy or false cause is assuming a causal relationship between two phenomena or events, which is not the case. An example of a spurious relationship can be seen by examining the relationship between the number of ice creams sold and the number of drownings in a city. When the rate of drownings in a city's swimming pools correlates with the highest rate of sales, the claim that selling ice cream causes drownings or vice versa would imply a spurious connection between the two. Warmer weather may have caused both (more ice cream sales and more swimming). In the study, the heat wave is an example of a hidden variable, which we call a confounding variable.

Spurious correlations can result from small sample sizes or incomplete or arbitrary follow-up endpoints. Researchers use rigorous statistical analysis to determine spurious relationships. Confirming a causal relationship requires a study that controls all possible variables [1].

An observational study of a collection of interactive processes known as "demand withdraw" concerning adolescent dating aggression was carried out. The results indicated a demand withdraw and demand avoid sequences led by either partner were positively associated with both partners' physical and psychological aggression (measured via a dual questionnaire method). A higher-quality demand (i.e., pressures for change that were specific and encouraged both members of the dyad to increase a given behavior) was inversely associated with aggression. The associations of demand withdrawal and demand avoidance sequences with dating aggression may be spurious. The sequences are a known correlate of dating aggression merely markers for hostility [2].

In another classical example, suppose we want to investigate the relationship between coffee consumption and heart attack. One of the possible situations is that drinking coffee is one of the causes of heart attack, but before deducing such an issue, one should also consider four other options that cause a connection between the two phenomena. Table 5.1 examines possible inferences after observing a relationship.

The first two factors of this table, that is, chance and bias, cause the creation of spurious

Table 5.1 Five possible inferences that may occur after observing the relationship between coffee drinking and heart attack in the studied sample

Possible options	Type of relationship	The reality of the target population	Causal pattern
1. Random error	Spurious	Drinking coffee and heart attack are not related	–
2. Bias (systematic error)	Spurious	Drinking coffee and heart attack are not related	–
3. Cause (cause-effect)	Real	Heart attack is one of the causes of drinking coffee	Drinking coffee → Heart attack
4. Confounding	Real	Drinking coffee is associated with an external factor that causes heart attacks	External cause → Heart attack; External cause → Drinking coffee
5. Cause (cause-effect)	Real	Drinking coffee is one of the causes of heart attack	Drinking coffee → Heart attack

associations. That is, the observed association is established only in the studied sample, but it does not exist in society, but when a real relationship (far from chance and bias) is observed, apart from the intended causal relationship, two other options are also likely to occur. In the discussed example, smoking is one of the known factors in the occurrence of heart attack, which is also related to drinking coffee. For this reason, smoking is one of the confounding factors in investigating the causal relationship between coffee drinking and heart attack.

Spectrum bias is another type of error that can lead to incorrect and unrealistic conclusions of a causal relationship. This error occurs when the accuracy of a test in a sample differs from that in the population due to the spectrum of disease (which affects sensitivity) or non-disease (which affects specificity). For example, in this bias, the sensitivity and specificity of a test can be affected by differences in patient characteristics in different settings because the severity of illness in each setting (e.g., primary care, emergency care, hospital setting) has a different mix of patients.

The response rate, meaning the proportion of eligible participants who answer a questionnaire or a specific question, can reduce the internal validity of the study and make the result subject to error. For example, the low response rate in a survey of a Muslim community (20% response rate) to a question about alcohol consumption showed that Muslims consumed less alcohol than non-Muslims in the same community, which is probably not a valid estimate of their actual consumption. Due to the prohibition of alcohol consumption in Islam, Muslims who may drink alcohol may choose not to answer the question because of accusations of irreligion or antisocial behavior.

In statistics, correlations can be spurious when variables have marginal and skewed distributions. It should be noted that the presence of a statistically significant association/correlation cannot necessarily confirm the true relationship [3]. Reasons for spurious correlation might be small sample sizes or arbitrary endpoints.

5.3 The Difference in Association and Causation

One of the common mistakes is to confuse association with causation. It is the same reason for the fall of the stone that occurs due to the gravity of the earth or the cause of quenching thirst in drinking water, but the explanation of the association is somewhat complicated. For example, in the summer season, the sales of cooling devices increase, and watermelon sellers are also more satisfied with summer, because it increases their sales. Now, if we do not consider the heat of the air, it can be said that there is a linear relationship between the sale of cooling devices and the sale of watermelons. In other words, with the increase of one, the other also increases! Therefore, a simple linear model is considered in this case, in which the number of sales of cooling devices will be a function of the number of watermelon sales. Something like the linear pattern of Ohm's law ($V = RI$)! And it can be wrongly concluded that the reason for the change in the number of sales of cooling devices was the change in the number of watermelon sales. Here is an important cognitive error. It means that there is a lack of understanding of the difference between causality and correlation. Here, an unknown cause-effect relationship is established from the simultaneous changes of two variables. The cause of both events is another event. But because both events were created under its influence, it is considered that one is the cause of the other!

5.4 Statistical Significance and Biological Relationship

A biological relationship is a connection between two individuals or organisms based on their shared genes, ancestry, or biological lineage. The most common biological relationship is genetic relatedness, which occurs when two or more individuals share DNA inherited from their biological parents. Examples of biological relationships include the following:

1. Parent-child relationship: Parents share roughly 50% of their genes with their biological children, making this one of the strongest biological relationships in humans.
2. Sibling relationship: Siblings share roughly 50% of their genes, depending on their parents' genetic makeup.
3. Grandparent-grandchild relationship: Grandparents share roughly 25% of their genes with their grandchildren, while grandchildren share roughly 25% of their genes with their grandparents.
4. Ancestral relationship: Humans also share biological relationships with their ancestors, such as great-grandparents, great-great-grandparents, and so on. In this case, the shared genetic material may be spread out more widely, depending on the number of generations involved.
5. Genetic relationship between species: Different species can also have biological relationships based on shared genetic material, such as between humans and other primates.

Understanding biological relationships can be important in fields such as genetics, evolutionary biology, and forensic science. Through genetic testing, researchers can examine the relationships between individuals or organisms to learn more about their ancestry, genetic predispositions, and other characteristics that are influenced by genetic factors.

In statistics, when there is a statistical association between two events, we call that relationship correlation. For example, the lower the temperature, the higher the sales of warm clothes. The relationship of this example is called positive correlation because when one variable increases, the other variable increases, and when one variable decreases, the other variable decreases, but sometimes some correlations are negative, so that when one variable increases, another variable decreases, for example, with an increase in the level of education, the amount of crime decreases. But the point that should be considered is that the existence of a correlation does not mean the existence of a cause-effect relationship. In the cause-effect relationship, the existence of one event causes the creation or disappearance of another event. In cause-effect relationships, the existence of a phenomenon causes the emergence or disappearance of another phenomenon. In many cases, the relationship of correlation is confused with the relationship of cause-effect. The difference between correlation and cause-effect is evident in examples such as does eating meat prevent cancer? Does dark color make pedestrians safer? Does basketball make you taller? Those who eat a lot of meat have a short life span due to increased blood fat and die before they get cancer. The relationship between dark colors and fewer accidents can be explained in another way. Those who buy dark colors are mainly conservative people in terms of personality types. Also, older people usually buy darker colors. In the example of basketball, it can be said that there is a cause-effect relationship to some extent but contrary to what this sentence shows. The more correct statement is that "those who are tall usually play basketball." Of course, playing basketball during growing age may have a small effect on increasing height, but it cannot be the reason why people are tall. Therefore, in many cases, correlation relationships should be examined more carefully so as not to be confused with cause-effect relationships.

In interpreting statistical analyses, it should always be kept in mind that defining the biological relationship of any change found should be of primary importance in the evaluation rather than a specific level of statistical significance. In practice, the biological effect is calculated using point estimates (statistics), and its uncertainty is expressed through interval estimates (e.g., confidence intervals). Using such point and interval estimates can help focus the discussion on the biological relevance of the results.

5.5 Controlling the Effect of Chance in Relationships

Controlling the effect of chance, or random variation, is an important aspect when examining relationships between variables. Chance refers to the possibility of a relationship occurring by coincidence, rather than due to a true cause-and-effect relationship.

There are several ways to control the effect of chance in relationships, including the following:

1. Random sampling: A random sample is a subset of a population that is selected in a way that every individual or element in the population has an equal chance of being included. This minimizes the effect of chance and ensures that the sample is representative of the population.
2. Statistical tests: Statistical tests are used to determine the likelihood that a relationship between two variables is due to chance, or whether it is statistically significant. If the relationship is statistically significant, it is more likely to be due to a true cause-and-effect relationship.
3. Matching: Matching is a technique used to ensure that individuals or groups in a study are matched on certain variables that may affect the relationship being studied. This reduces the effect of chance and ensures that the relationship is not confounded by other variables.
4. Controlling for confounding variables: Confounding variables are variables that may affect the relationship being studied. By controlling for these variables, the effect of chance is minimized, and the relationship between the variables is more likely to be due to a true cause-and-effect relationship.

Overall, controlling for the effect of chance is important in relationships as it allows researchers to determine whether the relationship is statistically significant and whether it is truly a causal relationship or simply due to chance.

Standardization is one of the necessary measures to control errors caused by spurious causal relationships. It is specific and detailed instructions for how to perform a measurement designed to maximize the repeatability and accuracy of the measurement. Most of the studies conducted in medical sciences are observational in which the researcher tries to find causal relationships between observations. These studies are prone to error in claiming causal relationships. Randomization as an approach to control errors is not possible in interventional studies on biological subjects due to ethical issues. The validity of the results of observational studies is lower than that of controlled studies because many of them are subject to selection bias.

Cardiology researchers try to compensate for this problem by using statistical methods, but that approach cannot always solve the problems caused by confounders. Suppose there is no relationship between drinking coffee and heart attack and 60% of people in society drink coffee. If a sample of 20 heart attack patients is selected, we expect 12 of them to consume coffee. Only due to chance, there may be 19 coffee drinkers in the sample of 20 people. In this case, if again due to chance, the number of coffee drinkers in the control group is 19 or more, an artificial relationship between coffee consumption and heart attack will be observed. These relationships that occur only due to random errors (chance) are known as type 1 errors. Figure 5.1 shows the role of smoking as a confounder concerning drinking coffee and heart attack.

Methods to reduce the role of random errors in inferences are possible when designing and analyzing the results (Table 5.2). Among these solutions are increasing the measurement accuracy and increasing the sample volume, which was studied in Chaps. 1 and 4. Calculating the probability value and building the confidence interval for the estimates are statistical methods of evaluating the role of chance in the observed relationships, which are widely used in the information analysis department. For example, observing a

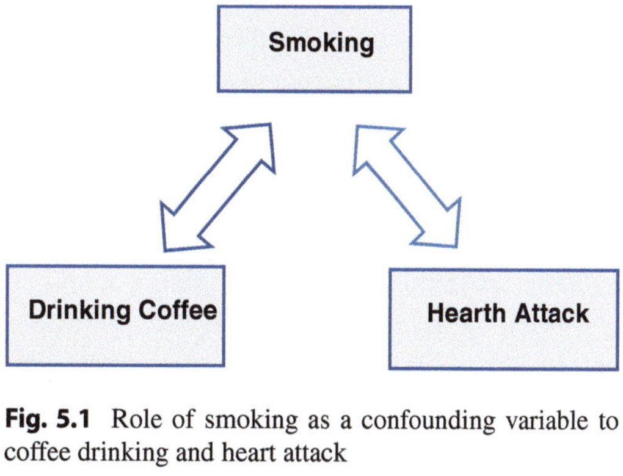

Fig. 5.1 Role of smoking as a confounding variable to coffee drinking and heart attack

Table 5.2 Methods of reducing the observation of spurious association in analytical studies

Sources of a spurious relationship	Control methods in the study design stage	Control methods in the data analyses stage
Random error	Increasing the sample size along with the solutions mentioned in the first and fourth chapters	Calculating and determining the probability value as one of the study documents
Bias	Deep attention to possible sources of difference between the research question and the study design, which includes the subjects under study, independent variables, and the outcome under study	Collecting additional data to investigate the role of potential distortions on the comparison relationships of the results obtained with the results of similar information

probability value equal to 0.1 indicates that a difference as big as that observed in the study between the subject groups in 10% of the cases is created only based on chance.

5.6 Controlling the Effect of Bias in Relationships

The appearance of a spurious association due to bias is much more complicated and misleading. The regular difference between the research question and what the researchers are investigating and finding the answer for is called bias. There are various solutions in the design and execution phase of the study, which can be used to minimize the bias (Table 5.2).

Different types of biases are known, and how to diagnose and control them are discussed in Chaps. 8 and 9. An interesting idea is to write the research question and the study plan together like in Fig. 5.2. Then the following three issues should be considered.

1. Are the samples examined in the study (e.g., cases and controls) a suitable representative of the target population?
2. Are the measurements and recording of background and independent variables valid enough?
3. Are the measurements and registration of the response variable valid enough?

The next step is to examine different solutions to prevent the occurrence of each of the potential biases. If the biases are easily preventable, the study design can be improved and the above three questions re-examined, and if they are not easily preventable, it should be worthwhile to conduct the study (comparisons and inferences made) despite the known potential biases. Usually, researchers encounter one or more potential sources of noise after collecting data. Some of these biases have been identified during the design of the study, but it is very difficult to prevent them, and some others are identified when it is too late to take measures to prevent their occurrence.

5.6.1 Effect Size

In any case, one of the common methods to control biases is to collect additional information to estimate the effect size of potential biases.

Effect size shows the significant size of the relationship between variables or the difference between groups. It is an essential factor when evaluating the strength or power of a statistical claim. It is a statistical concept calculated by dividing the difference between the means of two groups by standard deviation. Effect size can be measured in three ways: the odd ratio method, the standardized mean difference method, and the correlation coefficient method. A large effect size means that a research finding has practical significance, while a small effect size indicates that the practical applications of the study results are limited. For example, suppose the researcher discovers that the hospitalized control group is not adequately representative of the target population of people without complications of heart attack, because they have reduced coffee consumption due to chronic diseases. The size of this bias caused by the sampling method can be estimated by dividing the control group into two subgroups of patients who are required to reduce coffee consumption due to a specific type of disease (e.g., gastric ulcer) and patients who do not have such conditions. If both

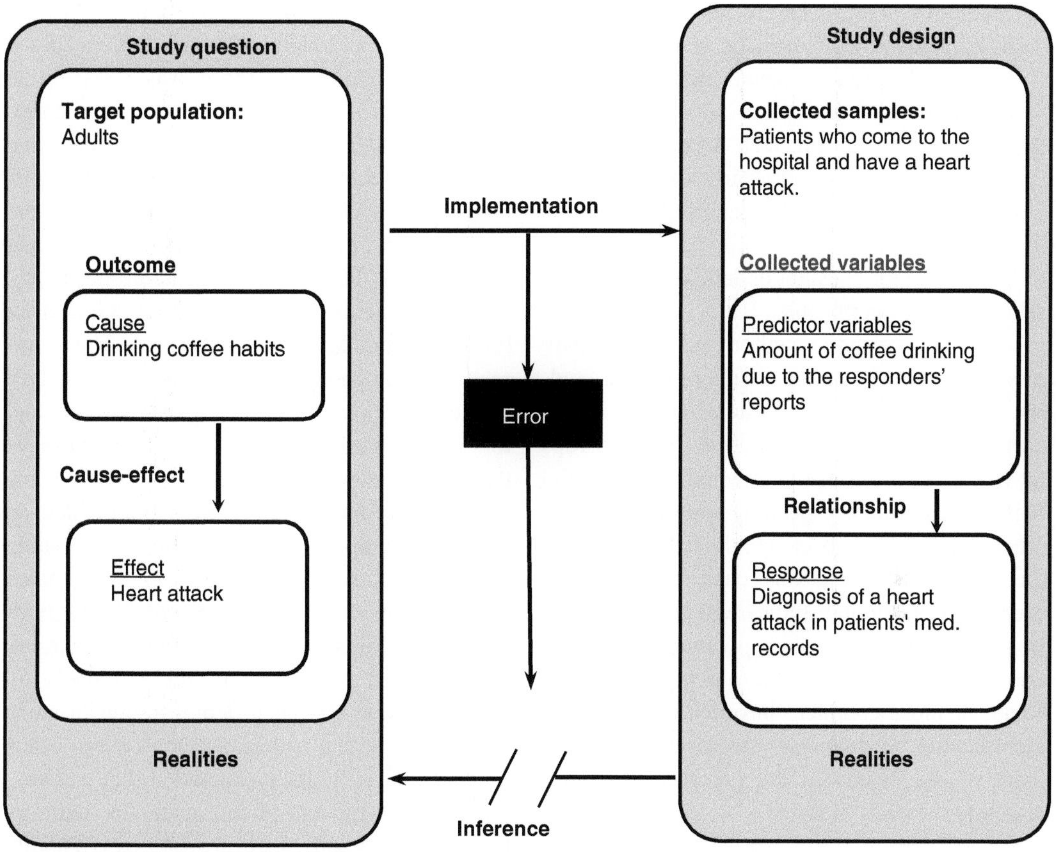

Fig. 5.2 Minimizing bias due to the comparison of research and study design

subgroups consume almost as much coffee as the subject group, the bias caused by the sampling method has little effect on the research findings. Also, when researchers are in doubt about the quality of collecting information about the amount of coffee consumption, one of the methods to investigate this bias is to select a subset of the subjects and witnesses of the study and re-examine their coffee consumption by an interviewer unaware of the group (case or control) patients. The degree of agreement of the results with the previous information determines the size of the bias effect caused by the low quality of the data.

Within Pearson's coefficient method, which utilizes values ranging between –1 and 1, the effect size can be interpreted in three ways. A value between 0 and 1 signifies a positive and direct relationship between the two variables, whereas a value between –1 and 0 indicates an inverse relationship with a negative value. When the result is 0, it suggests that there is no relationship between the two variables, represented as a zero value [4].

Under Cohen's *D*[1] effect size method, there are three interpretations [5]:

1. Small size (0.2): Such an effect between the two groups is negligible and cannot be spotted clearly.

[1]Cohen's *D* method determines standardized mean difference by dividing the difference between the mean values of two groups by the standard deviation value. It was introduced by the American statistician Jacob Cohen (April 20, 1923 to January 20, 1998). Cohen's *D* using a basic formula:

$$D = \frac{M_1 - M_2}{S_P}$$

where: M_1 and M_2 represent the sample means for the two groups being compared and S_P represents the pooled estimated population standard deviation.

Using SPSS version 27 or higher, you can estimate an effect size with your output for your independent samples *t*-test.

2. Medium size (0.5): This level of correlation is usually identified when the researcher goes through the data—medium size can have a reasonable overall impact.
3. Large size (0.8 or greater): A large effect can be observed easily and clearly—the impact is significant in real-world scenarios.

This indicator does not depend on the sample size and is very applicable.

Another common method is to compare research findings with the results of similar studies. If the results are consistent and similar to each other, probably the observed relationships have not been seriously affected by potential biases. This issue is especially appropriate when other studies have been conducted with other methods. Because in this case, the common sources of bias in the studies will be minimized. In general, in many cases, potential biases are one of the most important research problems. In Chap. 8, more complete information about the identification, evaluation of the effect, and adjustment of the results in the presence of biases affecting the study is stated.

5.7 Real Relationships Except for the Causal Relationship

When the non-artificiality of the observed relationships is ensured, other than the causal relationship, two other options, namely, the cause-effect relationship and the confounding effect, can occur.

5.7.1 Cause-Effect Relationship

There is always a possibility that what the researchers think of as the cause is a consequence or a complication that occurred as a result of what is called the effect. In other words, the real direction of the causal relationship should be the opposite of what the researchers have assumed. This is an important issue in cross-sectional and case-control studies. For example, in a cohort study, the relationship between serum uric acid (SUA) levels and anthropometric indices, blood cell count, and lipid profile was carried out. Results showed all studied factors were correlated with SUA level except VFL, BFM, and platelet-to-lymphocyte ratio. The highest correlation was with NC, BMR, hematocrits (HCT), and triglycerides (TG). The backward method revealed that TG, LDL, HDL, neutrophil, lymphocyte, platelet, HCT, BMR, and skinfold fat thickness were factors related to SUA. The occurrence of the cause-effect phenomenon in cohort studies is very rare because exposure to risk factors is measured many times before the onset of the disease. However, it is likely to occur in some diseases that have a long latent period and no detectable symptoms. Some findings of this study were derived cross-sectionally from a healthcare employee's prospective cohort study. These findings cannot demonstrate cause-effect relationships between studied factors and SUA levels [6]. This limitation has been demonstrated in some other studies and suggested that cause-effect models control it. They concluded that this cannot be used for causal inference. In addition, labeling causes and effects in a data set is a highly complicated task and needs to be emphasized that mislabeling in the data set may occur. Some methods to demonstrate a more logical cause-effect relationship can be grouped into expert judgments based on global insights, algorithms, and Bayesian or probabilistic methods. It is necessary to clarify the cause-effect relationships of uncertainties. The prioritization of uncertainties and risks and the structure of their cause-effect relationships enables us to effectively and logically concluded this study [7–9].

5.7.2 Types of Relationship

Relationships can be grouped under three general headings: (a) false relationship, (b) indirect relationship, (c) direct (causal) relationship:

1. One-to-one causal relationship
2. Multifactorial relationship

(a) ***False relationship***

Sometimes, the relationship obtained between a disease and the desired factor in a study may not be real. An example of an unrealistic relationship, such as a study in England that was conducted on 5174 home births and 11,156 hospital births, showed that perinatal death rates were 4.5 in home births and 8.27 in hospital births per 1000 births. In this study, perinatal death is more in hospital births! Such results are false or fabricated because, usually, the hospital attracts women who are at higher risk due to the presence of more equipment and specialists, while this is not the case in home births. The higher rate of perinatal death in the hospital is only for this reason and not because the care in the hospital is worse. Other factors may also be involved, such as the difference in age, number of pregnancies, quality of care during pregnancy, conditions in the home, general health, etc. between the two groups under investigation (home and hospital births). A false association occurs due to the wrong design of the study or the presence of bias in the study.

(b) ***Indirect relationship***

Many of the relationships that are initially considered to be causal are revealed by later studies to have been unreal relationships. A spurious relationship is a statistical relationship between two variables (target factor and disease or exposure and outcome) that is created due to the presence of another known or unknown factor. This third factor (i.e., the common factor) is also known as a "confounding" variable. A confounder is related to the independent variable and is a risk factor for the outcome. Since this confounding factor is common between the desired factor and the disease, it fully or partially justifies the relationship obtained between the two. Such confounding variables (such as age, sex, education, and social class) are potentially present in all studies and data and are a strong barrier to assessing relationships. An example of an indirect connection is the connection between coffee and pancreatic cancer. The importance of knowing the indirect relationship sometimes leads to a reduction in the risk of disease. Before the discovery of cholera disease, by examining the signs of the water well, it was determined that the source of the disease was a contaminated well. These indirect relationships help discover the etiology of diseases.

5.7.3 One-to-One Causal Relationship

In a one-to-one causal relationship, when a change in one variable causes a change in another, like variables, A and B have a causal relationship. Therefore, when there is a cause, a disease occurs, and vice versa, when there is a disease, there must be a cause. On the other hand, it can be said that this connection also conveys the concept of Koch's theory. Proponents of this theory believed that the cause must be necessary and sufficient for the disease to occur. But, many times, this is not the case, and the concept of being necessary and sufficient often does not fit in diseases. Consider a scenario involving a person exhibiting all the symptoms associated with Covid-19 but testing negative on a PCR diagnostic test, possibly due to test limitations. In this case, it is important not to dismiss the possibility of the disease solely based on the test result. The sufficiency of a single cause does not necessarily apply universally to all cases.

5.7.4 Multifactorial Relationship

Some noncommunicable diseases such as coronary heart disease are multifactorial. Smoking, high blood pressure, stress, and inactivity are predisposing factors for heart diseases. Multiple causal factors sometimes act cumulatively. Each factor may work alone, or when a person encounters several factors, it may have a synergistic or reinforcing effect, just like the synergistic effect of smoking and asbestos, which plays a role in causing lung cancer.

5.7.5 Adjusting the Confounding

Another option, when a real relationship is observed, is that the observed relationship is influenced by an external factor. How to identify confounding factors and ways to control them are discussed in Chaps. 6 and 7. It is possible to control or possibly eliminate the effect of confounding variables in two stages of design and data analysis. In the design stage, limitation, assimilation, and randomization in experimental studies are common methods to eliminate the effect of confounding variables. Table 5.3 shows the advantages and disadvantages of these methods.

Classification and multivariate analysis (modeling) of data are conventional methods to adjust the effect of confounding variables in the stage of analyzing the results. Table 5.4 examines the advantages and disadvantages of these methods.

Using the limiting method to control the confounding effect is very efficient and useful when the main purpose of the study is to investigate some subgroups of society. One of the important decisions in any study is the decision to perform assimilation. Usually, it is very effective to use the matching method to control background variables such as age, gender, and race that do not interact with other variables. This method can also be useful in cases where the sample size is small compared to the number of confounding variables in the study. Another important thing is to pay attention to whether it is easier to equate variables or to measure them, measuring some variables can be difficult or even impossible. Deciding on the analysis of the results by classification method or multivariate analysis can be delayed until the completion of the data. In this case, it is possible to check whether the factors are confounding and then decide on how to adjust the data [10].

Table 5.3 Adjusting the confounding effect in the information analysis stage

Strategy	Advantages	Disadvantages
Randomization	If the sample size is large enough, a random assignment will adjust all influencing variables (whether those that are measured by the researchers or those that are not measured or sometimes, the researchers do not know about their existence)	Except for experimental studies, it cannot be used in other studies
		To implement this method, many considerations such as ethical issues, cost, and time should be considered
Restriction	It is easy to understand and implement	It limits the generalizability of the results
Matching	The effect of some background variables such as age and sex (and with them the distribution of parameters related to those factors) are largely the same in the groups under study	It may be costly and time-consuming. Sometimes increasing the sample size is more efficient
	By adjusting the relative confounders for cases and controls in each category, the accuracy (statistical power) of the study increases	Since assimilation is done before conducting the study and the confounders are not known, it may have adverse effects on the analyzes and inferences
		It is not possible to calculate the relative risk or statistical modeling for the confounders based on which the assimilation has been done
		The analysis of these studies requires special methods
		There is a possibility of over-matching (matching for factors that are not confounding)

Table 5.4 Adjusting the confounding effect in the information analysis stage

Strategy	Advantages	Disadvantages
Stratification	It is easy to understand and implement	The number of classes may be very large compared to the sample size
		All the investigated variables must be nominal, this issue in the case of continuous variables (such as age, and blood pressure) can cause the loss of part of the information or inappropriate classification
Multivariate analysis	It is possible to adjust several confounders at the same time. It is possible to examine continuous variables	It is possible that the selected model is not suitable for examining the relationship between the response variable and the confounders of the study, in this case, the confounders are not properly controlled and adjusted
	These methods are very diverse and flexible	In case of choosing an inappropriate model or inaccuracy in modeling, incorrect estimates of the effect size of the disease risk factor are calculated
		It may be difficult to apply and understand the results

5.8 Criterion of Causality

In general, proving the relationship between cause-effect is called causation. Causality can be found anywhere in this world. For example, to know what is the cause of the disease? What is the cause of the disease? What factors affect the accident? The answers to the above questions are important for us in the sense that, by knowing them, we can prevent disease. All epidemiologic research has an essential role in showing whether the correlation is causal or not. There are various models in epidemiology to discuss causation, such as the wheel model, the network model of causality, etc., which will be presented later in this chapter. Part of epidemiology activities is limited to identifying the cause of diseases. In epidemiology, the cause is a factor that causes a change in the frequency of the disease, or the cause is a character without which the disease does not occur. For example, in cardiovascular disease, blood pressure is not the only cause, and this factor along with other factors such as increased cholesterol and lack of physical activity causes the inheritance of this disease; therefore, in epidemiology, diseases are multicausal. In epidemiological studies, descriptive studies show a clear face of disease in society, and by relating the disease to one or more factors (host factors, pathogen, and environment), they help to regulate causal hypotheses. Analytical and experimental studies test the hypothesis obtained from descriptive studies and prove or disprove the relationship between the target factor and the disease under study [11]. If we look at history, the cause of disease throughout history is as follows: (1) It has a superstitious aspect. (2) God's anger is mentioned in religious books. (3) Bile, soda, phlegm, and blood are mentioned. (4) Coldness and warmth are mentioned.

In the scientific literature, you can find many opinions and sources for causality criteria. The cornerstone of almost all these approaches is based on Hill's criteria. All of them agree on the principle of temporality but criticize other criteria.

5.8.1 Henle–Koch Criteria

The first time that the cause of the disease was scientifically noticed was by Koch in 1880. Robert Koch, a German physician and scientist, was one of the people who played an important role in the formation of the theory of pathogenic microbes.

Koch's causal hypotheses include the following:

(1) The microorganism must be found in the diseased; (2) The microorganism must be cultured from the diseased individual; (3); and finally (4)

1. The pathogen must be present in all cases of the disease but not in healthy individuals.
2. The pathogen must be isolated from the sick person and be able to cause the same disease in another host.
3. Inoculation of a healthy individual with the cultured microorganism must recapitulate the disease.
4. The pathogen must be re-isolated from the inoculated, diseased individual and matched to the original microorganism.

There are weaknesses in Koch's principles that can be pointed out. That pathogen will not be able to grow in artificial environments. Some pathogens are caused by several factors, and some pathogens such as *Staphylococci* can cause several types of diseases, and finally, some pathogens such as AIDS can only cause disease in humans.

The frequency of encountering the cause in patients is higher than in healthy people (case-control study). The frequency of new cases of the disease in people exposed to the cause is higher than in those not exposed (cohort study). In terms of time, the disease occurs following the cause, and if the cases of the disease are presented as a curve in terms of the incubation period, it should be symmetrical. Following exposure to the cause, there should be a range of responses in exposed individuals from mild to severe that is biologically meaningful. There should be a measurable response following exposure. In the experimental science of disease, the frequency of cases in exposed people is higher than in nonexposed ones. Eliminating or adjusting the presumed cause will reduce the frequency of the disease. Preventing and modulating the host's response to reduce disease cases (vaccine and medicine) [11–13].

All associations should be epidemiologically and biologically meaningful. In all the above cases, due to the multicausality of the diseases, the types of study designs, the society rather than the individual, the use of statistics in comparison, and finally the opinions of Evans show the relationship between the disease and the factors, and therefore, it does not always indicate the causality of the relationship. Statistical association means a strong association of two variables (e.g., the disease and the desired factor) to the extent that it cannot be attributed to chance alone. In other words, when we say that two variables are related, they happen together more than what is expected by chance, but correlation does not necessarily indicate causality.

Epidemiologists are interested in determining the "cause." Statistical correlation partially eliminates the chance of correlation. The relationship between two variables may be statistical or nonstatistical such as the high frequency of lung diseases on infected days compared to noninfected days. In the science of statistics, we show the relationship between two quantitative variables with correlation, and the intensity of the relationship is expressed by the correlation coefficient (−1 to 1). A positive correlation coefficient indicates a direct relationship and a negative correlation coefficient indicates an inverse relationship. It may be said that causation shows correlation, but it cannot be said that correlation shows causation. Always having a statistical relationship is not proof of its significance, and a slight difference may be significant due to the high sample size. A lack of statistical relationship may also occur due to a small sample size. The "degree" of the relationship between two features or variables (of qualitative nature) with the odds ratio (OR) from a case-control study or with the relative risk (RR) from a cohort study RR or OR varies from zero to infinity: between zero and one, there is an inverse relationship between two variables (disease and target factor or exposure and outcome). More than one, there is a direct relationship between two variables (disease and target factor or exposure and outcome).

5.8.2 Hill's Criteria for Causality

A statistical relationship is either causal or noncausal. The noncausal statistical relationship arises due to mistakes in different stages of the study (skewing or bias); Hill's criteria should be used to prove the causal relationship. Hill's criteria for judging the causality of the statistical relationship obtained between two variables (factor and disease or exposure and outcome) include the following:

- Strength
- Consistency
- Specificity
- Temporality
- Plausibility
- Biologic gradient
- Coherence
- Experimental evidence
- Analogy

5.8.2.1 Consistency

Consistency, which defines stable and consistent findings in different samples and in different times and places that are investigated by different researchers, is the existence of a relationship. The results of just one study are rarely enough to prove a "causal" relationship. More than 50 case-control studies and 9 cohort studies in different countries have shown the relationship between smoking and lung cancer. Exclusivity: The concept of specificity indicates a "one-to-one" relationship between the pathogen and the outcome. In the past, most discussions about smoking and lung cancer revolved around the nonspecificity of the relationship. That is, smoking not only causes lung cancer but causes various other diseases such as coronary heart disease, bronchitis, emphysema, cervical cancer, etc. This issue was raised for years as a debate against the causal relationship between smoking and lung cancer. Smoking is indeed related to many diseases, and this is a reflection of the nonspecificity of the relationship, but this argument cannot be strong enough to rule out causation. Proving specificity is very difficult not only in chronic diseases but also in some acute diseases, and one cause or factor can cause more than one disease, and secondly, most diseases are caused by several factors for which a one-to-one relationship cannot be shown. To justify the nonspecificity of the relationship between smoking and lung cancer, it can be stated that cigarette smoke is a collection of harmful substances such as nicotine, carbon monoxide, and other substances that can act in an increasing or strengthening and synergistic way. These different components of cigarette smoke are responsible for the occurrence of various diseases (lung cancer, emphysema). There are other factors other than smoking that increase the risk of lung cancer, such as occupational exposure to chromates, asbestos, nickel, uranium, and exposure to air pollution. Finally, it can be said that the specificity of the relationship confirms its causality, but its absence does not reject the causality.

Precedence of relationship: In a causal relationship, the factor (exposure) must precede the onset of the disease (consequence) in terms of time to justify the time required for the latent period of the disease. Temporal precedence is the basic necessity of the concept of causality. In some acute diseases, such as diarrhea caused by food or contaminated water, it is easy to discover the time precedence. But in many chronic diseases, due to the hidden onset and lack of knowledge about the details of the incubation period, it is difficult to obtain the chronological order between the disease and the desired factor.

5.8.2.2 The Power of the Relationship

The strength of the relationship is determined by the relative risk or odds ratio. The closer the relative risk or odds ratio is to one, the stronger the association. Of course, the weak relationship does not negate the possibility of causality. Biologically logical: If the existence of the relationship is confirmed biologically, that is, the existing relationship is in agreement with our current knowledge of the organs, tissues, and systems of the body, then the causal relationship is confirmed. For example, the connection between fatty foods and heart diseases is logical. But the connection between fatty foods and contracting Covid has no biological logic, and it states that the strength of the connection alone does not show the cause. Neglecting this criterion may cause errors in the conclusions of correlation studies. Of course, this criterion should not be applied with prejudice. That is, just because it is not logical from a biological point of view, one should not immediately reject the causality of the relationship between a factor and its resulting consequence, because this issue may be due to the limitation of current human knowledge. Biological gradient: Is there a dose-response or duration-response relationship? The amount-response relationship means that the incidence of the disease will increase with the increase in the amount of exposure to the agent. If the above relationship exists, the causal relationship is strengthened. The example of smoking and lung cancer: Value-response relationship plays a major role in accepting the relationship as a causal relationship. If there is no value-response relationship, it casts serious doubt on the causal hypothesis. Sometimes, exposure to a certain level has an increasing effect. But after that, it reaches a constant level or there is a threshold, and exposure to the agent after passing this threshold causes illness. Communication continuity: Continuity of the relationship between two variables (agent-disease) with the facts that are related to the subject. For example, historical evidence is related to the increase in tobacco use in the form of cigarettes and the increase in lung cancer. The difference in death rates from lung cancer in men and women is also associated with the recent increase in smoking in women. The death rate initially increased in men, and now, in women, it is increasing at a relatively faster rate. Being experimental: The relationship can be checked empirically. For example, if a factor is the cause of a disease, by removing that factor, the disease will also be removed. Stop exposure: If the exposure plays a role in causing the disease when the exposure is reduced or stopped, the risk of the disease should also be reduced or eliminated. But it should be noted that in some cases the effect of exposure may not be reversible, and the disease may occur when the exposure is stopped. The above criteria are used to verify causality in an association or relationship obtained between two variables (disease and factor). To judge or evaluate the relationship in terms of causality, all the above criteria must be used, and none of them alone are sufficient, and none alone is a necessary condition for inferring the existence of a causal relationship from statistical relationships, but each of them adds to the amount of evidence, and all together contribute to the statement of the probability of the relationship being causal.

5.8.3 Criteria from MacMahon et al.

Brian MacMahon, Thomas F. Pugh, and Johannes Ipsen are the authors of the world's first published Textbooks on Epidemiological Methods and Modern Epidemiology. The First Edition of B. MacMahon et al., 1960, had no criteria for causality. In the second version of this book (1970), they emphasize three causal criteria in Hill's version. They did not offer any criteria of their own and did not pay attention to the inclusion of the "dose-effect" relationship and the concept of "direction" [14].

The three main criteria that McMahon and colleagues emphasize as the main criteria of causality are as follows:

- Dependence on time or time sequence (events considered to cause must precede those considered to be affected).
- Strength of relationship + biological gradient (the stronger the relationship between two independent and dependent variables). If the suspected cause of exposure to a variable is quantitative, the existence of a dose-response relationship, that is, a relationship in which the frequency of the effect increases with the increase of the cause found is usually considered in favor of a causal relationship, although even in a causal relationship, such a relationship may not exist across the entire spectrum of causal exposures.
- Biological plausibility (e.g., a causal hypothesis based on epidemiological evidence is supported by knowledge of biology that makes it plausible, and evidence that the distribution of disease in populations follows the distribution of the hypothesized causal agent supports the causal hypothesis).

5.8.4 Criteria of Susser

Mervyn Wilfred Susser, a South African epidemiologist (1921–2014), believed that the process of causal analysis, central to all science, is most crucial where the subjects of study are least biddable. He presents environmental criteria of causation. The three obligatory points of this author, "association" (or "probability" of causality), "time order," and "direction of effect," are trivial, and two more special criteria, which are the development of "Popperian Epidemiology," that is, "survivability" of the hypothesis when it is tested by different methods (included in the refinement in Hill's criterion "consistency of association") and "predictive performance" of the hypothesis are more theoretical and hardly applicable for the practice of epidemiology and public health.

5.8.5 Evans Criteria

Alfred Spring Evans (1917–1996) developed unified "postulates" of the causality of infectious and chronic diseases together. In this approach, two epidemiological designs, case-control and cohort, are added to the list of Hill's and Susser's criteria. Such an extended approach would greatly enhance the evidence for causality. The Evans ten criteria list was completed in 1993 [15].

1. The prevalence of the disease should be significantly higher in those exposed to the putative cause than in cases and controls not so exposed [criterion "association"].
2. Exposure to the putative cause should be present more commonly in those with the disease than in controls without the disease when all risk factors are held constant ["case-control study"].
3. Incidence of the disease should be significantly higher in those exposed to the putative cause than in those not so exposed as shown in prospective studies [cohort study].
4. Temporally, the disease should follow exposure to the putative agent with a distribution of incubation periods on a bell-shaped curve [criterion "temporality"].
5. A spectrum of host responses should follow exposure to the putative agent along a logical biologic gradient from mild to severe [criterion "biological gradient"].
6. A measurable host response following exposure to the putative cause should regularly appear in those lacking this before exposure (i.e., antibody, cancer cells) or should increase in magnitude if present before exposure; this pattern should not occur in persons so exposed (surrogate endpoints) and "biological gradient."
7. Experimental reproduction of the disease should occur in higher incidence in animals or men appropriately exposed to the putative cause than in those not so exposed; this exposure may be deliberate in volunteers, experimentally induced in the laboratory, or demonstrated in a controlled regulation of natural exposure [criteria "biological plausibility" and "experiment"].
8. Elimination or modification of the putative cause or the vector carrying it should decrease the incidence of the disease (control of polluted water or smoke or removal of the specific agent).
9. Prevention or modification of the host's response on exposure to the putative cause should decrease or eliminate the disease (immunization, drug to lower cholesterol, specific lymphocyte transfer factor in cancer) [criterion "counterfactual experiment"].
10. The whole thing should make biological and epidemiologic sense [criteria "biological plausibility" and "coherence with current facts and theoretical knowledge"].

5.8.6 Individual Casualty in Medical Expertise

Causality can be conclusively established between a particular exposure as an entity and a particular disease as an entity. However, it is not possible to establish such a link conclusively between exposure and a particular disease of a given individual. For example, in legal investigations about the murder or death of a person, based on the results of epidemiological studies, the correct relationship between the agent or the cause of death and the incident cannot be presented for the court's decision. Ronald E. Gots presents principals for establishing individual causality in medicine probabilistic causality for the individual personally in medical and forensic practice [16].

He introduces the following principles of the methodology of causation analysis the individual level:

- Lack of alternative explanations criterion (Have other causes been properly considered and ruled out?)
- Has the exposure been confirmed?
- Strength of association (criterion "Was the exposure sufficient in duration and concentration?")
- Coherence with known facts from the natural history and biology of the disease (criterion "Was the clinical pattern appropriate?")
- Coherence with known facts from the natural history and biology of the disease (criterion "Is the morphological pattern appropriate?")
- "Temporality" criterion in philosophical terms (Is the temporal relationship appropriate?)
- "Temporality" criterion in epidemiological terms (Does the latent period of the disease correspond? Is the latency appropriate?)

A review of causal inference in forensic medicine has been explained in another article [17].

5.8.7 Inferring the Cause-Effect Relationship Based on Evidence

In the previous sections, the methods of identifying and evaluating the causal relationships of other relationships were investigated. In this part, we discuss how to evaluate the causal relationship based on the available evidence. In general, the main things to confirm the causality of a relationship are temporal relationship, stability (reproducibility and compatibility) of findings, and biological justification. In addition to these factors, other evidence such as dose-response relationship, the strength of correlation, interruption of exposure, specificity of correlation, and other explanations that can be presented can also be effective in inferring a causal relationship [1, 3, 5].

We know that if the agent plays a role in causing the disease, it must have been exposed before the symptoms of the disease appeared. In most cases, it is easier to show the temporal relationship in prospective cohort studies than in case-control or retrospective cohort studies. The temporal relationship between the exposure and the development of the disease is important not only in terms of the order of occurrence but also in terms of the time interval between the exposure and the onset of the clinical symptoms of the disease.

When the repetition of the study, with different methods and designs, results in observing consistent results, the possibility of observing accidental or distorted relationships due to distortions becomes weak. Real relationships, that is, causation, cause-effect, or bias, are usually stable. For example, if smoking and drinking coffee have a positive statistical relationship in society, we expect that the existence of a relationship between coffee drinking and heart attack will always be confirmed in various studies.

One of the important factors for the existence of a causal relationship is the existence of biological acceptability. If there is a causal structure that is scientifically justified for the observed relationship, then a strong reason and evidence for the causality of the relationship is provided. When a factor causes a disease, we expect that when exposure to that factor is reduced or completely stopped, the risk of contracting the disease will also decrease or disappear. The presence of a stronger relationship is stronger evidence in favor of observing a direct relationship. The relationships observed due to the presence of confounding factors, because they are indirect, are generally weaker than direct relationships such as causal relationships. In addition, stronger relationships often lead to the observation of a significant probability value, which reduces the likelihood that the relationship is due to chance.

The existence of a dose-response relationship is the positive evidence for the existence of a causal relationship. For example, the prevalence of lung cancer is higher in ordinary smokers than in normal people, and for professional smokers, the prevalence of cancer is higher than in both groups. Whenever it is possible, variables predicting the outcome should be measured continuously or in several classes, so that it is possible to observe the dose-response relationship. However, it is also possible to observe the dose-response effect in causal relationships or relationships distorted by confounders. For example, if people who smoke more often consume more coffee, it is possible to observe a dose-response effect in the relationship between coffee consumption and heart attack.

If the correlation is causal, we expect the observed findings to be consistent with the findings of other studies. For example, if smoking has a causal relationship with lung cancer, this relationship should be observed in both women and men in separate studies. To better understand how to make a causal inference, we will examine the relationship between *Helicobacter pylori* and gastric ulcers, which is discussed in the Gordis epidemiology book [11].

Studies that started in 1982 in the field of infection with *Helicobacter pylori*, a gram-negative bacterium, showed that this infection is related to chronic active gastritis. Later studies showed that this bacterium plays a role in causing gastrointestinal ulcers. In Table 5.5, possible evidence and inferences about the causality of the observed correlation have been collected. As can be seen, the available evidence strengthens the causality of the relationship. But the available evidence is still not enough to make a causal inference.

Table 5.5 Evaluation of the evidence presented for the existence of a causal relationship between *Helicobacter pylori* infection and duodenal ulcer

Temporality
Helicobacter pylori is associated with chronic spread. About 11% of patients with chronic gastritis become injured within 10 years. In a study in which 454 patients underwent endoscopy, after 10 years, 34 out of 321 people who were carriers of *H. pylori* (11%) had ulcers, and now only 133 people had ulcers due to this bacterial disease, which has been registered (0.8%)
Strength of association
H. pylori has been isolated from 90% of patients with duodenal ulcers. In at least one community with no reported cases of ulcerative colitis (from an aboriginal tribe in northern Australia who were isolated from other communities), *H. pylori* have never been isolated
Biological gradient (dose-response relationship)
The density of *H. pylori* in people with duodenum ulcers per square millimeter is higher than in patients who do not have this ulcers (pay attention to the strength of the relationship)
Consistency (reproducibility)
Many of the observations related to this finding are repeatable and have been repeated
Biological rationality/plausibility
Bacteria are attached to the primary cells of the small intestine and accompany them inside the intestine. *H. pylori* also induces signaling mediators. Mucous infected with *Helicobacter pylori* weakens and becomes more sensitive to harmful stomach acid
Coherence
The prevalence of *H. pylori* is the same in men and women. The incidence of intestinal ulcer, which was said to be higher in men than in women, has been reported the same in recent years
Experience (lack of exposure)
Eradication of *H. pylori* causes wound healing at the same speed as treatment with antihistamines. Eradication of *H. pylori* infection by using three drugs at the same time, causes the recurrence of intestinal ulcers after a long period of time, while the treatment with histamine antagonists has between 60% and 80% of recurrences
Specificity
The prevalence of *H. pylori* infection in patients with ulcers of the first part of the small intestine is 90–100%. This infection has been reported in some patients with stomach ulcers and healthy people
Other explanations
The results of studies show that smoking increases the risk of developing intestinal ulcers in patients infected with *H. pylori*, but this factor does not increase the risk in those for whom this infection has been eradicated

References

1. Soori H, Sharifi H, Asgarian SF. Causation in medical sciences [In Farsi language]. Tehran: Baghyatollah University of Sciences Publication; 2023. (ISBN: 978-964-2561-90-2).
2. Lorber MF, Mitnick DM, Tiberio SS, Heyman RE, Slep AMS, Trindade S, Damewood GN, Bruzzese JM. Demand-avoid-withdraw processes in adolescent dating aggression. Aggress Behav. 2023;49:274. https://doi.org/10.1002/ab.22070. PMID: 36645870.
3. Halperin S. Spurious correlations—causes and cures. Psychoneuroendocrinology. 1986;11(1):3–13. https://doi.org/10.1016/0306-4530(86)90028-4. PMID: 3704066.
4. Nuijten MB, van Assen MALM, Augusteijn HEM, Crompvoets EAV, Wicherts JM. Effect sizes, power, and biases in intelligence research: a meta-meta-analysis. J Intell. 2020;8(4):36. https://doi.org/10.3390/jintelligence8040036. PMID: 33023250; PMCID: PMC7720125.
5. Lakens D. Calculating and reporting effect sizes to facilitate cumulative science: a practical primer for t-tests and ANOVAs. Front Psychol. 2013;4:863. https://doi.org/10.3389/fpsyg.2013.00863. PMID: 24324449; PMCID: PMC3840331.
6. Soori H, Rezapoor P, Najafimehr H, Alirezaei T, Irilouzadian R. Comparative analysis of anthropometric indices with serum uric acid in Iranian healthy population. J Clin Lab Anal. 2022;36(2):e24246. https://doi.org/10.1002/jcla.24246. Epub 2022 Jan 16. PMID: 35037318; PMCID: PMC8842160.
7. Kesic MG, Savicevic AJ, Peric M, Gilic B, Zenic N. Specificity of the associations between indices of cardiovascular health with health literacy and physical literacy; a cross-sectional study in older adolescents. Medicina (Kaunas). 2022;58(10):1316. https://doi.org/10.3390/medicina58101316. PMID: 36295477; PMCID: PMC9609210.
8. Gultekin B, Demir S, Gunduz MA, Cura F, Ozer L. The logistics service providers during the COVID-19 pandemic: the prominence and the cause-effect structure of uncertainties and risks. Comput Ind Eng. 2022;165:107950. https://doi.org/10.1016/j.cie.2022.107950. Epub 2022 Jan 13. PMID: 35043031; PMCID: PMC8757651.
9. Lucendo AJ. Drug exposure and the risk of microscopic colitis: a critical update. Drugs R D. 2017;17(1):79–89. https://doi.org/10.1007/s40268-016-0171-7. PMID: 28101837; PMCID: PMC5318339.
10. Papadogeorgou G, Dominici F. A causal exposure response function with local adjustment for confounding: estimating health effects of exposure to low levels of ambient fine particulate matter. Ann Appl Stat. 2020;14(2):850–71. https://doi.org/10.1214/20-aoas1330. Epub 2020 Jun 29. PMID: 33649709; PMCID: PMC7914396.
11. Lindahl BIB, Nordenfelt LY. Health, disease, and causal explanations in medicine. Dordrecht: Springer; 2012.
12. Koterov AN, Ushenkova LN. Causal criteria in medical and biological disciplines: history, essence, and radiation aspects. Report 4, part 1: the post-hill criteria and ecolgical criteria. Biol Bull Russ Acad Sci. 2022;49:2423–66. https://doi.org/10.1134/S1062359022120068.
13. Kundi M. Causality and the interpretation of epidemiologic evidence. Environ Health Perspect. 2006;114(7):969–74. https://doi.org/10.1289/ehp.8297. PMID: 16835045; PMCID: PMC1513293.
14. Scheutz F, Poulsen S. Determining causation in epidemiology. Community Dent Oral Epidemiol. 1999;27(3):161–70. https://doi.org/10.1111/j.1600-0528.1999.tb02006.x. PMID: 10385353.
15. Evans AS. Causation and disease: a chronological journey. New York: Plenum Medical Book Company; 1993.
16. Gots RE. Medical causation and expert testimony. Regul Toxicol Pharmacol. 1986;6(2):95–102. https://doi.org/10.1016/0273-2300(86)90026-7. PMID: 2941828.
17. Meilia PDI, Freeman MD, Herkutanto, Zeegers MP. A review of causal inference in forensic medicine. Forensic Sci Med Pathol. 2020;16(2):313–20. https://doi.org/10.1007/s12024-020-00220-9. Epub 2020 Mar 10. PMID: 32157581; PMCID: PMC7245596.

Evaluation of the Role of Intervening Variables in Analytical Studies

6

Ever since men became capable of free speculation, their actions, in innumerable important respects, have depended upon their theories as to the world and human life, as to what is good and what is evil. This is true in the present day as at any former time. To understand an age or a nation, we must understand its philosophy, and to understand its philosophy we must ourselves be to some degree philosophers. There is here a reciprocal causation: the circumstances of men's lives do much to determine their philosophy, but, conversely, their philosophy does much to determine their circumstances.

—Bertrand Arthur William Russell (1872–1970)

6.1 Introduction

In many studies of medical sciences, to determine causal relationships, it is necessary to pay attention to the differences and similarities of the desired characteristics in the studied people. When the existence of a cause-effect relationship in any outcome is agreed upon by everyone, the error caused by correlation may be due to the lack of a proper definition of the variables under study. Familiarity with the types of variables and their significance in a study is essential. Variables can be defined and categorized based on their nature (quantitative-qualitative or continuous-discrete) and their role in research (independent-dependent-intervening and so on).

6.2 Variables and Relationship Pattern

Variables can be categorized based on the relationship pattern they have in a research model [1]. Usually, variables can be categorized into six categories:

- **Independent variable** (a variable that is manipulated by the researcher in experimental research to check its effect (or relationship) on another phenomenon).

  Example: To determine the relationship between a sedentary lifestyle and breast cancer, a sedentary lifestyle is an independent variable because it can increase the risk of breast cancer.
- **Dependent variable:** It is a variable on which the influence (or relationship) of the independent variable is examined. In other words, by manipulating the independent variable, the

H. Soori, *Errors in Medical Science Investigations*, https://doi.org/10.1007/978-981-99-8521-0_6

researcher tries to study the resulting changes in the dependent variable.

Example: In the example of determining the association between a sedentary lifestyle and breast cancer, breast cancer is the dependent variable because the effect or response is the independent variable.

- **Moderator variable:** This variable is the link between the independent and the dependent variables. It indirectly affects the direction or intensity of the independent and dependent variable relationship. In a statistical analysis, the effects of the mediating variable are analyzed as a direct effect. The moderator variable is sometimes called the second independent variable. It is a quantitative or qualitative variable that affects the direction and strength of the relationship between the independent and dependent variables. The third effect variable represents the observed relationship between an exposure and an outcome. Depending on whether there is a causal relationship, typically, a third variable takes the format of a mediator or a confounder. The moderating effect is a form of third variable in which the moderator and other variables have a mutual effect on the outcome.

  Example: In the relationship between a sedentary lifestyle and breast cancer, racial differences in the recurrence of breast cancer among affected patients can be a moderator variable.
- **Mediator variable:** It is a variable that can directly affect the direction of the relationship or the degree of relationship between independent and dependent variables. The effects of this variable can be seen and measured. The effect of the mediating variable is the product of the path coefficient of "*independent-mediating*" in "*mediating-dependent*," which is referred to as the indirect effect. For the calculation of hierarchical or ordinal regression, it is possible to determine the effect of several independent variables on a dependent variable in several steps.

  Example: Nutritional status and BMI have significant mediating effects of a sedentary lifestyle on breast cancer risk. Here, nutrition and inappropriate body mass index are defined as mediating variables.
- **Control variable:** If the mediating variable can be measured and the researcher wants to control its effects and remove it from the model, it is called a control variable. Because the effects of all variables cannot be investigated in one study, the researcher neutralizes the effects of some variables through statistical control or research controls. Such variables whose effects can be removed by the researcher are called control variables.
- **Intervening/confounding variable:** If the mediating variable cannot be measured and eliminated, it becomes an intervening variable. From a theoretical point of view, the intervening variable has an effect on the dependent variable, but it cannot be observed and measured to be considered as a moderating variable, nor can its effects be neutralized to be considered as a control variable [1].

6.3 Simpson's Paradox

In determining the causal relationships, not paying attention to some of the hypotheses may give us two completely contradictory answers to solve a problem. Sometimes, instead of the word contradiction, the term paradox is also used in such cases. Therefore, the meaning of contradiction is "Simpson' paradox."

Simpson's paradox (also known as the Yule–Simpson effect) refers to an association or effect found within multiple subgroups but which is reversed when data from these groups are aggregated. It could happen in observational study designs including cross-sectional, cohort, and case-control approaches [2, 3]. It is important because it reminds us that data is not what it seems. Therefore, it is not possible to reach a real inference or analysis easily by looking at a graph or table, but the process of information production and the factors affecting the results should be investigated and analyzed. In this way, the evidence may well indicate something that leads to confusion because not all information is available to us at that moment. Instead of relying on current information, it is better to research the subject and collect new data and information to reach more logical and effective results with the help of deep and scientific thinking. Data and information are powerful tools and weapons, and they can both help us and lead us astray.

Once we know about the quality and quantity of data production and how to collect them, we look for effective factors to discover cause-and-effect relationships. This work is not only considered a scientific research procedure, but it also warns us against obtaining deviant results from data and information. For this purpose, it is better to get help from the experiences of people who have expertise in the field and can better recognize cause-and-effect relationships.

Imagine that you and your wife are looking for a good restaurant for dinner. So, each of you searches for the most suitable restaurant for dinner tonight using virtual social network polls. Let's say you find the restaurant "A" that has a higher percentage of satisfaction among men and women than the restaurant your spouse found. Suppose that the name of the restaurant chosen by your wife is restaurant "B." Although restaurant A has a higher percentage of satisfaction among women and men than restaurant B, your wife claims that the restaurant she is looking for has more overall satisfaction (regardless of gender) than the restaurant you chose. Both of you have reached completely different conclusions based on the same source of information, and it seems that both of you are right, and each of you has a valid reason for your claim. What is the problem? What does this contradiction indicate? Who has reached the correct conclusion? Are the survey results wrong or is there a problem with the calculations? Logically, you have both reached the correct conclusion and unknowingly entered the world of the Simpson's paradox. Issues such as choosing the best or worst restaurant and choosing the right diet to lose weight or increase the risk of a particular disease are among the cases in which, based on the same data, people's conclusions may be completely contradictory.

Simpson's paradox occurs when a data set is divided into groups whose results are in the opposite direction to the way the data were grouped. In the example related to the restaurant that we mentioned above, it seems that the restaurant with a higher percentage of satisfaction among women and men should also have a higher overall satisfaction rate than the B restaurant. Using the following example, we show that this may not always be true. Table 6.1 shows the level of satisfaction for both restaurants by men and women. By combining the level of satisfaction of women and men in the last line, it is clear that the B restaurant has more satisfaction than the A restaurant.

Table 6.1 Level of satisfaction for both restaurants by men and women ($n = 1600$)

	Resturant A	Resturant B
Men	360/720 = 50%	100/300 = 3.33%
Women	72/80 = 90%	400/500 = 80%
Total	512/800 = 64%	500/800 = 62.5%

Although restaurant A has a higher percentage of satisfaction among women and men if we consider all people, regardless of their gender, the satisfaction level of restaurant B will be lower. How is such a thing possible? Where does this contradiction come from?

Because a different sample size of respondents was used to calculate percentages, Simpson's paradox appears. Each fraction has calculated the ratio of the number of satisfied users to the total number of users. In restaurant A, the men whose opinions were surveyed are much more than the women, and in restaurant B, this happened the other way around. Since there are fewer women than men who were asked in the Restaurant A survey, their satisfaction contributes less than men to the total percentage calculation. As a result, the total average has slightly increased compared to the average satisfaction percentage of men. On the other hand, the number of women who participated in the survey of restaurant B is more than the number of men. As a result, their share in calculating the total percentage is more than men. This is where Simpson's paradox occurred.

In such cases, it is better to decide according to which population or sample we want to calculate the percentages, by gender or by the total number of people. In any case, it may be necessary to combine the data in some way, but we must also pay attention to the method of collecting them (which is called the causal model). With this, we will no longer suffer from Simpson's paradox. Here, the question arises, what is the right approach to choosing a restaurant?

6.3.1 How Is Simpson's Paradox Controlled: Role of Confounding Factors

When there is a negative correlation (e.g., when an independent variable increases, the response variable decreases or vice versa), Simpson's paradox can also cause erroneous conclusions. Suppose that the hours of exercise per week and the probability of developing a disease are measured for two groups of patients. The first group is under 50 years old, and the second group is over 50 years old. The results show that, in both groups, the amount of sports activity has the opposite effect on the probability of disease progression. That is, with an increase in the number of hours of exercise, the probability of disease progression decreases. Now we combine these data and based on the integrated information in both groups, we measure the correlation coefficient between the number of hours of exercise and the probability of disease progression. In this case, we can see that the correlation coefficient of the two variables becomes positive. (As the number of hours of exercise increases, the probability of disease progression increases. So it is better not to exercise!) To avoid Simpson's paradox, which leads to conflicting results, we need to decide whether we need inferences and conclusions based on disaggregated data or whether we need to make the appropriate decision based on aggregated data. This explanation may be clear, but it does not specify when we need separation or aggregation. The answer to this question lies in the concept (of thinking causally). It means to know the origin and basis of the product information and understand what factor or factors have influenced the data that may be hidden from our view. In the above example, it is intuitively clear that the hours of sports training are not the only effective factor in improving or progressing the disease. Other factors such as diet, living environment, and heredity are also effective in the occurrence and progression of the disease. While in the diagram, only the probability of contracting the disease along with the hours of sports training is displayed. In this example, suppose that the probability of getting a disease is related to the two variables of exercise time and age. Meanwhile, the collected data indicate two types of factors for disease progression. Considering the relationship between the probability of disease and exercise hours the age factor has been neglected [2].

In this case, if we calculate the correlation coefficient between the probability of contracting the disease and age for both groups above 50 and below 50 years and draw a dot chart between these values, we will find that there is a difference between age and the probability of contracting the disease There is a strong correlation. This means that with increasing age, the probability of contracting the disease will also increase. In this way, it is clear that the probability of getting sick is higher for older people than for young people who do the same amount of exercise. To measure the effect of only exercise on the disease, we must consider the age constant and include the hours of exercise as a variable in the calculations.

Therefore, if we calculate the correlation coefficient between the probability of contracting the disease and age for both groups above 50 and below 50 years and draw a dot chart between these values, we will find that there is a difference between age and the probability of contracting the disease. There is a strong correlation. This means that, with increasing age, the probability of contracting the disease will also increase. In this way, it is clear that the probability of getting sick is higher for older people than for young people who do the same amount of exercise. To measure the effect of only exercise on the disease, we must consider the age constant and include the hours of exercise as a variable in the calculations. Separation of data into separate groups in such a case can be a method to fix one variable against the variability of another variable. By doing this, in our example, it is clear that for each age group (above or below 50 years), the hours of exercise training reduce the probability of getting the disease. This is what was seen in the initial charts. There, by dividing the data into two groups, the age factor of the control patients and the correlation between the number of exercise hours and the probability of contracting the disease were calculated. Simpson's paradox can be solved by recognizing the way of data collection and applying the causal model. In this way, data classification based on the factors that must be controlled will be the solution. The way we deal with questions and issues can be the solution to them. In the restaurant example, we want to identify which restaurant is preferred by both men and women. Since we do not have access to other factors that are involved in measuring the satisfaction of restaurant customers, we are forced to ignore them when we need more data to avoid Simpson's paradox.

In another example, suppose treatment methods A and B are two methods for treating kidney stones. The preliminary results show that method A seems to be better than method B in the treatment of small and large stones. But by inference based on aggregated data (regardless of stone size), treatment method B was better than A. Considering the stone size, treatment method A is more successful than method B in treating small stones, while the percentage of success of treatment method B is generally higher than method A. How is such a thing possible? Although treatment method A seems better than method B in the treatment of small stones, the presence of small stones in the kidney is not considered a serious problem. For this reason, doctors prefer to use treatment method B, which is less invasive (even with a lower success rate) because the patient's problem is not too serious. But the same doctors use treatment method A, which is more aggressive and of course more effective, to treat large kidney stones that cause serious problems for the patient. Therefore, if it seems that treatment method A has a lower success rate than method B, the reason is the serious condition of the patients who have been treated with method A. As a result, only the treatment method is not effective in the success of the treatment method, but also the worsening condition of the disease. It affects success. From the medical point of view, method A should be a better and more effective method than method B, but considering the number of treatments performed by method B, especially on patients with small kidney stones, it seems that method B has a higher percentage of more success. The effect or effect of this question is the treatment of the disease, which depends on the two factors of the treatment method and the size of the stone (severity of the disease). On the other hand, the choice of treatment depends on the stone size, which makes the stone size variable play a role as a confounding variable. To determine which treatment method is appropriate, we must control for the intervening variable using segregation rather than aggregation. In this way, based on the separation of the data, we find that treatment method A is more effective on the patient than treatment method B. Because it has a higher percentage of success in both groups of patients (small and large stones). So if the patient has a kidney stone, whether you have a large stone or a small one, you will choose treatment method A, because it has a higher success rate and thus the paradox is solved.

6.4 Confounding Variables

When we deal with the relationship between a risk factor and the disease, usually a third factor can be found that has an importance on the relationship between the risk factor and the disease. If this factor (at least relatively) can justify the observed relationship, a confounding phenomenon occurs.

For example, the relationship between the number of children and the prevalence of breast cancer may be observed in a sample of mothers that can be explained by the age of the mothers. Older mothers have more children, and increasing age also increases the risk of breast cancer. In this case, age is a third factor that explains the relationship between the number of children and the prevalence of breast cancer. Table 6.2 shows the hypothetical data of a risk factor and its outcome (patient/healthy).

As can be seen, the relative risk (presence of the risk factor versus its absence) is equal to 5.52, and this relationship is statistically significant ($P < 0.001$). In this case, it may be concluded that the risk factor is effective on the condition of the

Table 6.2 Status of the risk factor and the presence or absence of the disease in a hypothetical example

	Disease status		
Risk factor	Disease	Healthy	Risk
Exposed	81	29	0.7364
Not exposed	28	182	0.1333
Relative risk	5.52		

disease. Now suppose that the information related to the third variable, which is potentially confusing, is also collected. We denote this factor by C. Suppose the presence or absence of measurement feature C, and this information is given in Table 6.3.

A deeper look at the table makes it possible to justify this phenomenon. The confounding variable and the risk factor are interdependent, and the confounding factor alone is considered a risk factor for the disease because its relative risk is equal to it. In this case, when it was thought that the risk factor affected the disease, the distorting effect on the patient was observed. Table 6.4 shows the results of another hypothetical study. In this case, before considering the confounding effect, the potential risk factor is ineffective.

In Table 6.5, the risk and relative risk of contracting the disease for the same information, according to a hypothetical confounder, are shown.

As can be seen, at different levels of the confounding variable, the observed relative risks are greater than 1. The relative risk in both categories of confounding variable (presence or absence of confounder) is equal to 2.45 with a significant level of and. In this example, the existence of a confounding factor and lack of contact with the risk factor has a positive relationship. As in the previous example, in this data, the confounding factor is separately considered a risk factor. The relative risk of exposure to the confounder compared to no exposure is equal to

$$\frac{(105+195)/(105+195+5+305)}{(135+5)/(135+415+45+5)}=2.11$$

When there is complete confounding, the relative risks (or any estimate of the odds ratio for developing a disease) for different levels (not necessarily two levels) of the confounding variable are the same. This common value is different when the confounding variable is considered in the analysis of the results. The previous examples both show complete distortion. Complete confounding is rarely seen in the data. What is observed in reality is a degree of distortion that causes an overestimation or underestimation of the actual risk. However, if the risk estimate at different levels of the confounding variable is similar, or if the estimates in each category are almost the same as the total risk estimate, it can be argued that the confounding factor does not have much effect. The following table is obtained from real data related to 6 years of follow-up in the study of health and coronary heart disease (CHD) [4] (Table 6.6).

This information is related to the presence of CHD symptoms and housing conditions. As can be seen, the chance of CHD occurrence is higher in people who have rented housing. The question that comes to mind after observing this relationship is whether the inappropriate lifestyle of men who own a rented house can justify this relationship or not. Specifically, 57% of men who have rented houses and 37% of men who have owned houses smoke. We know that smoking is one of the risk factors for the occurrence of CHD. In Table 6.7, a three-way consensus table is shown for the simultaneous display of housing status, the occurrence of CHD, and smoking.

As can be seen from the table above, living in a rented house is still considered a risk factor even after adjusting for the confounding effect of smoking, although the relative risk has decreased slightly after adjustment. But due to

Table 6.4 Status of risk factor and disease in hypothetical data

	Disease status		
Risk factor	Disease	Healthy	Risk
Exposed	240	420	0.3636
Not exposed	200	350	0.3636
Relative risk	1.00		

Table 6.3 Status of the risk factor and disease to separate the hypothetical confounders in the data related to Table 6.2

	Existence of confounder			Absence of confounder		
Risk factor	Disease	Healthy	Risk	Disease	Healthy	Risk
Exposed	1	9	100%	80	20	0.800
Not exposed	20	180	100%	8	2	0.800
Relative risk	1			1		

Table 6.5 Three-way consensus table related to risk factor, disease status and exposure to a hypothetical confounder

	Existence of confounder			Absence of confounder		
Risk factor	Disease	Healthy	Risk	Disease	Healthy	Risk
Exposed	135	415	0.2455	105	5	0.9545
Not exposed	5	45	0.1000	195	305	0.3900
Relative risk	2.45			2.45		

Table 6.6 Housing status and occurrence of CHD in men

	CHD occurrence		
Housing status	Yes	No	Risk
Rental	85	1821	0/0446
Ownership	77	2400	0/0311
Relative risk	1.43		

Table 6.7 The data is given to separate the use and non-use of cigarettes

	Smokers			Non-smokers		
Housing status	CHD			CHD		
	Yes	No	Risk	Yes	No	Risk
Rental	33	923	0/0345	92	898	0.0547
Ownership	48	1722	0/0271	29	678	0.410
Relative risk	1.27			1.33		

the smallness of this reduction, it can be concluded that the confounding effect of smoking is small. Distortion in real data appears due to the existence of a relationship between variables or the way data is collected. For example, if the consumption of drugs and the use of alcoholic beverages are related to each other, then the effect of the disease related to the consumption of alcoholic beverages will be confused with the effect of drug consumption. Consider another example where an experimental study is designed to investigate the effectiveness of a preventive medicine against a disease, and the subjects are randomly given an effective medicine or a placebo. Let's suppose that in the group receiving medicine, the ratio of men is more than women, and in the group receiving placebo, the ratio of women is more than men. In this case, if the prevalence of the disease in question is higher in men than in women, there is a very high possibility that the preventive effect of the drug is estimated to be less than the actual value. This happens because the results are distorted by the gender effect. This type of confounding occurs due to the type of study design. In the worst case, all the people in the placebo group are women, and the people in the effective drug are men. In this case, the effect of the effective drug and the effect of gender is undetectable. Figures 6.1, 6.2, 6.3 and 6.4 show different situations where factor C can be a confounder or only a consequence. In these diagrams, the arrows indicate the relationship between the two factors under investigation regardless of other relationships between the discussed factors. Two-way arrows indicate a noncausal relationship, and one-way arrows indicate the direction of a causal relationship [5–7].

In general, drawing these diagrams is very useful for deciding whether a factor can be considered a potential confounder or not. The necessary conditions for being confounding are shown in Fig. 6.5.

Any variable that has the conditions in this chart should probably be considered a confounder. When we are not sure about the existence of one of the relationships, the best possible method is to assume the existence of a relationship during the design and data collection and to evaluate these assumptions after the data collection. For this reason, all known risk factors for a disease should usually be considered potential confounders. After completing the implementation stages of the study, there are various statistical methods to evaluate the effect of potential confounding variables. This issue will be fully investigated in the next chapter.

6.4.1 Features of the Confounding Factor

In general, the confounding factor must be related to both the exposure factor and the disease under study. However, this feature does not fully specify the confounding factor. There are cases where

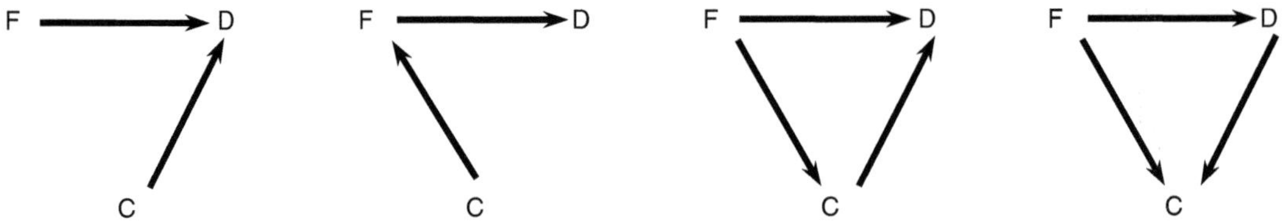

Fig. 6.1 Some situations where C is confusing for the F-D relationship

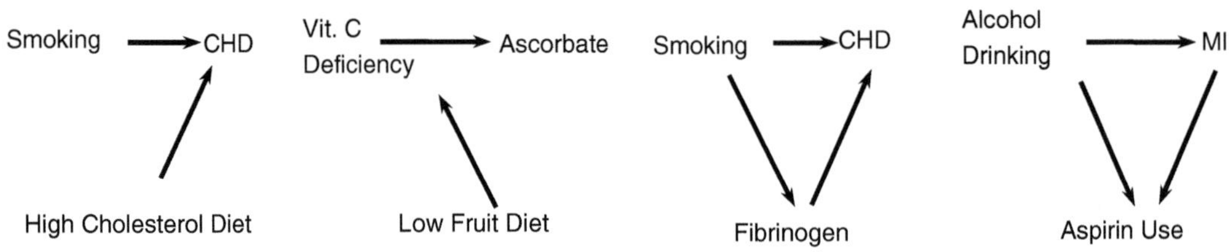

Fig. 6.2 Examples for Fig. 6.1

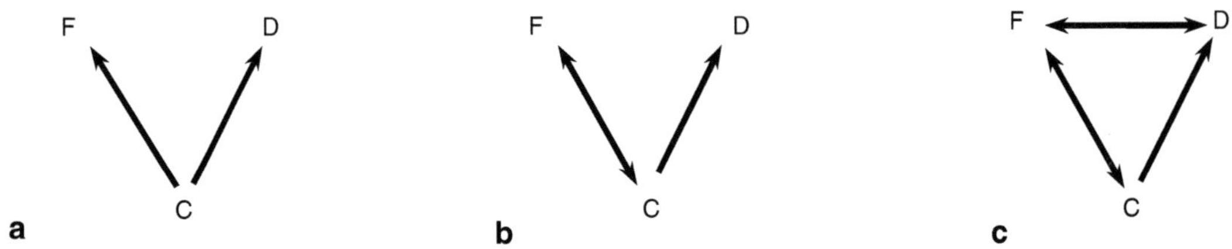

Fig. 6.3 Some situations where C is not confounding for the F-D relationship

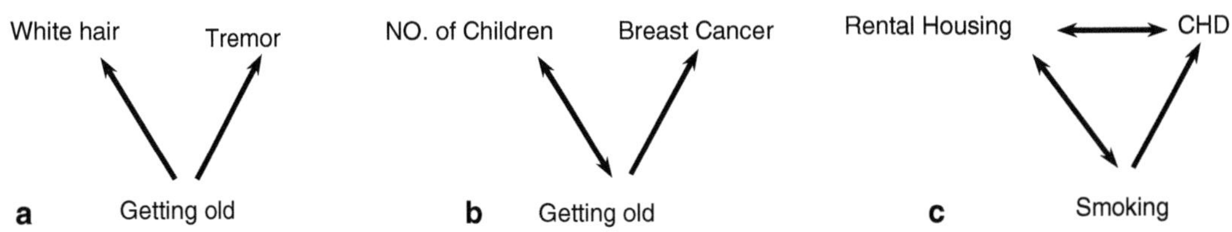

Fig. 6.4 Examples for Fig. 6.3

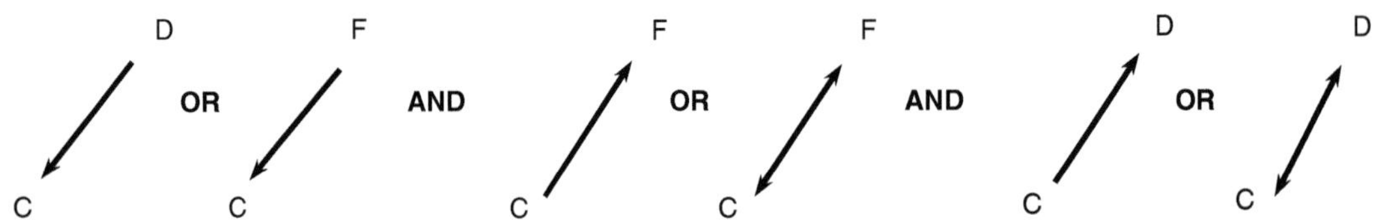

Fig. 6.5 Necessary conditions for C to be confusing in the F-D relationship

a variable has these correlations but is not considered confounding. This phenomenon can happen in different ways. The most common way of occurrence of this phenomenon is when the studied exposure has side effects. In this case, complications are also correlated with the disease due to the dependence on the exposure and the disease. For example, suppose that the frequency of soft drink consumption is related to the amount of pizza consumed and that soft drink consumption is one of the risk factors for bladder cancer. In this case, is the consumption of pizza considered a distraction? At first, the answer may seem positive because pizza consumption is related to both soda consumption and bladder cancer. But if pizza consumption is only one-sidedly related to bladder cancer due to dependence on soft drinks, it is not considered a confounding factor. The confounder must be an effective factor in the occurrence of the disease. That is, if pizza consumption is one of the factors affecting bladder cancer among people who do not drink soft drinks, then this factor can be considered a confounding factor.

6.4.2 Criteria Necessary for a Variable to Be Confounding

The following three criteria must be true for each variable to consider it a confounder:

1. Every confounding factor must be a risk factor for the disease. Any potential confounding factor must be one of the main causes of the disease or a prognosis related to one of the main causes of the disease. The relationship between the potential confounder and the disease must be direct. Indirect dependencies that originate from a relationship with one of the disease-causing exposures do not confuse. Using data to observe the relationship between potential confounders and disease can be a good guide. The relationship observed from the data structure does not determine the nature of the variables in terms of confounding, but the existence of a definite and theoretically proven relationship determines the nature of confounding. In studies with large sample sizes, where we face smaller sampling errors, we expect the relationship obtained from the data to be closer to reality. In the case of limited studies, the data may not be reliable enough.
2. The confounding factor must also be related to the exposure factor in the base population (population at risk which includes patients). The relationship between the potential confounder and the exposure factor should not be established secondary to the relationship between the exposure and the disease. For example, in cohort studies, the relationship between the potential confounding factors and exposure should exist at the beginning of the study and when the disease has not yet occurred. For this reason, in a cohort study, the relationship between exposure and confounders should be investigated by existing information and not by previous theoretical information. When experimental studies are designed, sometimes the effects of confounding factors in the study are ignored due to the random assignment of treatments to individuals. But randomization is a probabilistic process that may not completely neutralize the relationships between exposure and extraneous risk factors, especially if the total number of subjects under study is small. In general, it can be said that confounders may also exist in randomized studies, although their effects are smaller compared to nonrandomized studies. The confounding effect can be ignored in randomized studies with large sample sizes and proper design. In case-control studies, the aforementioned dependence must exist in the base population, which includes the cases. If the number of control group members is large enough and there is no selection error, a reasonable estimate of the relationship between the potential confounding factor and the exposure in the base population can be calculated. Otherwise, all efforts should be made to find out the degree of dependence between the potential confounder and the exposure in the population based on which the witnesses selected in the study are only representative of this population. Unfortunately, additional reliable information about possible relationships between risk factors in the population is rarely available. For this reason, in case-control studies, we usually have to provide an estimate of the relationship between exposure and confounders using the available data.
3. The confounding factor should not be affected by the relationship of exposure to the disease. In particular, the confounding factor cannot be an intermediate link in the causal path between exposure and disease. For example, consider the following pattern.

Cardiovascular disease → high blood pressure → smoking

Can high blood pressure be considered as a confounding factor? Certainly, high blood pressure is a risk factor for cardiovascular disease, and we know that it is related to the desired exposure (smoking), because the disease is caused by smoking. But high blood pressure in people who are not exposed (smoking) is also considered a risk factor because this complication is caused by reasons other than smoking. However, this factor cannot be considered an absolute confounder, because high blood pressure is a complication that is intermediate between smoking and cardiovascular disease.

Risk factors that occur as intermediate complications in the cause-and-effect loop are not considered confounders and should not be considered external risk factors. This point shows the precedence of the confounding factor of overexposure and disease. The researcher should investigate whether there is a causal mechanism and whether is it possible to reach the confounding factor through exposure or disease. Or that the factor that is called a distorter is only an intermediate link. If the factor in question is only an intermediate link, separate analysis methods are necessary to determine the nature of this action. Despite the above three conditions, most of the time we can define and diagnose the distortion. However, due to content and technical reasons, being limited to these three features in the diagnosis of the distorting factor may lead to a mistake.

In terms of content, the basis of confounding is based on the mixing or distortion of external effects with the effect of the factor investigated in the study. The first two characteristics are the logical result of this definition. It means the necessary conditions for a factor to be confounding. The third feature excludes situations where the potential confounding effect cannot be applied directly. From a technical point of view, it is possible that an agent has all three mentioned characteristics, but does not mix with the effect of the exposure agent. This happens when the potential confounder has no additional effect or complication on the disease among the exposure group, and there is only one relationship between this factor, the exposure, and its effect on the disease. For example, such a situation can happen when there are several potential confounders, each of which alone affects the incidence rate of the disease. But one of these factors is completely ineffective in the presence of other confounders, and the additional incidence rate in the exposure group is related to these other confounders.

6.4.3 Confounding Due to the Combination of Exposures

In the simplest case, distortion can be shown as a combination of the effects of different levels of exposure. In particular, the effect that is observed as an exposure effect can be the effect of an external factor combined with the desired exposure effect. The distortion of the inferences caused by the confounding factor can be very large and may lead to an overestimation or underestimation of the effect size of the original exposure. This issue depends on the relationship between the confounding factor with the exposure and the disease.

6.4.4 Substitute Confounder

Any external factor that causes a difference in the frequency of disease between exposed and nonexposed groups is called a confounder. Sometimes it is not possible to observe these factors alone, and only some surrogate variables can be observed and measured. For example, one of these surrogate factors is a calendar age. Increasing age has a strong relationship with the phenomenon of aging (accumulation of mutated and damaged cells that leads to disease). But increasing age in itself is not the pathological cause of these changes. The calendar age only shows the amount of life passed since birth. When a confounding factor is misclassified, it is very difficult and complicated to control it in the analysis of the results. Misclassification, when independent of exposure or disease classification, usually biases the results in favor of the null hypothesis. Incorrect classification can cause serious problems in the study. If the effect of the confounding factor is very strong and the relationship between exposure and disease is weak or zero, the incorrect classification of the confounding factor can cause extremely misleading results. For example, the existence of a strong causal relationship between smoking and bladder cancer, along with a strong relationship between smoking and drinking coffee, makes smoking a strong confounder in evaluating the relationship between coffee drinking and bladder cancer. But since the control of cigarette confounding depends on the correct information about the smoking pattern of the people under study, this information cannot be free of misclassification errors. Regardless of how the smoking pattern is measured, it can be concluded that in evaluating the relationship between coffee drinking and bladder cancer, the confounding effects cannot be completely controlled in the analysis of the results [6, 7].

6.4.5 Interaction

Interaction is an action that occurs between two or more entities, phenomena, or processes that interact. When the effect of a disease-related risk factor is different at different levels of a second risk factor, there is a mutual effect between the two risk factors under study.

When the incidence rate of the disease in the presence of two or more risk factors is different from the expected incidence rate of the effect of each risk factor alone, the interaction effect has occurred. This effect may be more than we expect, in which case the interaction positive honors is called (synergism-positive interaction), or if it is less than our expectation, it is called antagonism-negative interaction. Steps to discover an interaction [8–10].

To discover a one-to-one interaction, we must answer the following questions:

(a) Is there a correlation between exposure and disease (or other conditions)? If the answer is yes.
(b) Is this correlation the result of a confounding factor? After layering.
(c) Is the strength of correlation the same in all two layers that we have formed based on the third variable?

Yes → there is no interaction.

No, there is an interaction.

To better understand the interaction, you should know that the effect of simultaneous exposure to two factors either follows the cumulative model or the multiplicative model.

What is the cumulative model? For example, if 12 cases of the disease occur as a result of exposure to factor x, 18 cases of the disease occur as a result of exposure to factor y, and the disease occurs in 6 people without exposure to x or y, if the exposure model is cumulative We expect that there will be 24 people who are exposed to both x and b. In this way, the 3 people who got sick without any exposure represent the background risk that exists in any case, with this account, probably out of the 12 people who got sick. Six people who have become ill from x include the same background risk, and the remaining six people represent the risk attributed to x. Regarding factor y, it can be concluded that out of 18 people who are sick, 6 people are due to background risk, and the other 12 people are due to exposure. In relation to factor y, the analysis reveals that out of 18 individuals who are ill, 6 cases can be attributed to background risk, while the remaining 12 cases are attributable to exposure. Consequently, individuals who have been exposed to both factors y and x must contend with the risk associated with exposure to x, the risk associated with exposure to y, as well as the underlying background risk. Hence, the imputed risk for exposure to both x and y is calculated as the sum of the imputed risk for y, the imputed risk for x, and the background risk.

$$6+12+6=24$$

When these risks are added together, the exposure model follows the cumulative model. What is the multiplicative model? Now imagine that exposure to factor x triples the underlying risk of 6 for disease and exposure to factor y increases the underlying risk of 6 by 10 times. In this model, we expect the relative risk for simultaneous exposure to x and y to be equal to 360:

$$6\times10\times6=360$$

To determine the type of interaction, it is necessary to know the biology of the disease and how the pathogen works at the cellular and molecular levels.

Likewise, when there is no mutual effect between two risk factors at different levels of the other risk factor, the effect of each risk factor becomes the same (homogeneous). One of the famous examples in this field is the effect of smoking on the chance of heart attack and the death rate in the first 6 months after the first heart attack. Since smoking is one of the known factors in the occurrence of the first heart attack, this issue causes that there is a mutual effect between smoking and the history of heart attack (having/not having) [11].

6.4.6 Interaction Effect

Mutual effects is a situation where the effect of one variable on another variable depends on the size and value of the third variable. The main effect is the effect that an independent variable has on the dependent variable, regardless of the effect of other independent variables. That is, any change in the main variable will cause a change in the test response. An interaction effect occurs when the effect of an independent variable on the dependent variable changes depending on the level of another independent variable. This term is mostly used for experimental design methods. According to the number of main variables, interactions are classified as two-level interactions, three-level interactions, etc. When the interaction effects are too large, the main effects have little practical meaning.

To find interaction in a causal relationship, one must have a factorial design, in which two (or more) independent variables are "crossed" with each other so that there are observations at any combination of levels of the two independent variables.

Statistical tests for interaction are dependent on the *measurement scale*—additive or multiplicative. In statistics, interaction is a deviation from conditional independence, where ratio measurements such as relative risks or odds ratios evaluate the effects of risk factors on a multiplicative scale, as they represent the degree to which the risk of disease (for relative risk) or odds (for odds ratio) multifolds in affected individuals. The interaction varies depending on which of these measurement scales is used. For example, when considering factors A and B, interaction on a multiplicative scale is defined as a different RR for factor A across classes defined by factor B, whereas on an additive scale, the interaction is defined as a different RD for factor A is defined in width strata defined by factor B. Using these two different measurement scales can lead to fundamental conclusions in interaction studies [12].

The statistical tests for interaction are often referred to as subgroup analyses, implying any comparison of effect between treatment groups across subsets of patients with specific characteristics that could be potentially relevant effect modifiers. There are different methods to control effect modifiers and interaction such as *exploratory analyses* for differential responses from early clinical trial data or from clinical trials that failed to establish treatment efficacy in its intended population, *inferential analyses and supportive analyses* aim at investigating the consistency of treatment effect across subgroups for a clinical trial that has established treatment efficacy in its intended overall population (see [13] for more information) [13].

To simplify the present issue, we assume that the studied risk factors have only two levels. We define these two levels with the names of endangered and those that are not endangered. Figure 6.6 shows the different modes of interaction and the mode where there is no interaction. It is possible to have three different types of interaction: opposite direction, same direction, and one-way. As can be seen, the lack of interaction creates parallel lines in the figure of interactions. But in the practice of observing such lines, it rarely happens and typical changes in the calculated chances cause minor changes or even fundamental changes. In this case, these changes cause the lines of the graph to cross, while there is no mutual effect. For this reason, it seems very logical to test the data to detect the existence of interaction.

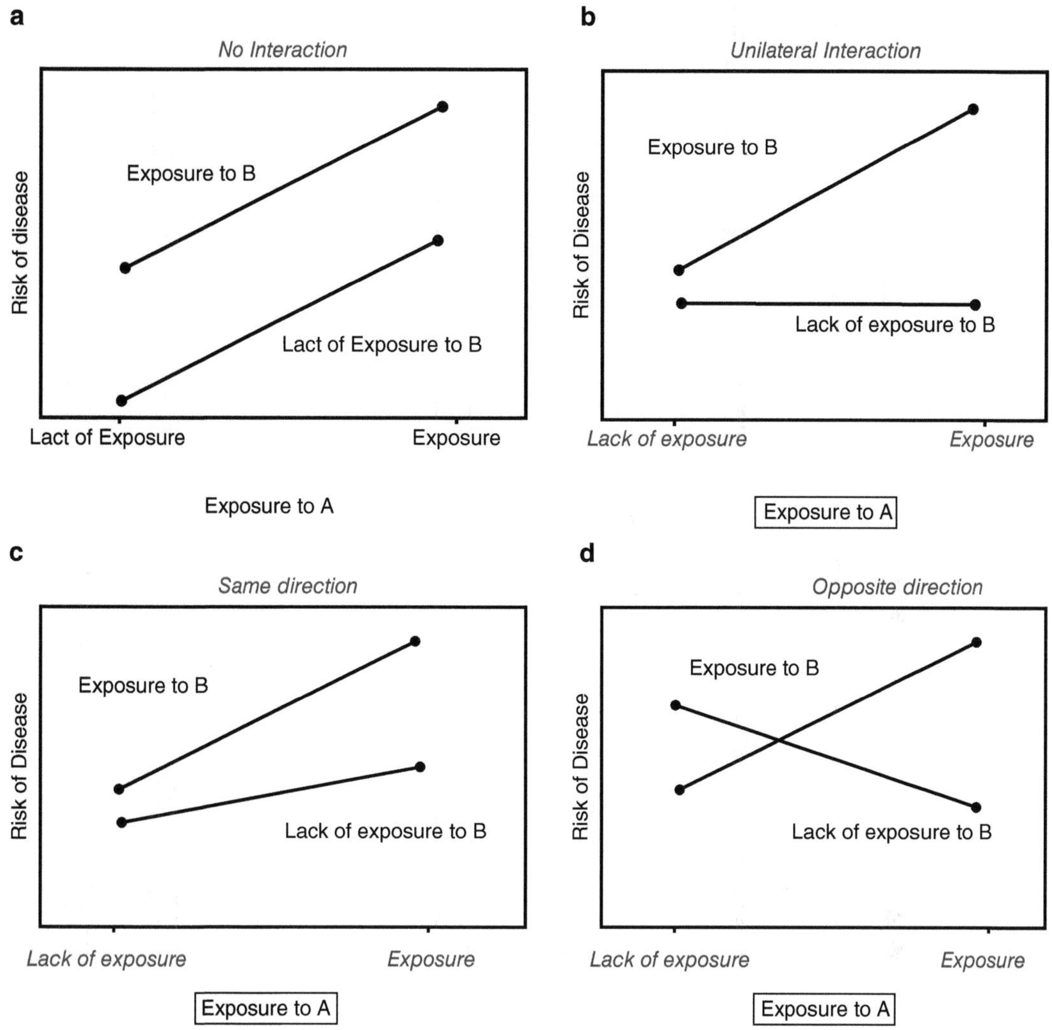

Fig. 6.6 Different modes of interaction between risk factors A and B

References

1. Elwood M. 'Confounding', critical appraisal of epidemiological studies and clinical trials. 4th ed. Oxford: Oxford Academic; 2017. https://doi.org/10.1093/med/9780199682898.003.0007. Online ed. Accessed 3 Mar 2023.
2. Marang-van de Mheen PJ, Shojania KG. Simpson's paradox: how performance measurement can fail even with perfect risk adjustment. BMJ Qual Saf. 2014;23:701–5. https://doi.org/10.1136/bmjqs-2013-002883.
3. Rojanaworarit C. Misleading epidemiological and statistical evidence in the presence of Simpson's paradox: an illustrative study using simulated scenarios of observational study designs. J Med Life. 2020;13(1):37–44. https://doi.org/10.25122/jml-2019-0120. PMID: 32341699; PMCID: PMC7175433.
4. Woodward M. Epidemiology: study design and data analysis. 3rd ed. Boca Raton: Chapman and Hall/CRC; 2013.
5. Malta DC, Mascarenhas MD, Porto DL, Duarte EA, Sardinha LM, Barreto SM, de Morais Neto OL. Prevalence of alcohol and drug consumption among adolescents: data analysis of the National Survey of School Health. Rev Bras Epidemiol. 2011;14(Suppl 1):136–46. https://doi.org/10.1590/s1415-790x2011000500014. PMID: 22002150.

6. Breslow N, Borgan Ø, Gail MH, Scott AI, Chatterjee N, Wild CF. Handbook of statistical methods for case-control studies. Boca Raton: CRC Press LLC; 2020.
7. Rothman K, Greenland S, Lash TL. Modern epidemiology. 3rd ed. Philadelphia: Lippincott Williams & Wilkins; 2008.
8. Nigra AD, Teodoro AJ, Gil GA. A decade of research on coffee as an anticarcinogenic beverage. Oxidative Med Cell Longev. 2021;2021:4420479. https://doi.org/10.1155/2021/4420479. PMID: 34567408; PMCID: PMC8460369.
9. Szklo M, Nieto FJ. Epidemiology: beyond the basics. Burlington: Jones & Bartlett Learning; 2014.
10. Simundić AM. Bias in research. Biochem Med. 2013;23(1):12–5. https://doi.org/10.11613/BM.2013.003. PMID: 23457761; PMCID: PMC3900086.
11. Schwartz S. Modern epidemiologic approaches to interaction: applications to the study of genetic interactions. In: Institute of Medicine (US) Committee on Assessing Interactions Among Social, Behavioral, and Genetic Factors in Health, Hernandez LM, Blazer DG, editors. Genes, behavior, and the social environment: moving beyond the nature/nurture debate. Washington, DC: National Academies Press (US); 2006. https://www.ncbi.nlm.nih.gov/books/NBK19918/. Accessed 22 Apr 2023.
12. Institute of Medicine (US) Committee on Assessing Interactions Among Social, Behavioral, and Genetic Factors in Health, Hernandez LM, Blazer DG, editors. Genes, behavior, and the social environment: moving beyond the nature/nurture debate. Washington, DC: National Academies Press (US); 2006. Chapter 8, Study design and analysis for assessment of interactions. https://www.ncbi.nlm.nih.gov/books/NBK19921/. Accessed 22 Apr 2023.
13. Christensen R, Bours MJL, Nielsen SM. Effect modifiers and statistical tests for interaction in randomized trials. J Clin Epidemiol. 2021;134:174–7. https://doi.org/10.1016/j.jclinepi.2021.03.009. PMID: 34016442.

Methods of Controlling Confounding in Medical Sciences Studies

7

Francis Bacon believed that empirical observation and experimentation were essential to scientific research. He emphasized the importance of controlling variables in experiments to ensure that the results were accurate and reliable. While he did not specifically discuss confounding variables in medical sciences studies, his views on the importance of rigorous methods in experimentation and observation can be applied to the control of confounding variables in medical research. Bacon's emphasis on careful observation and experimentation can be seen as a precursor to modern methods of controlling confounding variables in medical sciences studies.

—Francis Bacon (1561–1626)

7.1 Introduction

In biomedical studies, there are different strategies including randomization, restriction, matching, stratification, multivariable regression analysis, and propensity score analysis to control the confounding effect that can be used alone or together. In general, the confounding control methods are divided into two categories: control methods during design and control methods during data analysis. Randomization and limitation are methods of control or elimination of confounding during study design. Matching is a method that is used both within the consider plan stage and in the analysis phase. Stratification, multivariate analysis, and propensity score analysis are confounding control methods when analyzing data.

7.2 Methods of Controlling Confounding When Designing the Study

To control confounding when designing a study, three methods, randomization, restriction, and matching can be used. Randomization is used only in intervention studies, but restriction and matching can be used in the design of all analytical studies.

7.2.1 Randomization

Randomization is the foremost advocated strategy to adjust confounding. It could be a crucial viewpoint of biomedical research to guarantee the validity and reliability of study results. It

H. Soori, *Errors in Medical Science Investigations*, https://doi.org/10.1007/978-981-99-8521-0_7

involves the random assignment of participants to different treatment groups or interventions, which helps to control for potential confounding variables and minimize bias. The unique power of randomization is due to the almost equal distribution of risk factors and different exposures in the groups under investigation. Randomization, if the study volume is large enough, ensures the same distribution of data of all commonly known confounding variables and even unknown risk factors in the comparison groups. In smaller samples or even in large samples where chance causes the unbalanced distribution of risk factors in groups, it is possible to control these factors by using appropriate adjustment methods in the data analysis stage.

7.2.2 Restriction

The restriction is a method of controlling confounding variables in biomedical research. It involves limiting the study population to a specific group or set of criteria. It can also be used to exclude individuals with certain medical conditions or risk factors that may confound the study results.

Restriction may limit the generalizability of the study results. The restriction is one of several methods that can be used to control confounding variables in biomedical research, and it should be used in conjunction with other methods to ensure the validity and reliability of study results.

As mentioned before, if the potential confounding factor is the same in the comparison groups, the effect of confounding becomes neutral. Accordingly, one of the methods to control the confounding is to limit the criteria for the inclusion of people in the study, so that the studied people fall into only one or more specific categories of the potential confounding factor. For example, if race and gender are two potential confounding factors, one of the ways to control these factors is to limit the study to non-white men or white women.

7.2.3 Matching

Matching involves selecting study members who are comparable in certain characteristics, such as age, sexual orientation, or therapeutic history, and allocating them to different treatment groups or interventions. By matching, researchers can reduce the impact of these variables on the study outcome and increase the precision of the analysis.

There are two types of matching: individual or one-to-one matching and frequency matching. Individual matching involves selecting a control participant who is similar to a case participant in specific characteristics. Frequency matching involves selecting a control group with the same distribution of certain characteristics as the case group. Matching can be done using various statistical techniques, such as stratification and pairing.

In case-control studies, matching is said to be the same selection of cases and controls in terms of some confounding variables. Matching and limiting are two common methods of controlling confounders that are applied in the sampling stage. In these methods, only cases and witnesses are compared with each other that are similar in terms of certain confounders. Since there is a possibility of the presence of samples of all levels of confounding variables in the study, matching is considered a generalized state of the restriction method. Matching is usually done for groups of two members (even). For example, in examining the amount of coffee consumption and the incidence of heart attack, each of the cases (patients with heart attack complications) can be matched with one or more of the witnesses in terms of the amount of cigarette consumption (for example, does not smoke, ten cigarettes per day, and more than ten cigarettes per day). In this case, coffee consumption in each of the cases is compared only with matched control(s). Another method of matching group assimilation. In this method, for each level of the confounding variable (smoking in the previous example), there are some identical cases and witnesses for comparison. In the previous example, if the ratio of cases to controls is 2 to 1 and 10 cases smoke more than 20 cigarettes per day, it is necessary to select 40 controls with the same amount of cigarette consumption per day to match the case group of 20 people. According to the method of individual and group assimilation, it is clear that group matching is easier than individual assimilation. But the similarity of people in comparison groups is more in individual assimilation. Another point is that individual matching needs special statistical methods, but the analysis of the results in the group matching method is no different from the usual methods. The number of variables used for matching should be the least necessary. The increase of matched variables makes the criteria for choosing suitable control subjects harder and the study becomes ineffective in practice. The main application of matching is in a case-control study, but it is also used in other studies.

7.2.3.1 Advantages and Disadvantages of Matching

Some advantages of matching are:

- Homogenization is an effective method in preventing confounding by background factors such as age and gender, these factors have a strong and determining effect on many diseases. Usually, matching is done for factors that do not interact with other factors and do not play a mediating role in the causal model.
- Matching is appropriate in controlling confounders whose quantity cannot be measured and controlled by other methods. For example, matching the children of the same family or, ideally, twins can control all unmeasurable genetic and environmental factors.
- Matching due to balancing the number of cases and witnesses at each level of the confounding factor increases the accuracy of comparisons (increasing power). This issue is very important when items are rare or access to them is limited.
- Matching can be used as a method to perform available sampling. For example, in a study about shock syndrome caused by poisoning, the studied patients were asked to introduce some of their friends as a control group, but this type of sampling increases the risk of over-matching [1]. Some disadvantages of this method are:
- In the studies that use assimilation, it is not possible to investigate the effect of the matching variables. For example, if the age of the people in the two groups being compared is the same, it is no longer possible to investigate the effect of age on the desired outcome. In other words, variables should be selected for matching whose confounding effect is well known.
- Sometimes matching requires additional time and cost to find matching groups for each item. For example, in case-control studies, the higher the matching criteria, the lower the possibility of accessing more sources of witnesses to find suitable people, and the cases for which no suitable witnesses can be found are excluded from the study.
- Since matching is considered a sampling strategy, the decision about matching should be made at the beginning of the study. This issue requires an initial analysis of the effect of the confounders for which matching was done.
- If the matched variable is an intermediate factor in the causal chain, serious problems arise in the inferences. For example, if we have the desire to investigate the effects of alcohol consumption on heart attack and conduct the study based on equalizing HDL serum levels, we will be unaware of the mediating effect of alcohol in increasing HDL.
- The analysis of matched data requires statistical methods and the use of normal statistical methods for paired data is incorrect. These methods are very specialized and are not available in much statistical software.
- Another disadvantage of matching is the possibility of over-assimilation. This happens when matching is done for factors that are not confounding. Over-matching reduces the statistical power of studies. As a result, a real relationship is hardly statistically significant. For example, in the case of the study of shock syndrome caused by poisoning, the use of

matching may cause unintentional matching of factors such as the residential area of cases and controls, the brand of food products consumed, and other factors such as these. However, it is important to note that overmatching does not distort the relative risk estimate (of course, if special methods of analyzing the matched data are used), but it causes a decrease in the significance level. For this reason, when a meaningful relationship is obtained from a matched study, overmatching does not affect the results [1].

7.3 Methods of Restraining Confounding During Data Analysis

In analytical studies, the main goal is to evaluate the relationship between the disease and factors such as environmental exposures, demographic variables, health indicators, genetic traits, etc. Even if the study aims to investigate a simple relationship between a disease and an exposure, other influential factors affect this relationship. Stratification and multivariate analysis (modeling) are statistical methods that are widely used to control the effect of these influencing (confounding) factors, calculate the effect of exposure after adjusting the confounders, and find patterns of dependence between the disease and predictive variables.

Stratification studies that have potential sources of confounding are to classify them. Stratification includes simple and comprehensible methods for evaluating the existence and the degree of influence of the confounding factor. Stratification methods are a type of statistical analysis used in biomedical research to classify study participants into different categories or groups based on specific characteristics or variables. These methods are useful for controlling confounding variables and analyzing study outcomes in a structured and systematic way. Table 7.1 shows a hypothetical example of a case-control study that examines the relationship between gender and malaria infection. As can be seen in this table, in crude analysis, the risk of contracting malaria in men (OR = 1.71) is higher than in women. If this relationship is causal, the observed dependence should not be influenced by other factors that are related to gender and disease. One of these factors is the job. People who live in open environments all the time (such as farmers and workers) are more likely to be exposed to malaria vector mosquitoes. Therefore, if the ratio of men who work in open environments is more than women, the obtained relationship can be justified by the type of job.

Table 7.1 Analysis based on the stratification method to evaluate the relationship between gender and malaria disease

	Healthy	Disease	Total
Raw analysis:			
Male	68	88	156
Female	82	62	144
Total	150	150	300
	Risk ratio = 1.7		
Stratified analysis based on job:			
People who are in the open space most of the time due to work issues			
Male	15	53	68
Female	3	10	13
Total	18	63	81
People who are mostly indoors due to work issues			
Male	53	35	88
Female	79	52	131
Total	132	87	219
	Risk ratio = 1.00		

Based on Table 7.1, stratified estimates are different from raw estimates. In the example above, it is possible to calculate the dependence between gender (exposure) and malaria (disease), separately for two job categories. The risk ratios calculated in each category are almost equal and different from the raw estimate, as a result, the confounding hypothesis of the occupational category for the relationship between gender and malaria is strengthened. Also, due to the closeness of the risk ratios obtained from the two occupational categories, this hypothesis that there is no real relationship between gender and malaria is strengthened [2].

With the help of stratification, we are also able to identify mutual effects. In the previous example, the risk ratios of the two classes are very close. It is possible to calculate the adjusted odds ratio based on job category. How to calculate this odds ratio, which is known as the weighted average method, is explained in this chapter. Table 7.2 shows another example of a case-control study in which the effect of oral contraceptive pills (OCP) on increasing the risk of heart attack has been investigated.

As shown in the first part of the table, the risk of a heart attack in women using OCPs is approximately 70% higher than in women who do not use OCPs. However, the possibility of distorting the results by age was noticed by the researchers. Age is one of the known factors that directly increases the risk of heart attack and has an inverse relationship with the exposure studied in this study [3].

The stratified analysis of the results according to age is given in the second part of Table 7.2, except for the age group of 35–39 years, in all categories, the risk ratios are much larger than the raw estimate of the risk ratio. This issue strengthens the confounding hypothesis of age with the opposite effect.

Table 7.2 Stratification analysis of the relationship between oral contraceptive pills (OCP) and heart attack in women

	Heart attack +	Heart attack –
Raw analysis:		
Taken oral contraceptive pills	29	135
Not taken oral contraceptive pills	205	1607
	234	1742
	Risk ratio = 1.7	
Analysis stratified by age:		
• Age 25–29		
Taken oral contraceptive pills	4	62
Not taken oral contraceptive pills	2	224
	Risk ratio = 7.2	
• Age 30–34		
Taken oral contraceptive pills	9	33
Not taken oral contraceptive pills	12	390
	Risk ratio = 8.9	
• Age 35–39		
Taken oral contraceptive pills	4	26
Not taken oral contraceptive pills	33	330
	Risk ratio = 1.5	
• Age 40–44		
Taken oral contraceptive pills	6	9
Not taken oral contraceptive pills	65	362
	Risk ratio = 3.7	
• Age 45–49		
Taken oral contraceptive pills	6	5
Not taken oral contraceptive pills	93	301
	Risk ratio = 3.9	

7.3.1 Assumptions

Analysis by stratification method is almost without presupposition. The only condition of this method is that the categories are meaningful from a scientific and logical point of view. This issue is synonymous with data homogeneity in terms of the confounding factor. In Table 7.1, the assumption of homogeneity of the relationship between gender and malaria disease in two job categories is accepted, and in Table 7.2, the assumption of homogeneity of the relationship between OCP pill consumption and heart attack in age groups is accepted. If this assumption is not suitable in any of the previous two examples, more accurate categories (for example, more accurate and detailed separation of jobs or shorter age ranges) are needed for analysis by stratification method.

Adjusting the indicators requires more assumptions. In general, all methods of index adjustment are based on accepting statistical models, which summarize the dependence between the variables under investigation. Sometimes the assumed statistical models are simple, such as the models whose adjustment is done based on the stratification method (such as the Mantel-Haenszel method). In this method, the weighted average of the specific odds ratios of each category is calculated as a summary of the overall odds ratio estimate. As mentioned before, homogeneity of data (absence of interaction effect) is the main condition of this type of analysis. These simple methods are very efficient when the number of confounders is small and the stratification of variables does not cause a loss of information. In more complex cases, multivariate adjustment methods are performed based on regression models. In these methods to examine relationships, multiple factors are adjusted simultaneously. In these models, when the effect of one factor on the disease is investigated, all other confounding factors are under control at the same time. In these models, it is possible to investigate the effect of confounders in a continuous mode (without stratification). Many health indicators, such as disease and death rates, are related to background variables such as age and gender. For example, older societies have higher crude death rates than societies with a younger demographic composition. In these cases, using raw rates is misleading. This issue applies to other and potentially confusing indicators related to them. This part is dedicated to the introduction of methods based on stratification to control the main confounding variables and make the compared groups compared with each other.

7.3.2 Standardization by the Direct Method

Direct standardization is a method that is usually used to adjust age in comparing death and disease rates between different areas or different periods. But the common use does not mean that this method is used only for age adjustment. The easy use of statistical models by software has limited the use of this method in analysis, but due to its simple and understandable logic, this method is still considered one of the main methods of data analysis.

Table 7.3 shows how this method works to compare the incidence rate of two groups A and B (for example exposed and not exposed to the desired potential confounder).

- For each confounding category, the incidence rate is calculated in two groups (columns 4 and 7).
- Members of the reference population are specified in each category of the confounding variable (column 8).
- The number of expected cases from the reference population is calculated by multiplying the incidence rates of each category of groups A and B by the number of members of the reference population (columns 9 and 10).
- The ratio of cases of each group from the total number of the reference population determines the adjusted or standardized incidence rate of each group. The standard rate indicates that if the two groups A and B had a structure completely similar to the structure of the ref-

Table 7.3 Using the direct standard method to compare the incidence rate (I) in the two study groups

	Group A			Group B			References population		
Potential confounding variable	N	Case	Incidence	N	Case	Incidence	N	Expected cases using group A incidence	Expected cases using group B incidence
(1)	(2)	(3)	(3)/(2) = (4)	(5)	(6)	(6)/(5) = (7)	(8)	(4) × (8) = (9)	(7) × (8) = (10)
Class 1	DA_1	XA_1	IA_1	DB_1	XB_1	IB_1	W_1	$IA_1 \times W_1$	$IB_1 \times W_1$
Class 2	DA_2	XA_2	IA_2	DB_2	XB_2	IB_1	W_2	$IA_2 \times W_2$	$IB_2 \times W_2$
Class 3	DA_3	XA_3	IA_3	DB_3	XB_3	IB_3	W_3	$IA_3 \times W_3$	$IB_3 \times W_3$
–	–	–	–	–	–	–	–	–	–
Class K	DA_K	XA_K	IA_K	DB_K	XB_K	IB_K	W_K	$IA_K \times W_K$	$IB_K \times W_K$

erence population in terms of confounders (for example, they had the same age distribution as the reference population), they would have incidence rates of I_A^* and I_B^*.

The relationship based on which the standardized rates are calculated is a type of weighted average of the specific rates of each group. The desired weights in this method are the number of people in the reference society in each category. With the help of standardized rates, adjusted attributable risk or adjusted relative risk can be calculated as follows:

$$\text{Adjusted attributable risk } \text{AR} = I_A^* - I_B^*$$

$$\text{Adjusted relative risk } \text{PR} = \frac{I_A^*}{I_B^*}$$

In this table, DA_i and DB_i are the number of samples in the *i*th category from groups A and B, XA_i and XB_i is the number of events in groups A and B, and IA_i and IB_i are the incidence rates in groups A and B.

Table 7.4 shows the use of the direct standardization method in calculating adjusted rates of coronary artery occlusion disease (CHD). In this study, the entire population aged 25–64 in the northern areas of Glasgow was investigated. Table 7.4 shows the number of CHD cases by age and socioeconomic class (completely deprived = 1 to completely privileged = 4) [4].

7.3.3 Indirect Standard Method

Indirect standardization is also commonly used to remove the effect of age in studies related to pathogenic mortality. In this method, the expected number of events under investigation (e.g., death) in each category of potential confounders (e.g., different occupational exposures) is calculated using reference community rates (standard rates). The ratio of the total number of expected events in each group provides an estimate of the relative risk or adjusted odds ratio.

Table 7.5 shows how to calculate these estimates. When this estimate is used to analyze death data, it is known as the Standardized Death Ratio (SMR). The terms standardized incidence rate (SIR) and standardized prevalence ratio (SPR) are also common. Indirect standardization is very appropriate when the number of events in each of the exposure categories is small, or when no events have occurred in some categories. In this situation, the direct standard method is not effective. One of the important points in using this method is to use the appropriate reference population. The reference population is usually a separate population from the individuals under study, although it is also common to use pooled data as a reference population. But it is very important to note that when different studies have different reference populations, the resulting standardized rates may not be comparable.

$$\text{Standard mortality ratio SMR} = \frac{\text{Observed deaths}}{\text{Expected deaths}} = \frac{\sum_i XA_i}{\sum_i [M_i \times nA_i]}$$

7.3.4 Mantel-Haenszel Method for Estimating Modified Indices

When we want to summarize the adjusted odds ratio or relative risk for a nominal confounder, the Mantel-Haenszel method is usually used [5–7]. Table 7.6 shows Mantel-Haenszel's notations. Based on this notation, the adjusted odds ratio for nominal data is as follows:

$$\text{OR}_{\text{MH}} = \frac{\sum_i \frac{a_i d_i}{N_i}}{\sum_i \frac{b_i c_i}{N_i}}$$

Calculating OR_{MH} is very simple. In the table (7.1), the raw chances of contracting malaria were calculated separately, which shows that men have a higher risk of contracting it. But the calculation of stratified chances based on the job showed no correlation between infection rate and

Table 7.4 Occurrence of coronary artery occlusion by age groups and socio-economic categories in the northern areas of Glasgow and the reference population of England in the age range of 25–64

Socio-economic class									
	1		2		3		4		
Age group	No. events	Samples	No. events	Samples	No. events	Samples	No. events	Samples	Reference population
25–29	0	4784	0	4972	0	4351	0	4440	12,982,900
30–34	0	4210	0	4045	0	3232	1	3685	10,772,120
35–39	1	3396	4	3094	1	2438	5	2966	8,087,920
40–44	6	3226	7	2655	9	2241	10	2763	7,619,500
45–49	7	2391	13	2343	17	3360	15	2388	6,921,860
50–54	16	2156	11	2394	19	2708	24	2566	69,755,040
55–59	17	2182	28	2597	43	2968	28	2387	7,195,140
60–65	25	2054	44	2667	53	2802	56	2380	7,130,160
Total	72	24,399	107	24,767	142	23,100	139	23,575	57,984,640
Rate per 1000	2.95		4.32		6.15		5.90		

Table 7.5 Using indirect standardization to calculate the standardized mortality rate with the reference population

Study 1				Reference population
Potential confounder	Number	Observed deaths	Death rate	Expected deaths when population A has the same mortality rate as the reference population
(1)	(2)	(3)	(4)	(2) × (4) = (5)
Class 1	nA_1	XA_1	M_1	$M_1 \times nA_1$
Class 2	nA_2	XA_2	M_2	$M_2 \times nA_2$
Class 3	nA_3	XA_3	M_3	$M_3 \times nA_3$
–	–	–	–	–
Class K	nA_k	XA_k	M_k	$M_k \times nA_k$
Total		$\sum_i XA_i$		$\sum_0 [M_i - nA_i]$

Table 7.6 Notations used to calculate the adjusted odds ratio by the Mantel-Haenszel method—the first category of confounding

	Controls	Cases	Total
Exposed	b_i	a_i	M_{1i}
Not exposed	d_i	c_i	M_{2i}
Total	n_{2i}	n_{1i}	N_i

sex. Using the adjusted odds ratio with the Mantel-Haenszel method gives a summary estimate of the correlation between sex and the incidence rate. How to calculate OR_{MH} is as follows:

$$OR_{MH} = \frac{\sum_i \frac{a_i d_i}{N_i}}{\sum_i \frac{b_i c_i}{N_i}} = \frac{\frac{53\times 3}{81} + \frac{35+79}{219}}{\frac{10\times 15}{81} + \frac{52\times 53}{219}} = 1.01$$

To compute the OR_{MH} regarding the association between heart attack and oral contraceptive pill (OCP) consumption, the calculation procedure is outlined using data from Table 7.2. To follow the necessary steps and determine the OR_{MH} value, refer to equation and Table 7.2.

$$OR_{MH} = \frac{\sum_i \frac{a_i d_i}{N_i}}{\sum_i \frac{b_i c_i}{N_i}} = \frac{\frac{4\times 224}{292} + \frac{9\times 390}{444} + \frac{4\times 330}{393} + \frac{6\times 362}{442} + \frac{6\times 301}{405}}{\frac{2\times 62}{292} + \frac{12\times 33}{444} + \frac{33\times 26}{393} + \frac{65\times 9}{442} + \frac{93\times 5}{405}} = 4.0$$

7.3.5 Mantel-Haenszel Method for Analyzing Matched Studies (McNemar Method)

The odds ratio in matched case-control studies is calculated by dividing the number of pairs in which cases have exposure and controls without exposure by the number of pairs in which cases have no exposure and controls have exposure. Thus, in 2 × 2 consensus tables like what is seen in Table 7.7, the odds ratio is equal $\frac{b}{c}$.

7.3.6 Limitations of Adjustment Methods Based on the Stratification

Any of the methods discussed in the previous sections to control confounding variables can be used to control multiple confounding variables. For this purpose, all possible combinations of the set of confounding variables should be separated as desired categories. Table 7.8 shows a hypothetical example of this situation. This method of analysis for multivariate adjustment has the following limitations and disadvantages.

- The calculated adjusted indices are only used to estimate the relationship between the exposure and the desired response. For example, to evaluate the relationship between OCP consumption and heart attack, the confounders of age and level of education may be adjusted. If it is necessary to evaluate the relationship between the level of education and heart attack, all the steps must be repeated from the beginning.
- These methods are only used to adjust nominal confounders (such as gender and race). When we are dealing with continuous variables, their stratification is inevitable, the way of classifying variables can be a matter of taste and lead to different results.
- When the number of confounders is large, the number of classes increases and the data may be scattered so that the results become unreliable.
- Limited generalizability: Matching and stratification methods may reduce the sample size and limit the generalizability of the study results to a broader population. This is because they often involve selecting participants who meet specific criteria, which may not be representative of the overall population.
- Potential for bias: Matching and stratification methods can be prone to selection bias if the selection of participants is not random or if the matching or stratification is not done properly. This can lead to biased results and affect the validity of the study.
- Difficulty in finding matched participants: It can be challenging to find matched participants, especially in large studies or studies with specific inclusion criteria. This can result in reduced sample size and decreased statistical power.
- Inability to control for all confounding variables: Matching and stratification methods can only control for known confounding variables, and there may be unknown or unmeasured confounding variables that cannot be controlled using these methods.

Table 7.7 How to display results in paired studies

	Controls		
Cases		Exposed	Not exposed
	Exposed	*a*	*b*
	Not exposed	*c*	*d*

$$Paired\ odds\ ratio = \frac{b}{c}$$

7.3.7 Regression Model to Control Confounders at the Same Time

Stratification methods are a type of statistical analysis used in biomedical research to classify study participants into different categories or groups based on specific characteristics or variables for controlling confounding variables.

One example of a stratification method is discriminant analysis, which is used to determine the relationship between a set of independent variables and a categorical dependent variable.

Table 7.8 Hypothetical example of how to perform direct adjustment to simultaneously control gender, race, and level of education

Gender	Race	Years of schooling	Class	Rates related to group A	Rates related to group B	Weights obtained from the reference population
Male	Black	<12	1	–	–	–
		≥12	2	–	–	–
	White	<12	3	–	–	–
		≥12	4	–	–	–
Fe male	Black	<12	5	–	–	–
		≥12	6	–	–	–
	White	<12	7	–	–	–
		≥12	8	–	–	–

Stratification methods can be useful in biomedical research for identifying patterns and relationships between different variables and outcomes.

There are different types of stratification methods, including cluster analysis, discriminant analysis, and logistic regression. Cluster analysis involves grouping participants based on similarities in their characteristics or behaviors, while discriminant analysis is used to determine the relationship between a set of independent variables and a categorical dependent variable. Logistic regression is a statistical method used to predict the probability of an event occurring based on a set of predictor variables.

They can be particularly useful in identifying subgroups of participants who may respond differently to a particular treatment or intervention. This information can then be used to tailor treatments or interventions to specific subgroups of patients, leading to more effective and personalized healthcare.

Considering the limitations and problems caused by stratification-based methods, the multiple regression method is usually more efficient. In this method, the simultaneous effect of all exposures, while adjusted for potential confounders, is presented in the form of a model. In this method, it is also possible to examine continuous variables [7]. Another advantage of these methods is the possibility of predicting the desired estimates by using the model made for the variables.

7.3.8 Propensity Score Analysis

Propensity score analysis is a powerful method to control for confounding variables in medical sciences research, and it can provide more accurate estimates of treatment effects compared to traditional regression models. It involves calculating the probability of a participant receiving a specific treatment or intervention based on their characteristics and then using this score to control for confounding variables in the analysis. Can be useful in situations where randomization is not feasible or ethical, such as in observational studies or in situations where the treatment assignment is based on clinical decision-making.

Further discussion of these topics is postponed to Chap. 8.

References

1. Rothman KJ, Greenland S, Lash TL. Modern epidemiology. 3rd ed. Philadelphia, PA: Lippincott Williams & Wilkins; 2008.
2. Hernán MA, Robins JM. Causal inference: what if. Boca Raton, FL: Chapman & Hall/CRC; 2020.
3. Akbarzadeh M, Sharifi N, Zare N. Investigation of the relationship between myocardial infarction, angina pectoris, and venous thrombosis and some risk factors in the women suffering from cardiovascular diseases with a history of contraceptive pills consumption. Int Cardio Res J. 2016;10(2):e10286. https://doi.org/10.17795/icrj-10(2)86.
4. Austin PC, Stuart EA. Moving towards best practice when using inverse probability of treatment weighting (IPTW) using the propensity score to estimate causal treatment effects in observational studies. Stat Med. 2015;34(28):3661–79. https://doi.org/10.1002/sim.6607.
5. VanderWeele TJ, Shpitser I. On the definition of a confounder. Ann Stat. 2013;41(1):196–220. https://doi.org/10.1214/12-AOS1058.
6. Soori H, Rahimi M, Mohseni H. Association between job stress and work-related injuries: a case-control. Iran J Epidemiol. 2006;1(3–4):53–8. http://irje.tums.ac.ir/article-1-198-en.html. Accessed 22 Ap 2023.
7. Zhang J, Yu KF. What's the relative risk? A method of correcting the odds ratio in cohort studies of common outcomes. JAMA. 1998;280(19):1690–1. https://doi.org/10.1001/jama.280.19.1690.

8 Data Analysis for Controlling Errors in Medical Science Investigations

Data is like garbage. You'd better know what you are going to do with it before you collect it.

—Mark Twain (1835–1910)

8.1 Introduction

Usually, every research includes data collected from various variables such as background variables, confounding variables, parameters related to the desired outcome or event, measurements related to the follow-up of the people under study, and the occurrence of possible complications. Before analyzing information, it is necessary to design a written program for analysis, review the quality of data, perform preliminary studies such as charts, descriptive statistics, and agreement tables, remove unimportant data, analyze one variable, and finally model (simultaneous analysis of variables). Otherwise, there is not enough confidence in obtaining reliable and repeatable results.

8.2 Designing a Written Program for Analysis

Usually in every research proposal there is a section explaining how to analyze the results. Providing the details of the analysis in this part is very useful and helpful to guide the plan. Important points are different depending on the type of study. In randomized trials, due to the precise nature of these studies, the analysis program should be mentioned with precise details. This issue can include how to investigate the main and side effects, statistical methods used, and instructions on making adjustments for basic variables. In observational studies where the descriptive aspect and the expression of relationships between parameters are important, the main hypotheses are usually very useful and directional. In another part of the analysis program, a list of independent variables, responses, and potential confounders that must be collected to answer the questions should be prepared.

8.3 Data Quality Review

It is important to verify the accuracy of the data and to control the quality of the dataset or information base before performing the analysis. The first step is to review the primary forms to determine missing data or items excluded from the study. The next step is to search the data to find outliers. In continuous data, this issue starts with the distribution of data dispersion and in ordinal variables with the preparation of agreement tables and the evaluation of the frequencies related to each house. In cases where the volume of data and the number of variables are large, the importance of this issue doubles. The next step is

H. Soori, *Errors in Medical Science Investigations*, https://doi.org/10.1007/978-981-99-8521-0_8

to evaluate the compatibility of the information. For example, if the type of cancer and gender are recorded, it is inconsistent to observe women with prostate cancer. In the case of continuous variables, it is very useful to draw a scatter diagram. For example, drawing charts of weight and height or weight and age helps to find inconsistent cases. Some other remote data are identified with this method. Possible errors, wherever possible, should be eliminated by checking the recorded data with original values. Sometimes, errors can be fixed. In most cases, it is necessary to introduce special codes to register errors, and missing, remote, or incomplete data. There are special statistical methods for missing cases, the use of which requires consultation with statistics experts.

8.4 Descriptive Statistics

After completing the data quality verification phase, it is possible to describe the information. It is better to start drawing fullness and scatter plots. In addition to the final control of data accuracy, this issue provides an intuitive understanding of what happened in the research. In many cases, separate investigation of the investigated subgroups (supposedly, patients and healthy people) is mandatory. To evaluate each research question, it is necessary to determine the response variable and the exposure variables. In observational studies, control of confounders plays an essential role in the validity of the studies. For this purpose, it is necessary to determine potential confounding variables and background before starting the study.

8.4.1 Mean

The mean value of a series of numbers is usually the arithmetic mean of the numbers, referred to as the mean value for short. The average is calculated by adding the numbers and dividing them by their number:

$$\text{Mean} = \overline{X} = \frac{\Sigma x}{n}$$

In this relation, X represents the numerical values of the desired variable and the sign of the sum of n numbers with each other.

8.4.2 Variance

In most statistical analyses, variance or standard deviation is the most appropriate criterion for representing the spread of data.

Variance tells how much data is spread out. First, you add all the differences from the average to find the answer. Then, you take each difference and square it. Finally, you add up all the squared differences and divide by the number of data points. A high variance indicates that there is considerable variability in the data points, with large deviations from the mean. Conversely, a low variance suggests that the data points are closely clustered around the mean value, with minimal deviations. The variance is calculated as follows.

$$\text{Variance}: S^2 = \frac{\Sigma(x-\overline{x})^2}{(n-1)}$$

8.4.3 Standard Deviation

One of the problems with interpreting variance is that its unit is square, the main unit of data. For example, if the unit of the weight observations is grams, the unit of the variance is grams to the power of 2. In most cases, we want to reset the unit variance to the original scale by taking the square root of it. This new criterion is called standard deviation. The standard deviation measures how far the data is from the mean. A low standard deviation indicates that the data is clustered around the mean, while a high standard deviation indicates that the data is more spread out. The standard deviation is calculated as follows.

$$\text{Standard deviation}(\text{sd}): S = \sqrt{\frac{\Sigma(x-\overline{x})^2}{(n-1)}}$$

and or

$$\text{Standard deviation}: S = \sqrt{\frac{\sum x^2 - \frac{(\sum x)^2}{n}}{(n-1)}}$$

8.4.4 Normal Distribution

The normal distribution is an important concept in many areas of statistics, also known as the Gaussian or bell-shaped distribution. In many cases, the frequency distribution of the data in the form of symmetric and bell-shaped distributions seems appropriate. In practice, such an experimental distribution is considered equal to the normal distribution. Figure 8.1 shows a picture of the normal distribution obtained from height measurements of adult men. It is not difficult to find many distributions that are not similar to the normal distribution. Income distribution, life span, and the growth of a tumor are examples of this. In such cases, transformation (for example, transformation by taking logarithms from the data) helps to normalize the data.

The importance and widespread use of the normal distribution is not only due to the approximate similarity of the experimental frequency distributions with the normal distribution, but also to some mathematically favorable properties of this distribution. This distribution plays a very important role in statistical analysis. One of these important features is derived from the central limit theorem. According to this case, regardless of the initial shape of the experimental frequency distribution, if the sample size is large enough, the average frequency distribution of the sample will be equal to the normal distribution. Normal distribution is determined by knowing the mean (μ) and standard deviation (σ) of the population. The mathematical relation of this distribution is as follows:

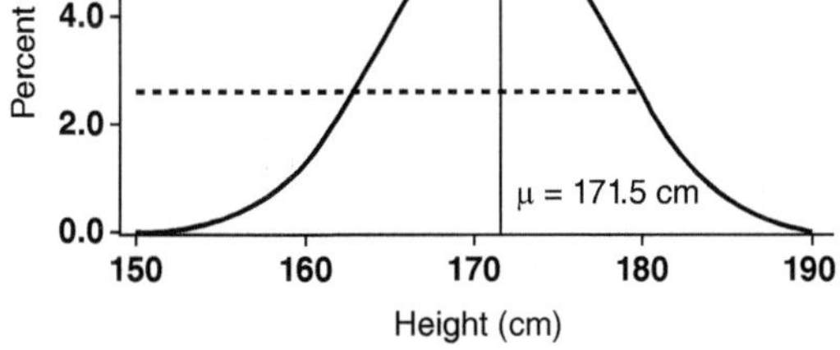

Fig. 8.1 Approximate normal shape for height distribution of adult men

$$Y = \frac{1}{\sqrt{2\pi\sigma^2}} \exp\left(\frac{-(x-\mu)^2}{2\sigma^2}\right)$$

8.4.5 Standard Normal Distribution

If the distribution of the variable is normal, changes in variable unit do not change the distribution. So, for example, if height is measured in centimeters, inches, or meters, the distribution of the size variable is still normal. Changing the mean causes the normal curve to shift in the horizontal axis, and changing the standard deviation changes the width of the curve.

According to this feature, all normal distributions can be converted to the standard normal distribution, which has a mean of 0 and a standard deviation of 1. This issue is obtained by dividing the data from the sample mean and dividing them by the standard deviation of the sample. This relationship can be shown as follows:

$$\text{SND}: Z = \frac{x-\mu}{\sigma}$$

In this relationship, x is the main variable with mean (μ) and standard deviation (σ) and Z is the standardized variable (SND). This is done for the normal distribution of Fig. 8.1. The resulting standard normal distribution is shown in Fig. 8.2.

8.4.6 Confidence Interval

Indicators such as mean (μ) and standard deviation (σ) of society parameters are under investigation.

In general, every indicator of society is called a parameter. Parameters have a fixed but unknown value. What happens in applied research is choosing a suitable sample from the community and estimating the desired parameters. In this way, $\overline{X}$ and S are point estimates of the parameters of the society, i.e., μ and σ. Another type of estimate

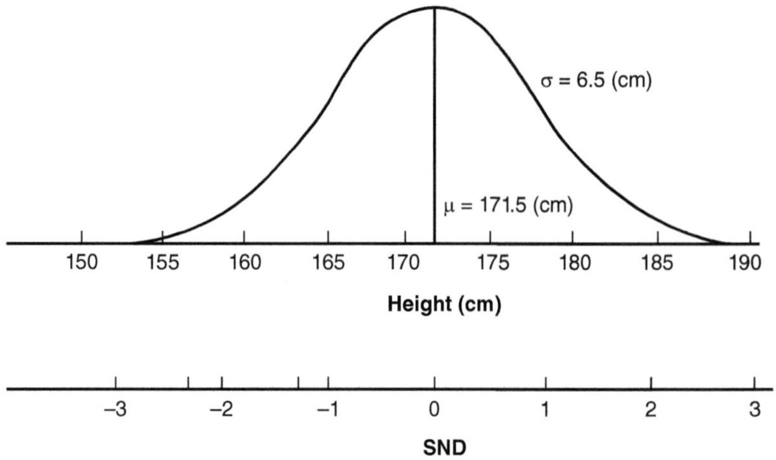

Fig. 8.2 The relationship between the normal distribution in the original scale and the standardized normal distribution

is the interval estimate. Distance estimates are a method to show the accuracy of parameter estimation. For this purpose, the standard error of each estimate should be calculated first. The general relationship for calculating the confidence interval is as follows:

$$\text{Confidence Interval} = (\text{Point Estimate}) \pm (\text{Confidence Coefficient}) \times (\text{Estimation Standard Error})$$

The interval estimate for the population mean parameter is calculated as follows:

$$\bar{X} \pm t_{n-1} \frac{S}{\sqrt{n}}$$

In this regard, t_{n-1} the desired confidence coefficient is at a fixed and predetermined level (for example, 95%), from the student's *t*-distribution with degrees of freedom $n - 1$. The t distribution can be considered as a substitute for the normal distribution when the sample size is small.

8.4.7 Agreement Tables and Measurement of Exposure Effect

The most useful way to summarize the relationship between two ordinal variables is to set up a table like Table 8.1. These tables are called 2 × 2 agreement tables.

Calculating the indicators of pathogenicity, exposure, risk, chance and the like is much easier for such tables. For example, if we want to find the ratio of the disease in each exposure group and in general in Table 8.1, these ratios are as follows:

Proportion of disease in exposure group $P_1 = \frac{d_1}{n_1}$
Proportion of disease in non-exposed group $P_0 = \frac{d_0}{n_0}$
Disease proportion in all people $P = \frac{d}{n}$

are calculated.

In the same way, 8*t* can be calculated from this table.

$$\text{Prevalence} = \frac{\text{Number of patients at a point in time}}{\text{Total population}}$$

$$\text{Cumulative incidence} = \frac{\text{Number of new cases in a period of time}}{\text{Number of healthy people in the population}}$$

Table 8.1 A 2 × 2 agreement table along with symbols related to showing the relationship between a two-mode response variable and two-level exposure variable

Outcome			
Exposure	With outcome (d)	Without outcome (h)	Total
Group 1 (exposed)	d_1	h_1	n_0
Group 2 (not exposed)	d_0	h_0	n_0
Total	d	h	n

Table 8.2 Famous indices for comparing two ratios

Comparing indicator	Equation for calculation
Risk difference (AT)	$P_1 - P_0$
Relative risk (RR)	$\frac{P_1}{P_0}$ and/or $\frac{\frac{d_1}{d_1+h_1}}{\frac{d_0}{d_0-h_0}}$
Odds ratio (OR)	$\frac{d_1 \times h_0}{d_0 \times h_1}$ and/or $\frac{\text{odds}_1}{\text{odds}_0} = \frac{\frac{d_1}{h_1}}{\frac{d_0}{h_0}}$

8.4.8 Comparing Two Ratios with Each Other

In many cases we want to compare two key figures from two subgroups of a population. These ratios can be the comparison of the number of improved cases caused by the new drug compared to the standard drug, the ratio of pathogenicity in two different geographic climates, etc. In this section we present different statistical methods for these comparisons.

- Risk difference (attributable risk)
- Relative risk
- Odds ratio

How to calculate each of these indicators is shown in Table 8.2.

The 95% confidence interval for the risk difference is calculated as follows:

$$\text{AT}: P_1 - P_0 \pm 1.96\sqrt{\frac{P_1(1-P_1)}{n_1} + \frac{P_0(1-P_0)}{n_0}}$$

In this regard, P_1 the estimation of the disease ratio in the exposed group and P_0 the estimation of the disease ratio in the non-exposure group are. The 95% confidence interval for the relative risk is calculated as follows:

$$\log(\text{RR}): \log\left(\frac{P_1}{P_0}\right) \pm 1.96\,\text{se}(\log \text{RR})$$

in this regard as: se(log RR)

$$\text{se}(\log \text{RR}) = \sqrt{\frac{1}{d_1} - \frac{1}{d_1+h_1} + \frac{1}{d_0} - \frac{1}{d_0+h_0}}$$

it will be counted. In this case, the upper and lower limits of the 95% confidence interval are calculated as follows:

$$L_{\log} = \log \text{RR} - 1.96\,\text{se}(\log \text{RR})$$

$$U_{\log} = \log \text{RR} + 1.96\,\text{se}(\log \text{RR})$$

that in all the above relationships, the logarithm is based on a Napier's number.[1] To find the confidence interval in the main unit, it is necessary to raise the obtained limits to the power of e means:

$$L = \exp(L_{\log})$$

$$U = \exp(U_{\log})$$

The 95% confidence interval for the odds ratio is calculated as follows:

$$\log(\text{OR}): \log\left(\frac{\text{odds}_1}{\text{odds}_0}\right) \pm 1.96\,\text{se}(\log \text{RR})$$

in this regard se (log OR) is calculated as:

$$\text{se}(\log \text{OR}) = \sqrt{\frac{1}{h_1} + \frac{1}{d_1} + \frac{1}{h_0} + \frac{1}{d_0}}$$

In this case, the upper and lower limits of the 95% confidence interval are calculated as follows:

$$L_{\log} = \log \text{OR} - 1.96\ \text{se}(\log \text{OR})$$

$$U_{\log} = \log \text{OR} + 1.96\,\text{se}(\log \text{OR})$$

[1]The logarithm in the fixed base e or Napier number ≈ 2.718 is called the natural logarithm. This logarithm is very useful in pure mathematics, especially differential and integral calculus.

Table 8.3 Smoking status by gender

Smoking status			
Gender	Smoker	Non-smoker	Total
Male	2279	2241	4520
Female	1562	2559	4161
Total	3841	4840	8681

Table 8.4 Smoking status and occurrence of cardiovascular diseases during follow-up

Cardiovascular cases within the study follow-up			
Smoking status	Yes	No	Total
Smoker	166	1176	1342
Non-smoker	50	513	563
Total	216	1689	1905

Like the confidence interval for RR, it is necessary to raise the obtained limits to the square of e means:

$$L = \exp\left(L_{\log}\right)$$

$$U = \exp\left(U_{\log}\right)$$

Example: Suppose the smoking variable is collected as smokers and non-smokers based on gender in Table 8.3.

In this case, the proportion of smokers in men and women is equal:

$$P_0 = \frac{2279}{4520} = 0.5042$$

$$P_1 = \frac{1562}{4161} = 0.3754$$

And the 95% confidence interval for the difference in the risk of smoking in men and women is calculated as follows:

$$\text{AT} = 0.5042 - 0.3754 \pm 1.96 \frac{0.5042(1-0.5042)}{4520} + \frac{0.3754\sqrt{1-0.3754}}{4161}$$

which will be equal to 0.0207 ± 0.1288 or (0.108, 0.150).

Example: Table 8.4 was obtained from a multicenter study to investigate risk factors for cardiovascular diseases in men in different cities in the United States [1].

In this study, the estimated risk of contracting the disease for smokers is $P_1 = \frac{166}{1342} = 0.1237$ and for non-smokers it is $P_0 = \frac{50}{563} = 0.0888$. In this case, the relative risk of cardiovascular diseases in smokers compared to non-smokers is calculated as RR = (0.1237)/(0.0888) = 1.393, and the standard error for the logarithm of the relative risk is equal to:

$$\sqrt{\frac{1}{166} - \frac{1}{1342} + \frac{1}{50} - \frac{1}{563}} = 0.1533$$

is calculated and we have:

$$L_{\log} = \log\left(1.393\right) - 1.96 \times 0.1533 = 0.310$$

$$U_{\log} = \log\left(1.393\right) + 1.96 \times 0.1533 = 0.6319$$

And finally, the upper and lower limits of the 95% confidence interval for RR are as follows:

$$L = \exp\left(0.0310\right) = 1.031$$

$$U = \exp\left(0.6319\right) = 1.881$$

As a result, the researchers are 95% sure that the confidence interval contains the real relative risk of the society. Example: For the data in Table 8.5, the 95% confidence interval for OR is as follows:

Chances (odds) of heart disease in smokers compared to non-smokers:

$$\text{OR} = \frac{\frac{166}{1176}}{\frac{50}{513}} = 1.448$$

The standard error of this estimate is as follows:

$$\sqrt{\frac{1}{166} + \frac{1}{1176} + \frac{1}{50} + \frac{1}{513}}$$

is calculated and finally the 95% confidence interval for OR will be as

$$\left(1.04, 2.02\right)$$

8.5 Modeling

In statistics, modeling involves using mathematical or statistical techniques to describe a relationship between variables or to make predictions about future events based on past data. Many different types of models are used in statistics, including linear regression models, time series models, and machine learning models. The choice of model depends on the type of data and the research question to be addressed.

In this chapter, we briefly introduce four famous models for multivariate analysis. Linear regression is used when analyzing continuous results (e.g., blood pressure and weight). Poisson regression is used to fit rates when there are multiple potential confounders. Logistic regression used for serial outcomes (like disease incidence and death) and Cox regression are used in analysis of survival data [2]. The relationships and details of the calculation, interpretation and evaluation of these models have been studied in many statistical books. In this section, these relationships are omitted and only their applications are examined.

Table 8.5 shows how these models are symbolized.

8.5.1 Linear Regression

There are many instances where researchers wish to examine the concurrent relationship of a continuous scale outcome with a few independent variables. This problem is possible by using the multiple linear regression method. Linear regression is a statistical technique used to model the relationship between two continuous variables, considering one variable as the dependent variable and the other variable as the independent variable. The goal of linear regression is to find the best fitting straight line that describes the relationship between the two variables.

In linear regression, the dependent variable is modeled as a linear function of the independent variable, plus a random error term. The main applications of multiple regression are to estimate the effect size of an exposure when the effect of other factors is controlled. For example, if two exposure groups are different in terms of factors such as age, sex, and social class that affect the outcome under study, it is very important to adjust the effect of these factors to make the exposure groups comparable. Another reason for using models is to increase the accuracy of the estimation of the exposure effect due to the

Table 8.5 Symbolization and interpretation of regression coefficients in multiple regression models

Regression model	Equation	Interpretation of coefficients (b)
– Linear	$Y = b_0 + b_1X_1 + b_2X_2 + \cdots + b_kX_k$	When all the desired confounders in the study are under control at the same time, for each unit of increase in the X_1 variable, the average of the studied outcome (Y) increases by b_1
– Poisson	$\log(\text{rate}) = b_0 + b_1X_1 + b_3X_3 + \cdots + b_kX_k$	When all the desired confounders in the study are under control at the same time, for each unit of increase in variable X_1, the logarithm of the rate of the studied outcome (Y) increases by b_1
– Logistic	$\log(\text{odds}) = b_0 + b_1X_1 + b_2X_2 + \cdots + b_kX_k$	When all the desired confounders in the study are under control at the same time, for each unit of increase in variable X_1, the logarithm of the chance of the outcome under study (Y) increases by b_1
– Cox	$\log(\text{hazard}) = b_0 + b_1X_1 + b_2X_2 + \cdots + b_kX_k$	When all the desired confounders in the study are under control at the same time, for each unit of increase in variable X_1, the logarithm of the risk of the outcome under study (Y) increases by $b1$

reduction of the standard deviation of the estimates. For example, in a study to investigate the lung volume of 7.10-year-old children, the maximum amount of air breathed in 1 s (FEV1) was measured by a spirometer. The variables of age, height, and any respiratory disease in the last year were measured as factors related to the desired outcome. Figure 8.3a, b show the distribution of FEV1 with age and height for 630 children [3].

As can be seen from the graphs, there can be a strong linear relationship between FEV1, age and height. This problem is confirmed by testing the regression coefficients. Table 8.6 shows the results of fitting the linear regression model to these data.

According to Table 8.6, the best linear model for these data is as follows:

$$FEV_1 = -2.3087 + 0.0897 \times Age + 0.0250 \times Height$$

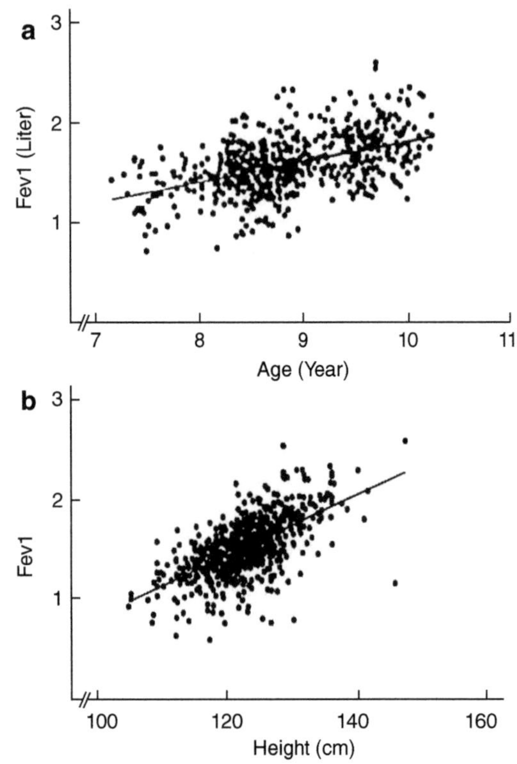

Fig. 8.3 FEV1 scatter chart along with age (**a**) and height (**b**) of 636 children

8.5.2 Poisson Regression

In this section, we introduce the Poisson regression model for rate comparison. The important point of this model is to compute the estimate on a logarithmic scale. Because of this, the coefficients must be converted to a real scale for analysis. In this model, the rate of the examined outcome in the study groups is calculated after adjustment for confounding factors. It is used to model the relationship between a count response variable and one or more predictor variables. It is commonly used when the response variable represents how often an event occurs in a fixed interval of time or space. The Poisson regression model assumes that the response follows a Poisson distribution and that the logarithm of the expected value of the response is a linear function of the predictor variable.

Table 8.7 shows a simple form of this model for comparing two groups.

The base rate is the infection rate in one of the exposure groups with which the rates obtained from other groups are compared. The exposure rate ratio shows the effect of exposure on the disease rate and is calculated as follows:

Table 8.6 Computer output of estimating multiple regression coefficients for measuring FEV1

FEV_1	β	Standard deviation	*P* value	95% confidence interval
Constant value	−2.3087	0.0812	0.000	−2.6645 to−1.9529
Age	0.0897	0.0157	0.000	0.0214 to 0.02385
Height	0.0250	0.0018	0.000	0.0558 to 0.1206

Table 8.7 Poisson regression model equations for comparing two exposure groups

Exposure	Outcome rate	Log rate
Exposed	Basic rate × exposure rate ratio	Log (basic rate) + log (exposure rate ratio)
Not exposed	Basic rate	Basic rate

$$\text{Exposure ratio} = \frac{\text{Morbidity rate in exposed group}}{\text{Morbidity rate in not exposed group}}$$

The following example shows the use of Poisson regression in the study of cardiovascular disease risk factors:

A study is conducted to investigate the relationship between smoking status and the incidence of cardiovascular disease (CVD) among a group of 1000 adults aged 40–70 years. The participants are followed up for 10 years, during which time 150 cases of CVD are identified [4].

The study collects data on several potential risk factors for CVD, including age, sex, body mass index (BMI), blood pressure, cholesterol level, and smoking status. The smoking status variable is coded as 0 for non-smokers and 1 for smokers.

A Poisson regression model is used to examine the association between smoking status and the incidence of CVD, after adjusting for the other risk factors. The model is specified as follows:

$$\log(\text{CVD incidence rate}) = \beta_0\beta_1(\text{smoking status}) + \beta_2(\text{age}) + \beta_3(\text{sex}) + \beta_4(\text{BMI}) + \beta_5(\text{blood pressure}) + \beta_6(\text{cholestrol level})$$

The model estimates the incidence rate ratio (IRR) for smoking status, which represents the relative risk of CVD for smokers compared to non-smokers, after adjusting for the other risk factors. The results show that the IRR for smoking status is 2.0 (95% confidence interval: 1.5–2.7), indicating that smokers have twice the risk of CVD compared to non-smokers, after adjusting for age, sex, BMI, blood pressure, and cholesterol level.

The Poisson regression model also allows for the examination of the effects of the other risk factors on CVD incidence. The results show that older age, male sex, higher BMI, higher blood pressure, and higher cholesterol level are all significantly associated with an increased risk of CVD, after adjusting for smoking status.

This example reveals the use of Poisson regression to examine the relationship between smoking status and the incidence of CVD, after adjusting for other risk factors. The Poisson regression model provides estimates of the incidence rate ratio for smoking status, as well as the effects of other risk factors on CVD incidence, and can be a useful tool in the study of cardiovascular disease risk factors.

8.5.3 Logistic Regression

The most well-known model for multivariate analysis of qualitative data is the logistic regression model. This model is also computed on a logarithmic scale such as Poisson regression, and the logarithm of the odds ratio of exposure in each of the study groups compared to a baseline group (and adjusting for potential confounders at the same time) is calculated. The odds ratio can be defined as follows.

$$\text{Exposure odds ratio} = \frac{\text{Odds in exposed group}}{\text{Odds in not exposed group}}$$

In Table 8.8, these relationships are shown on a logarithmic basis, similar to what is used in the logistic model for the comparison of two exposure groups [5].

A study was conducted in Sierra Leone about river blindness. In this study, people were classified based on whether they lived in villages located in Savanna (pastures) or forest areas. The subjects of this study were examined according to the presence and absence of Onchocerca volvulus (mf) microfilariae under the skin. Table 8.9

Table 8.8 Logistic regression model equations for comparing two exposure groups

Exposure	Outcome odds	Log odds
Exposed	Basic odds × exposure odds	log(exposure odds) + log (basic odds)
Not exposed	Basic odds	Log (basic odds)

Table 8.9 Number and percentage of people infected with river blindness by place of residence

	Exposure to *Onchocerca volvulus*			
Place of residence	Exposed	Not exposed	Total	Odds of infection
Tropical forest	$d_1 = 541$ (%71.7)	$h_1 = 213$ (%28.3)	754	$\frac{541}{213} = 2.540$
Savana	$d_0 = 281$ (%51.3)	$h_0 = 267$ (%48.7)	548	$\frac{281}{267} = 1.052$
Total	822	480	1302	

Table 8.10 Relationship between age groups and mf

	Exposure to *Onchocerca volvulus*			
Age group	Exposed	Not exposed	Odds of infection	Odds ratio in comparison with the base group
5–9	46	156	$\frac{46}{156} = 0.295$	1
10–19	99	119	$\frac{99}{119} = 0.832$	$\dfrac{\frac{0}{832}}{\frac{0}{295}} = 2.821$
20–39	299	125	$\frac{299}{125} = 2.392$	$\dfrac{\frac{2}{392}}{\frac{0}{295}} = 8.112$
≥40	378	8	$\frac{373}{80} = 4.725$	$\dfrac{\frac{4}{725}}{\frac{0}{295}} = 16.02$
Total	822	480		

shows the prevalence of this outcome in two groups [6].

In this study, we would like to investigate the effect of age on the relationship between disease prevalence and place of residence. Table 8.10 shows the relationship between age and exposure to mf.

Table 8.11 shows the computer output of this model.

Place of residence (1 = tropical forest, 0 = savannah) Age group: (0 = 5–9 years, 1 = 10–19 years, 2 = 20–39 years, 3 = more than 40 years)

8.5.4 Analysis of Survival Data

The analysis and modeling methods presented in the previous sections are based on the assumption that the incidence rate will remain constant during the study. However, in some longitudinal studies designed on the basis of the follow-up of the subjects studied, it may not be appropriate to accept this assumption. Example: The risk of death after heart surgery is very high and decreases over time after the recovery period. The rate of tumor recurrence changes over time after diagnosis and treatment. The methods

Table 8.11 Computer output for mf contamination model with place of residence and age groups

	Odds ratio	Z	$P > \|z\|$	95% confidence interval
Place of residence	3.083	8.181	0.000	2.354–4.038
Age groups:				
Age group (1)	2.599	4.301	0.000	1.683–4.016
Age group (2)	9.765	10.944	0.000	6.493–14.69
Age group (3)	17.64	13.295	0.000	11.56–26.93
Constant value	0.147	−9.741	0.000	0.100–0.27

referred to as survival analysis are designed to study such events without accepting the assumption that the infection rate is constant over time [7].

The two main indicators when analyzing this data are: Risk is represented by $h(t)$ and represents the instantaneous rate of occurrence at time t. The survival function is represented by $s(t)$ and shows the survival curve of the people under study. Life table, Kaplan-Meier and Nelson-Allen methods are the most famous descriptive methods for estimating and describing survival data. Example: In a randomized trial study to determine the effectiveness of azathioprine on biliary cirrhosis, 284 patients were enrolled and followed for 12 years. Out of these 284 patients, 248 patients had complete information on all basic variables. Of these, 31 patients had internal cholestasis (a feature that indicates more acute disease), 24 of them died, and 7 patients had an incomplete follow-ups. The information on these patients is shown in Table 8.12 [8].

The first death happened on the 19th. So the risk of death in the first 19 days is equal. The probability of survival until this day is in the form and function of survival in the form. The next death occurred on the 48th day. At this time, 30 patients are at risk, and the risk of death in this period is equal. The probability of survival until this day is equal and the function of survival is equal. The values of these indicators are fully shown in Table 8.12.

Figure 8.4 shows the Kaplan-Meier estimate of the survival function for two groups with internal cholestasis and without internal cholestasis.

These groups can be statistically compared by performing the log-rank test. One of the main assumptions in many descriptive and analytical methods of survival is the proportionality of risk over time. In other words, we assume this relationship throughout the study period Fixed $\frac{h_1(t)}{h_0(t)}$ is established

8.5.5 Log-Rank Test

The log-rank test is a statistical hypothesis test used to compare the survival distributions of two or more groups. It is commonly used in medical research and clinical trials to compare time-to-event data, e.g., B. the time to death or the time to recurrence of an illness. To compare the survival times in two different groups, the common method is to compare the hazard ratios in the two groups. The log-rank test is also based on this. In this method, the number of deaths that occurred in each period is compared with the expected number of deaths when the hazard ratio is equal to one (two groups have the same survival times).

For the simultaneous comparison of hazard rates adjusted for confounding variables, many parametric and semi-parametric models have been proposed, the most famous of which are the Cox and Weibull regression models.

Table 8.12 How to calculate the Kaplan-Meier estimate of the survival function for 31 patients with biliary cirrhosis with internal cholestasis

Date (day) t	Number at risk when the outcome occurs n_t	Number of deaths (time: t) d_t	Number of cases censored at follow-up (time t) c_t	Risk of death $r_t = d_t/n_t$	Probability of survival $s_t = 1 - r_t$	Survival function s_t* $S(t) = S$ ($t_{previous}$)
19	31	1	0	0.0323	0.9766	0.9677
48	30	1	0	0.0333	0.9667	0.9355
69	29	1	0	0.0345	0.9655	0.9032
150	28	1	0	0.0357	0.9643	0.8710
177	27	1	0	0.0370	0.9630	0.8387
193	26	1	0	0.0385	0.9615	0.8065
201	25	1	0	0.0400	0.9600	0.7742
245	24	1	0	0.0417	0.9583	0.7419
251	23	1	0	0.0435	0.9565	0.7097
256	22	1	0	0.0455	0.9545	0.6774
302	21	0	1	0	1	0.6774
341	20	1	0	0.0500	0.9500	0.6435
395	19	1	0	0.0526	0.9474	0.4097
421	18	1	0	0.0556	0.9444	0.5758
464	17	1	0	0.0588	0.9412	0.5419
578	16	1	0	0.0625	0.9375	0.5081
582	15	0	1	0	1	0.5081
586	14	0	1	0	1	0.5081
688	13	1	0	0.0769	0.9231	0.4690
828	12	0	1	0	1	0.4690
947	11	1	0	0.0909	0.9091	0.4263
1159	10	0	1	0	1	0.4263
1219	9	1	0	0.1111	0.8889	0.3790
1268	8	1	0	0.1250	0.8750	0.3316
1292	7	0	1	0	1	0.3316
1693	6	1	0	0.1667	0.8333	0.2763
1881	5	1	0	0.2000	0.8000	0.2211
1940	4	1	0	0.2500	0.7500	0.1658
1975	3	1	0	0.3333	0.6667	0.1105
2338	2	0	1	0	1	0.1105
2343	1	1	0	1	0	0

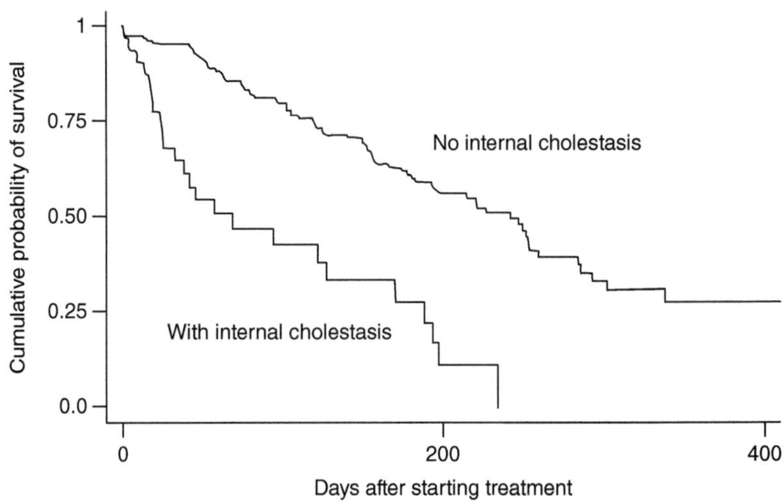

Fig. 8.4 Kaplan-Meier estimation of the survival function $S(t)$ for two groups of patients with biliary cirrhosis

8.6 Choosing the Right Method for Data Analysis

The main purpose of this chapter is to present the statistical methods required to analyze the effect of a group of variables on the response variable, which may include confounding variables and exposure or treatment. Choosing the right data analysis method depends on several factors, including the type of data, the research question, and the goals of the analysis (Table 8.13).

Table 8.13 Summary based on the purpose of the study and the type of variables under study

Continuous variables
One exposed group
The mean of the outcome, the confidence interval for the mean
– Large sample size:
using methods based on normal distribution
– Small sample size:
using methods based on t distribution
– Non-normality of data:
use of transformation to normalize data, use of non-parametric methods (methods based on ranks, bootstrap method)
Two exposed group
The difference between the means, the confidence interval for the difference between the means
– Large sample size:
using methods based on normal distribution
Small sample size: using methods based on t distribution
– Non-normality of data:
using transformation to normalize data
– Inequality of standard deviation of two groups:
use of Fisher-Behren test, Welch test non-parametric methods (methods based on ranks, bootstrap method, robust estimation methods)
Paired measures: tests for paired data
More than two exposed groups
One-way analysis of variance
Simple linear regression
– Continuous or rank exposure variables.
Simple linear regression
Pearson's correlation coefficient
Spearman's rank correlation coefficient, Kendall's correlation coefficient
Investigating nonlinear relationships
– The presence of confounding or accompanying variables.
Multiple regression
Two-way or multi-way analysis of variance
Using direct standardization methods
Ordinal variables with two categories

Table 8.13 (continued)

One exposed group
Ratio, confidence interval for ratio
Hypothesis test to check the value of the ratio
Chance, confidence interval for chance
Two exposed group
– Criteria for estimating the effect of exposure:
The difference in ratios
Risk ratio odds ratio
Chi-square test for 2 × 2 agreement tables
Accurate tests for small samples
More than two exposed groups
Chi-square test for $r \times 2$ agreement tables
Logistic regression
– Continuous or rank exposure variables.
Chi-square test to check the trend
Logistic regression
– The presence of confounding variables.
Mantel-Haenszel method
Logistic regression
Poisson regression
Direct standardization method
– Matched or paired data.
Comparison of ratios
Odds ratio and McNemar test
Conditional logistic regression
Ordinal variables with more than two categories
Chi-square test for $r \times c$ tables
Multimodal logistic regression
Rank logistic regression
Survival rates and times
One exposed group
Rate, confidence interval for rate
– Survival analysis:
Life table
Kaplan-Meier estimates for the survival curve
Two exposed group
– Methods based on rates:
The difference in rates
Ratio of rates
Poisson regression
– Survival analysis:
Hazard ratio (log-rank test)
Cox regression
Examining the proportionality of hazards
More than two exposed groups
Poisson regression
Cox regression
– Continuous or rank exposure variables
Poisson regression
Cox regression
– Presence of confounding or associated variables:
Mantel-Haenszel method
Poisson regression
Direct standardization method
Indirect standardization method

8.7 Data Analysis Based on the Type of Study Design

Each of the study types considered so far has different goals and structures that should be considered when analyzing the data. Notwithstanding the descriptive data, not complex in data analysis, we will review randomized clinical trials and observational studies in this section.

8.7.1 Randomized Clinical Trials

The important points for choosing a statistical method in the analysis of this type of data are:

- The type of answer to be considered.
- Need to adjust for base variables.
- The need to make a comparison between the studied subgroups.
- Longitudinal data.

Two key points in the analysis of randomized trials, in addition to the previous ones, are the existence of cluster data and crossover designs.

Table 8.14 shows how to choose the right method for analyzing these data.

8.7.2 Longitudinal and Crossover Studies

The important points for choosing the appropriate statistical method for analyzing these studies are:

- Type of sampling plan.
- The number of measurements (once, continuously, or repeatedly over time).
- Type of response and exposure variable.

Table 8.15 shows data analysis method in crossover and longitudinal studies. It also shows how to choose the right method to analyze these data.

8.7.3 Case-Control Studies

Each of the study types considered so far has different goals and structures that should be considered when analyzing the data. Notwithstanding the descriptive data, not complex in nature in data analysis, we will review randomized clinical trials and observational studies in this section. Table 8.16 shows appropriate methods for analyzing case-control studies.

Table 8.14 Data analysis method in randomized trial studies

Type of method(s)				
	Continuous	Nominal	Rate	Survival time
Data description	Mean and standard deviation	Table 2 × 2 or $r \times 2$	Number of events, rate, and person-time (with confidence interval) in each group	Number of events and person-time in each group Kaplan-Meier curve
Effect size	Difference between means *t*-test	Risk difference, odds ratio, risk ratio Z-test, Chi-square	Rate ratio, *Z*-test	Log-rank test Mantel-Cox test
Adjustment of basic variables	Multiple linear regression	Mantel-Haenszel method logistic regression	Mantel-Haenszel method Poisson regression	Cox regression
Determining the difference in treatment effect in subgroups	Adding the interaction effect in regression models			In addition to the interaction effect, the test of proportionality of risks in groups
Special cases	Study of cluster randomized trial and crossover designs			

Table 8.15 Data analysis methods in crossover and longitudinal studies

Methods				
Type of exposure	Continuous	Nominal	Rate	Survival time
Dichotomous	Difference between means *t*-test	Odds ratio, risk ratio, Chi-square	Rate ratio, *Z*-test	Log-rank test Mantel-Cox test
Categorical	Mean between groups Analysis of variance Regression	Odds ratios based on baseline group Logistic regression	Rate ratios based on base group Poisson regression	Risk ratios based on the base group Cox regression
Ordinal	Mean increase in each group Linear regression	Increasing the logarithm of the odds in each group Logistic regression Chi-square test for trend	Logarithmic increase of the rate in each group Poisson regression	Logarithmic increase of hazard in each group Cox regression
Continuous	Linear regression	Logistic regression	Poisson regression	Cox regression
Adjustment for confounders	Multiple linear regression	Multiple logistic regression Mantel-Haenszel test	Multiple Poisson regression Mantel-Haenszel test	Multiple Cox regression
Specific cases	Cluster data (repeated measures in longitudinal studies, multiple measurements over time for each individual, cluster sampling)			

Table 8.16 Study of appropriate methods for case-control data analysis

Design	Exposure variable	Adjustment for confounding variables
Simple random (case-control without matching)	Tables 2 × 2 show the condition of simultaneous exposure and disease, odds ratio, Chi-square test	Logistic regression Mantel-Haenszel method
Matching to a group (multiple cases and controls)	2 × 2 agreement tables on each stratum Mantel-Haenszel test Odds ratio Chi-square test	Analysis by stratification method Logistic regression based on simultaneous control of matched and confounding factors
Individual matching (paired)	Table 2 × 2 shows the agreement between case-control pairs according to the risk factor Odds ratio based on pairs McNemar test	Analysis by stratification method Logistic regression based on simultaneous control of matched and confounding factors
Paired controls at the same time for each case	Odds ratio by mantel-Haenszel method Chi-square test Stratification based on matched groups	Analysis by stratification method Logistic regression based on simultaneous control of matched and confounding factors

References

1. Pooling Project Research Group. Relation of blood pressure, serum cholesterol, smoking habit, relative weight, and ECG abnormality to incidence of major coronary events: final report of the pooling project. J Chronic Dis. 1978;31(4):201–306. https://doi.org/10.1016/0021-9681(78)90012-4.
2. Vittinghoff E, McCulloch CE. Relaxing the rule of ten events per variable in logistic and Cox regression. Am J Epidemiol. 2007;165(6):710–8. https://doi.org/10.1093/aje/kwk052.
3. Kumar R, Gupta N, Gupta P. Comparison of lung function in children aged 7.10 years from urban and rural areas of Haryana, India. Indian J Chest Dis Allied Sci. 2017;59(1):13–7. https://doi.org/10.4103/ijc.IJC_132_15.
4. Gepner AD, Piper ME, Johnson HM, Fiore MC, Baker TB, Stein JH. Effects of smoking and smoking cessation on lipids and lipoproteins: outcomes from a randomized clinical trial. Am Heart J. 2011;161(1):145–51. https://doi.org/10.1016/j.ahj.2010.09.032.
5. Bland JM, Altman DG. Multiple significance tests: the Bonferroni method. BMJ. 1995;310(6973):170. https://doi.org/10.1136/bmj.310.6973.170.

6. McMahon E, Faal H, Colebunders R, et al. Epidemiology of onchocerciasis in a rain forest area of Sierra Leone. Trans R Soc Trop Med Hyg. 1998;92(4):389–93. https://doi.org/10.1016/s0035-9203(98)90720-9.
7. Hosmer DW Jr, Lemeshow S, May S. Applied survival analysis: regression modeling of time-to-event data. New York: John Wiley & Sons; 2008.
8. Lindor KD, Dickson ER, Baldus WP, Jorgensen RA, Ludwig J, Murtaugh PA. Ursodeoxycholic acid and azathioprine for the treatment of primary biliary cirrhosis: a pilot study. Hepatology. 1993;18(4):863–8. https://doi.org/10.1002/hep.1840180415.

Identification and Control of Bias in Medical Sciences Investigations

9

The most important thing in science is not to avoid making mistakes, but to learn from them.

—George Bernard Shaw (1856–1950)

9.1 Introduction

Biases can be defined as systematic errors in the design or implementation of the study. Systematic errors can be from the methods of selecting people under study, the way of collecting information about the degree of reaching the desired result, and the method of evaluations from the way of choosing the people to be studied. As discussed later in this section, many biases can affect the results. One of the important topics is to distinguish bias from random errors (sample errors). Random errors occur due to the size of the sample compared to the entire population. The remarkable point about biases is that it happens because of the type of study chosen, but depends on how the study is designed and conducted. If the design and implementation of a study are without bias, the study is considered valid because (the averages) are correct. A study that has an incomplete design or implementation is called biased (invalid). However, due to the existence of sample variations, a study with bias may be very close to the truth.

Whenever bias exists, if an infinite number of the same study is performed, it is on average far from the truth. For example, when the average hazard ratio in a large (theoretically unlimited) number of case-control studies is equal to 2, while there is no correlation, the methods used are biased. This definition is of no use in practical studies that are not willing to evaluate it. For this reason, it is necessary to recognize bias through a detailed and critical evaluation of the study design, methods, and programs used in the study. Bias prevention and control consist of two stages.

- Ensuring the appropriateness of the study plan based on the desired principles and hypotheses.
- The stages of monitoring and precise executive control include measurements, data collection, and analysis.

Biases in medical sciences investigations could be presented in different categories. Some categorized them as selection bias, information bias, confounding bias, publication bias, reporting bias, performance bias, and detection bias. The number of biases is increasing in medical sciences investigation and here we include the five major ones, namely, information bias, selection bias, response bias, sampling bias, and cognitive bias. Someone may have a different categorization such as information bias and selection bias.

H. Soori, *Errors in Medical Science Investigations*, https://doi.org/10.1007/978-981-99-8521-0_9

9.2 Why Is Research Bias a Problem?

Bias can lead to inaccurate or misleading results. It refers to any systematic error in the design, conduct, analysis, or reporting of a study, which can distort the true relationship between variables or lead to incorrect conclusions. Bias can weaken the validity of logical inquiry, dissolve open belief in science, and lead to negative results for people and society. Subsequently, it is basic for analysts to distinguish and control their inclination to create high-quality inquiries that are exact, dependable, and dependable. In medical research, bias can lead to the development of ineffective or harmful treatments, or the failure to identify effective treatments.

9.2.1 Generalizability and Comparability

Generalizability and comparability are important concepts in medical sciences investigations as they relate to the ability to apply research results to a wider population and to make valid comparisons between different studies.

Generalizability is the degree to which the results of a study can be considered representative of the broader population or phenomenon of interest. It could be defined as the external validity of a study.

Generalizability depends on factors, including the representativeness of the study sample, the similarity of the study setting to real-world situations, the validity and reliability of the study measures, and the appropriateness of the statistical analyses used. We need to carefully consider these factors, and the strengths and limitations when designing and conducting studies, and when interpreting and communicating our findings.

Bias can affect generalizability in several ways. For example, selection bias can lead to a distorted sample that is not representative of the target population, which can limit the generalizability of the results. Information bias can also affect generalizability if there are errors in the measurement or recording of data, which can lead to incorrect conclusions about the target population.

Comparability refers to the ability to make valid comparisons between different groups or conditions. Comparability is essential in medical research to accurately assess the effectiveness of treatments, interventions, or diagnostic tests. Comparability can be achieved through careful study design, including randomization, blinding, and appropriate selection of study participants.

To maximize generalizability, and comparability and minimize bias, it is important to use appropriate study designs, sampling techniques, and measurement protocols. This can include using random sampling to ensure a representative sample, using standardized measurement tools to reduce measurement bias, and using appropriate statistical analysis techniques to control for confounding variables.

9.3 Information Bias

Information bias is caused by the incomplete definition of research variables or defects in the data collection process. This error is caused by the incorrect classification of the amount of exposure or desired outcome in certain sections of the people under study. Collecting data about the amount of exposure in the people under study is one of the sources of creating this bias. This problem mainly occurs in case-control studies. For this reason, most of the examples in this field are related to case-control studies. Two important categories of this type of bias are memory bias and interviewer bias. There are different types of information biases including recall bias, reporting bias, interviewer bias, observer bias, measurement bias, and surveillance bias.

9.3.1 Recall Bias

Recall bias occurs due to incorrect or incomplete recall of past exposures. This bias is one of the most important types of bias in exposure measurement. Specifically, in case-control studies, when subjects are asked to recount their previous exposures, errors in recalling previous events cause misclassification of exposure levels. When the manner or quality of the memory bias is the same in cases and controls, it is called undirected bias, and when the manner or quality of this bias is different in cases and controls, it is called directed bias. The effect of memory bias was investigated experimentally in the "Nurses' Health" cohort study [1]. In this study, the participating members were asked to record their ability to tan their skin at the beginning of the study and during the follow-up in the group of cases, who were diagnosed with skin cancer and people without complications (controls). The results showed that the actual value of the skin tanning ability was overreported in cases compared to the time before the disease. While the information about the control group remained constant over time.

For example, a study might ask participants who have been injured in road traffic accidents to recall the circumstances surrounding the accident, such as the speed of the vehicle at the time of the accident. However, participants may have difficulty accurately recalling this information, especially if they were injured or traumatized in the accident. As a result, the data collected may be subject to recall bias, which can lead to inaccurate conclusions about the relationship between speed and injury severity.

9.3.2 Interviewer Bias

When the condition of the patient or the health of the subjects under study in a case-control study is known to the researchers responsible for collecting the data, bias related to observation, such as interviewer bias, has a high probability of occurrence. One of the ways to create this type of bias is when the interviewer encourages them to recall past encounters during the interview with the cases, and by doing so, he violates the rules of the interview mentioned in the research instructions. For instance, an interviewer who believes that distracted driving is the primary cause of road traffic accidents may ask leading questions or show a bias towards participants who report distracted driving as a cause of their injury [2]. This can influence the participant's responses and lead to inaccurate or biased data.

How to evaluate and diagnosing this bias is very difficult. The best way to prevent it is to provide special measures in the design phase of the study. Ensuring the high quality of the research, providing complete details of the executive instructions, training the subjects under study, standardizing the way of data collection, and monitoring the data collection are the general methods of preventing these biases. One of the practical ways to remove this bias is to blind the disease status to the team responsible for collecting information. Many times, it is impossible or very difficult to use this method. In these situations, the use of a wide-spectrum questionnaire that includes questions about the health status of cases and controls can keep the main research questions hidden to a large extent. This topic is very useful in psychological studies. Biases related to outcome measurement are likely to occur in case-control and cohort studies. Lack of accurate and complete definition of the intended outcome (disease) or error in the data collection stage causes this bias.

9.3.3 Hawthorne Effect (or Observer Effect)

The Hawthorne effect is a phenomenon in which research participants change behavior or performance simply because they are aware of what is being observed or studied. This effect can lead to artificially exaggerated or distorted results and thus may affect the validity of research studies.

The Hawthorne effect was first identified in a series of studies conducted in the 1920s and 1930s at the Hawthorne factory in Chicago. Researchers observed that workers were more productive during the study, regardless of changes in working conditions.

To minimize the Hawthorne effect in research studies, researchers can employ several strategies for research methods. Additionally, researchers can explain the purpose of the study and ensure that participants' performance and behavior will not be evaluated, monitored, or judged.

For instance, a study might evaluate the impact of a safety campaign on reducing the number of road traffic injuries. However, the study participants may be more cautious and drive more safely simply because they know they are part of a study and their behavior is being observed. This can lead to an overestimation of the effectiveness of the safety campaign and may not accurately reflect the actual impact of the intervention.

9.3.4 Performance Bias

Performance bias is an important consideration in research studies, and researchers should carefully consider strategies to minimize its impact on the validity of study results. Performance bias is a potential source of research study bias that occurs when differences in the care or treatment of participants in different study groups lead to differences in the outcome rather than the intervention itself. This is the case if participants or healthcare providers are aware of the intervention being studied and modify their behavior or care based on that knowledge.

To minimize performance bias in research studies, blinding is used so that neither participant providers are aware of which group they belong to (i.e., intervention or control) can do. This can be achieved through single-blind, double-blind, or triple-blind study designs. Additionally, using objective outcome measures that are not subject to interpretation can help minimize performance bias. For example, in studies examining the efficacy of new drugs to treat road traffic injuries, performance bias occurs when providers provide different levels of care to intervention and control groups based on their knowledge of the treatment under study. There is a possibility. To minimize this potential bias, the study design should include blinding both participants and providers in the intervention group and use objective outcome measures such as the number of hospitalizations and duration of hospitalization. Included.

9.3.5 Regression to the Mean (RTM)

Regression to the mean is a statistical phenomenon that can bias certain types of studies.

Bias occurs when subjects are selected based on extreme values of a variable, and subsequent measurements of the same variable tend toward the population mean.

Subjects are selected based on their hypertension readings, and after taking their medication, their blood pressure is measured again.

Due to regression to the mean, the second reading should be lower than the first reading even without medication simply because the first reading was extreme. A second reading that is lower than the first may give the false impression that the drug had a beneficial effect when in fact the lower reading is due to regression to the mean. To address mean-biased regression, researchers can use a variety of study designs and statistical techniques, including Randomization, Paired Measurements, and Adjusted Baseline Values. To address mean-biased regression, researchers can use a variety of study designs and statistical techniques, including Randomization, Paired Measurements, and Adjusted Baseline Values. By accounting for regression to the mean, researchers can obtain more accurate estimates of treatment effects and avoid drawing erroneous conclusions from study results [3].

9.4 Selection Bias

Selection bias occurs when the results of a trial are affected by systematic differences in the way people are selected or rejected for a trial, or when interventions are assigned only to people who agree to participate in the trial. Prevention of this type of bias is the main reason for using randomized clinical trials to compare and evaluate different interventions. With proper randomization, all participants in the study are given the same chance to attend each of the study groups. In other words, if the trial is properly randomized, the investigators and study participants cannot influence the allocation of groups. However, a completely randomized method of dividing participants into different groups does not protect randomized clinical trials from selection bias. Selection bias can be applied when some people who might have been eligible for selection are excluded from the study due to the knowledge of the group in which they are placed. For example, the team responsible for selecting patients to participate in the MS trial believes that depressed patients are less likely to respond to a new drug. In the trial, a questionnaire was not designed to determine the depression of the participants, and this team has access to a sequence of random numbers to allocate patients to the groups under study. The team responsible for the selection can consciously or unconsciously create an obstacle in receiving the new drug by depressed patients and cause biases. Bias is applied in at least two ways: first, the depressed patients who are placed in the group receiving the new drug are coordinated with the exclusion criteria, or in most cases, they are placed in the placebo group. Second, the information related to the trial is provided to the depressed patients who are in the group receiving the new drug. So, they refuse to agree to participate in the trial. At the end of the trial, if the investigator's guess is correct and depressed patients have a lower response to the new drug, the trial shows an exaggerated effect of the new drug's effect in the treatment of MS. Documentary documents confirm that if the sequence of randomization of the participants during the preparation of the consent form to participate in the trial is not hidden from the reviewers, the effect of new interventions can be magnified.

9.4.1 Common Types of Selection Bias

9.4.1.1 Sampling or Ascertainment Bias

Sampling bias or ascertainment bias is a type of bias that occurs when the selection of research participants does not accurately represent the target population of interest. This can lead to biased estimates of exposure-outcome associations and affect the generalizability of study results.

For example, a study looking at the association between coffee consumption and cardiovascular disease could introduce sample bias if only coffee drinkers were included and non-coffee drinkers were excluded. The study results are representative of coffee drinkers only and do not consider potential health effects in non-coffee drinkers, so they may not be generalizable to the general population.

9.4.1.2 Attrition Bias

Attrition bias occurs when there is a differential loss of participants during a study, leading to a biased sample. An example of attrition bias in the context of road traffic injuries could be a longitudinal study that follows individuals who have been injured in a road traffic accident over a period.

For example, a study might follow individuals who have been injured in a road traffic accident for 1 year to evaluate the long-term impact of the injury on their quality of life. However, if a large number of participants drop out of the study before the 1-year mark, the remaining sample may not be representative of the broader population of individuals who have been injured in road traffic accidents.

9.4.1.3 Self-Selection (or Volunteer) Bias

Volunteers are usually healthier than the general population, exercise more and consume less coffee and cigarettes. Also, it is possible that these people may express the effect of the treatment or the consequences of the treatment more precisely or by mentioning more details for certain reasons (for example, concern about their health). They are interested in participating in the study and the information obtained from them cannot be generalized to the general population. For example, a study might recruit participants who have been injured in a road traffic accident by posting a call for volunteers on a social media platform. However, individuals who are more likely to respond to the call for volunteers may have different characteristics or experiences compared to those who do not respond. This can lead to a biased sample that is not representative of the target population and can limit the generalizability of the study results.

9.4.1.4 Survivorship Bias

Survivorship bias is a type of selection bias that occurs when the analysis of a dataset includes only subjects who survived or succeeded, ignoring subjects who did not survive or did not succeed. This bias can lead to misleading conclusions about group characteristics and performance by not considering those who did not survive or did not succeed.

An example of survival bias in road traffic injury studies is when studies include only patients who survived their injuries and were discharged from the hospital, excluding patients who died from their injuries. This can bias estimates of the efficacy of a particular intervention or treatment. This study considers only survivors who may have different characteristics or outcomes than those who did not survive. For example, if a study finds that a particular intervention is associated with improved outcomes for survivors, this may not necessarily be the case for those who did not survive.

9.4.1.5 Non-response Bias

Non-response bias is a type of bias that occurs when participants who do not respond to a survey or study are systematically different from those who do. This can lead to biased estimates of exposure-outcome associations and affect the generalizability of study results. An example of nonresponse bias in a road traffic injury study would be if the study sent surveys to patients who were discharged from the hospital after a road traffic injury, but a large proportion of these patients did not respond to the survey. If people who did not respond were more likely to be seriously injured or in poorer health than those who did, this could introduce a non-response bias. This can lead to skewed estimates of the prevalence or severity of road traffic injuries because this study only includes respondents who may have different characteristics or outcomes compared to non-responders.

9.4.1.6 Undercoverage Bias

Undercoverage bias occurs when a survey or the sample used in a survey is not representative of the target population because some members of the population are not sampled or are unlikely to be sampled. An example of underreporting bias in road traffic injury studies is when the study includes only patients treated at a particular hospital or trauma center and excludes patients treated at other hospitals or those who did not see a doctor. This could lead to underreporting bias, as the study only considered patients treated at a specific hospital and may not be representative of all road traffic injury patients in the population. For example, if a study finds that a particular intervention was associated with improved outcomes for road traffic injury patients treated at a particular hospital, this does not necessarily mean that patients or physicians treated at other hospitals may not apply to undiagnosed patients.

9.4.1.7 John Henry Effect

The John-Henry effect is a type of bias that occurs when the control group perceives that it did not receive the intervention or treatment offered to the intervention group. The control group can then change their behavior to achieve similar outcomes as the intervention group, leading to an underestimation of the true effect of the intervention.

An example of the John Henry effect in car accident studies would be a study comparing the effectiveness of two different treatments for car accidents. If the control group knew they were not on the "new" treatment, they might be more cautious about following road safety rules or more adherent to the treatment plan, leading to similar outcomes to the intervention group. This may underestimate the real difference in efficacy between the two treatments.

9.5 Sampling Bias

Sampling bias is a type of bias that occurs when certain individuals or groups are likely to be included or excluded from a research sample, and as a result, do not accurately reflect the population of interest. An unrepresentative sample is generated. This can lead to biased estimates of exposure-outcome associations and affect the generalizability of study results. Various biases, including the following, are included in the sampling bias group.

9.5.1 Self-Selection Bias

Self-selection bias is a type of bias that occurs when self-selecting studies or surveys based on individual characteristics, attitudes, or behavior, results in unrepresentative samples that do not accurately reflect the population of interest. You get This can lead to biased estimates of exposure-outcome associations and affect the generalizability of study results. For example, if a study examining the effectiveness of a smoking cessation program found that individuals who were motivated to quit were more likely to enroll in the program, this could introduce a self-selection bias. It may not generalize to the general population because it is representative only of individuals who are motivated to quit and does not consider the potential smoking prevalence and attitudes of individuals who are unmotivated to quit.

9.5.2 Sampling Bias in Non-probability Samples

Self-selection bias is a type of bias that occurs when self-selecting studies or surveys based on individual characteristics, attitudes, or behavior, results in unrepresentative samples that do not accurately reflect the population of interest. You get This can lead to biased estimates of exposure-outcome associations and affect the generalizability of study results. For example, the study examining the effectiveness of a smoking cessation program it may not generalize to the general population because it is representative only of individuals who are motivated to quit and does not consider the potential smoking prevalence and attitudes of individuals who are unmotivated to quit.

9.5.3 Pre-screening or Advertising Bias

Pre-screening or advertising bias is a type of bias that occurs when study participants are recruited in a way that systematically favors a particular group so that it does not accurately reflect the population of interest. A non-representative sample is obtained. This can lead to biased estimates of exposure-outcome associations and affect the generalizability of study results. For example, if a study examining the efficacy of a new drug for a particular disease was recruited via advertisements specifically targeted to those who had responded well to previous treatments, this could lead to pre-screening or advertising bias. The results of the study represent only those who are likely to respond well to treatment and do not consider the potential consequences of those who have not responded well to previous treatments, and therefore cannot be generalized to the general population.

9.5.4 Healthy User Bias

Healthy user bias is the type of bias that occurs when people who are healthier, more health conscious, and have more access to healthcare are more likely to participate in research or receive certain treatments, resulting in an inaccurate and non-representative sample. It reflects the population of interest. This can lead to biased estimates of exposure-outcome associations and affect the generalizability of study results. For example, studies looking at the effectiveness of a new drug for a particular condition could bias study leads if people who are healthier or have better access to medical care are more likely to participate in the study or receive the drug may occur healthy users. The results of this study are representative only of people who are healthier or have better access to healthcare and do not consider the potential consequences of those who are sicker or have less access to healthcare. It is not possible to generalize to the general population.

9.6 Response Bias

Response bias is a type of bias that occurs when research participants provide inaccurate or misleading information due to factors such as social desirability, memory, or misinterpretation of questions. This can lead to biased estimates of exposure-outcome associations and affect the generalizability of study results. Various biases, including the following, are included in the response bias group.

9.6.1 Common Types of Response Bias

9.6.1.1 Acquiescence Bias

Acquiescence bias is a type of response bias that occurs when survey participants tend to agree or say yes to survey questions. This is regardless of whether you believe the opinion to be true. This can lead to inaccurate responses and biased estimates of exposure-outcome associations. For example, in studies examining the effectiveness of new treatments for disease, participants may say, "I feel better after treatment" or "The treatment is effective" because they want or lack to please the researcher. I tend to agree with statements such as it may lead to acceptance of critical evaluation of treatment.

9.6.1.2 Demand Characteristics

Demand characteristics are research cues or features that can influence participant behavior or responses, leading to biased estimates of exposure-outcome associations. These cues may include study design, question formulation, or researcher behavior. Participants may change their behavior and reactions to try to match the perceived expectations of the researcher or to present themselves in a favorable light. For example, in a study examining the effects of a new treatment for a particular condition, if participants knew they were receiving a new treatment and researchers knew they had high hopes for that treatment, this can influence their behavior and responses.

9.6.1.3 Social Desirability Bias

Social desirability bias is a type of response bias in which people answer questions in ways that others rate them positively. Also occurs when trying to answer a question in a socially acceptable way. In these situations, people are more likely to provide answers that are considered socially acceptable than to provide accurate answers. For example, someone may be more likely to report that they engage in healthy behaviors, such as exercising regularly, than to report that they do not.

9.6.1.4 Courtesy Bias

Courtesy bias is a type of response bias in which people answer questions politely or respectfully instead of correctly. It occurs when people are motivated to answer in a friendly and polite manner, leading them to answer questions in a socially acceptable way rather than truthfully. You are more likely to give a positive answer, even if you do not like it. One way to reduce politeness bias in your survey is to make sure your questions are unambiguous. It is also important to create a safe and comfortable environment in which respondents feel safe and honest. Finally, it is important to ensure that the survey is anonymous so that respondents are not influenced by external factors or social pressures when submitting their responses.

9.6.1.5 Question-Order Bias

Question order bias is a type of answer bias that occurs when the order of questions influences the answer. This is because following certain patterns makes people more likely to give certain answers. For example, if a survey starts with a question about a person's income, they are more likely to answer higher than their actual income. Randomizing the order of questions in a survey is important to reduce question order bias. To reduce bias in question order, it is important not to ask similar questions in a row. Additionally, it is important to avoid asking questions that might influence the answers to subsequent questions. For example, if the survey begins with questions about personal income, it is important not to immediately ask about spending habits. It is also important to make sure your questions are clear and easy to understand so that your respondents are not subject to confusion or misunderstanding.

9.6.1.6 Extreme Responding

An extreme response is a form of reaction bias in which people answer questions in extreme ways. This can occur when people are motivated to provide exaggerated answers, inducing them to answer questions in ways that are more extreme than their true beliefs and opinions, they are more likely to say "strongly agree" or "strongly disagree" than a more neutral response. To reduce extreme responses, it is important to ensure that survey questions are crafted neutrally and have a balance of possible responses.

For example, consider the survey question "How satisfied are you with the product or service you received?". This question does not lead to extreme responses as it allows respondents to be more neutral in their responses.

9.7 Cognitive Bias

Cognitive bias is a type of bias that occurs when people make judgments and decisions based on mental shortcuts and assumptions. This can occur when people rely on their beliefs and experiences instead of evaluating evidence objectively. These include confirmation biases, which are more likely to be accepted, and availability heuristics, which overestimate the likelihood of easily recalled events. Cognitive biases can lead to distorted thinking and inaccurate reasoning. It can also lead to biased decisions, as people are more likely to make decisions based on their beliefs and experiences than on objective evidence. To mitigate cognitive biases, it is important to consider multiple perspectives, recognize your biases and assumptions, and look for evidence that challenges existing beliefs. Cognitive biases can lead to distorted thinking and inaccurate conclusions. It can also lead to biased decisions, as people are more likely to base their decisions on their beliefs and experiences than on objective evidence. To reduce cognitive biases, consider multiple perspectives. It is important to be aware of your biases and assumptions and look for evidence that challenges existing beliefs.

Various biases, including the following, are included in the cognitive bias group.

Some common types of cognitive bias are:

9.7.1 Anchoring Bias

Anchoring bias is a type of cognitive bias in which people rely too much on their first point of reference when making decisions. This can lead to decisions based on first reference points rather than objective evidence. To mitigate anchor bias, it is important to consider multiple perspectives and evidence and recognize your biases and assumptions. For example, if you were asked to estimate the number of traffic injuries in a particular region, you would likely overestimate that number if you were given a higher starting point than the actual number. This can lead to inadequate allocation of resources and a lack of focus on the actual risk factors associated with road traffic injuries. To reduce anchor bias, it is important to consider multiple perspectives and evidence and recognize your biases and assumptions.

9.7.2 Framing Effect

The framing effect is a type of cognitive bias in which people's decisions are influenced by how information is presented. This can happen when people are presented with the same information in different ways and make different decisions based on how the information is organized. For example, a winner and a loser he is more likely to choose the option labeled winner when asked to choose between two options. To mitigate the framing effect, it is important to consider multiple perspectives and evidence and recognize your biases and assumptions. Several strategies can be used to reduce the impact of framing effects.

First, it is important to make sure that the information is presented objectively, without prejudice or prejudice. Thinking from multiple perspectives is also important. That means taking the time to consider all available evidence before making a decision and being prepared to change your mind if new evidence emerges.

9.7.3 Actor-Observer Bias

Actor-observer bias is bias in which we attribute other people's behavior to our personality traits and personalities, and our behavior to external factors. This can lead to distorted thinking and inaccurate conclusions. For example, some people attribute their mistakes to external factors such as bad luck, while others attribute the mistakes of others to their character and personality. To mitigate actor and observer bias, it is important to consider multiple perspectives and evidence and recognize your biases and assumptions.

9.7.4 Availability Heuristic (or Availability Bias)

The availability heuristic is a type of cognitive bias that overestimates the likelihood of events that people can easily recall. This can happen when you rely on your experience or memory rather than evaluating the evidence objectively. For example, if you have recently experienced or heard of a car accident, you are more likely to overestimate your chances of being involved in a car accident. To reduce availability heuristics, it is important to consider multiple perspectives and evidence and recognize your biases and assumptions.

9.7.5 Confirmation Bias

This bias can lead to distorted thinking and inaccurate conclusions. For example, they are more likely to accept evidence that supports their existing beliefs while ignoring evidence that contradicts them. To reduce confirmation bias, it is important to consider multiple perspectives and evidence and recognize your biases and assumptions. Additionally, before making a decision, it is important to take the time to review all available evidence and change your mind if new evidence emerges.

9.7.6 Halo Effect

In this bias, people's overall impression of someone or something influences their judgments and decisions about that person or thing. This can lead to distorted thinking and inaccurate conclusions. For example, people who have an overall positive impression of a person are more likely to agree with that person in all situations. To mitigate the halo effect, it is important to consider multiple perspectives and evidence and recognize your biases and assumptions. Additionally, before making a decision, it is important to take the time to review all available evidence and change your mind if new evidence emerges.

9.7.7 The Baader-Meinhof Phenomenon

The Baader-Meinhof phenomenon is a type of cognitive distortion in which one suddenly becomes aware of something after recently knowing it. This can occur when people are more likely to notice something they have heard or seen recently than to objectively evaluate the evidence. The Baader-Meinhof phenomenon can lead to distorted thinking and inaccurate conclusions. To mitigate the Baader-Meinhof phenomenon, it is important to consider multiple perspectives and evidence and be aware of your biases and assumptions. To mitigate the Baader-Meinhof phenomenon, it is important to consider multiple perspectives and evidence and be aware of your biases and assumptions. Additionally, pay attention to the context of the information presented and avoid making assumptions based solely on recent experience or memory.

9.7.8 Pygmalion Effect

It is a type of cognitive bias in which people's expectations of someone or something influence their behavior and performance. This can occur when you act on given expectations other than objectively evaluating evidence. To mitigate the Pygmalion effect, it is important to consider multiple perspectives and evidence and be aware of your biases and assumptions. Additionally, before making a decision, it is important to take the time to review all available evidence and change your mind if new evidence emerges.

9.8 Misclassification

Information biases lead to misclassification of the exposure or outcome under investigation. For example, when memory bias is created in a case-control study, some exposed individuals are classified in the non-exposed group and some non-exposed individuals are classified in the exposed group. This issue is likely to occur in cohort studies in the form of incorrect diagnosis of the investigated outcome. In such cases, people with complications are considered healthy and people without complications are considered patients.

For example, a study might classify road traffic injuries as minor or severe. However, there may be variability in the classification of severity across different healthcare providers, hospitals, or regions. This can lead to misclassification of the severity of the injury, which can affect the accuracy of the conclusions drawn from the study.

If the misclassification is non-differential, meaning it occurs equally between groups, it may lead to an underestimation of the true effect. On the other hand, if the misclassification is differential, meaning it occurs differently between groups, it may lead to either an overestimation or underestimation of the true effect.

In general, this network has two categories of directed misclassification and undirected misclassification. Non-directional misclassification occurs when the exposure misclassification rate is independent of the outcome categories under study (or vice versa).

Table 9.1 shows a hypothetical example of the effect of undirected misclassification when there are two categories [4]. In this example, exposed members are classified as non-exposed members. In practice, this error probably occurs in both directions. This bias occurs in case-control studies when the sensitivity and specificity of the tests are less than 100%. For this reason, attention to sensitivity and specificity in studies (especially screening studies) can be very useful. Directional misclassification occurs when the amount of misclassification is not the same in the groups being compared. Undirected misclassification generally underestimates the amount of true association between exposure and outcome, but directional misclassification causes bias in both directions.

The effect of this type of bias is shown in Table 9.2.

Identifying and measuring the effect of misclassification bias in medical studies is of great interest. Some studies have shown that this bias can even cause a complete bias of the real relationship between the exposure and the investigated outcome. In cases where the true odds ratio or relative risk is close to 1, the occurrence of non-directional classification bias can completely invalidate the true relationship. For example,

Table 9.1 A hypothetical example of the effect of misclassification without direction for two categories with exposure and without exposure with an error rate of 30%

Exposure	Cases	Controls
Exposed	50	20
Not exposed	50	80
Odds ratio	$\frac{\left(\frac{50}{50}\right)}{\left(\frac{20}{80}\right)} = 4$	
30% error in exposure classification		
Exposed	50 − 15 = 35	20 − 6 = 14
Not exposed	50 + 15 = 65	80 + 6 = 86
Odds ratio	$\frac{\left(\frac{35}{65}\right)}{\left(\frac{14}{86}\right)} = 3.3$	

Table 9.2 Hypothetical example of the effect of directional misclassification on exposure detection in controls in a case-control study when the true odds ratio is 4

Sensitivity	Specificity	Exposure among controls	Observed odds ratio
0.9	0.85	0.2	2.6
0.6	0.85	0.2	1.9
0.9	0.95	0.2	3.2
0.9	0.6	0.2	1.9
0.9	0.9	0.368	3.0
0.9	0.9	0.2	2.8
0.9	0.9	0.077	2.2

when the exposure has a prevalence of 16% and the true odds ratio is 1.3, the incidence of non-directional misclassification bias can show an estimated odds ratio equal to 1 (when the sensitivity and specificity are both equal to 70%). Directional misclassification causes bias in any direction. Usually, data are not available to compare and evaluate classifications; But when there is such a situation, comparisons will be very useful. However, the comparison of samples is not enough in terms of the correctness of classification only in the case of the response variable and should be applied to all the important variables that have potential sources for the occurrence of this type of bias. For example, recording interviews with study subjects is a useful method that makes it possible to review the answers. Evaluating measurement tools, using objective tools to measure exposure and outcome, such as the use of sonography and CT scan devices, make researchers confident about the results. In cases where the sensitivity and specificity of measurement tools are known in advance, it is possible to calculate and report adjusted indices for the relative risk measure (for example, modified risk ratio).

More advanced statistical methods are needed to calculate adjusted indices when outcome assessment and exposure measurement have misclassification errors.

In this part, we will examine biases that are the result of combined errors in selection and information. These biases are more common in studies related to patient monitoring, cross-sectional studies, and screening studies than in other studies.

9.9 Other Types of Biases

9.9.1 Referral to the Center Bias

The reputation or reputation of a medical center may cause certain patients or more serious cases of that disease to visit that center and as a result, it will cause congestion. For example, most cases of severe disease in the cities refer to that center due to the lack of necessary facilities or the centrality of a special treatment center in Tehran. If only the patients referred to that center are examined, the severity of the disease may be overestimated. Such a problem may also occur in patients referred to referral centers. Access to disease diagnosis centers or information about some special diagnosis centers may also cause swelling.

For example, a study might recruit participants who have been injured in a road traffic accident from a specialized trauma center that primarily serves individuals with more severe injuries. This can lead to a biased sample that does not accurately reflect the broader population of individuals who have been injured in road traffic accidents.

9.9.2 Conformity Bias

Conformity bias is a type of cognitive bias in which we are more likely to conform to the beliefs and opinions of others than to objectively assess the evidence. This can lead to distorted thinking and inaccurate conclusions. For example, some people are more likely to accept the majority opinion than to consider another point of view. To reduce fit bias, it is important to consider multiple perspectives and evidence and recognize your biases and assumptions. To reduce conformity bias, it is important to consider multiple perspectives and evidence and recognize your biases and assumptions. This bias can lead to distorted thinking and inaccurate conclusions. For example, they are more likely to accept evidence that supports their existing beliefs while ignoring evidence that contradicts them. To reduce confirmation bias, it is important to consider multiple perspectives and evidence and recognize your biases and assumptions. Additionally, before making a decision, it is important to take the time to review all available evidence and change your mind if new evidence emerges.

9.9.3 Quo Bias

Quo bias is a type of cognitive bias that tends to accept the status quo rather than objectively assess the evidence. This can lead to distorted thinking and inaccurate conclusions. For example, someone is more likely to accept the status quo than consider possible alternatives. To reduce status quo bias, it is important to consider multiple perspectives and evidence and recognize your biases and assumptions. Additionally, before making a decision, it is important to take the time to review all available evidence and change your mind if new evidence emerges.

9.9.4 Sponsor Bias

Sponsor bias is a type of bias in which people's opinions and decisions are influenced by sources of information. This can occur when people are more likely to accept information from sources who have a legitimate interest in the outcome rather than objectively assessing the evidence. Rather than considering your point of view, you are more likely to accept the opinion of the company that makes a particular product.

9.9.5 Affinity Bias

Affinity bias is a type of bias that makes people more likely to accept information from people they have an affinity with than objectively assess the evidence. For example, we are more likely to accept the opinions of family and friends than to consider alternative points of view. To mitigate affinity bias, it is important to consider multiple perspectives and evidence and recognize your biases and assumptions. Several strategies help mitigate the effects of this bias in group decision-making. First, make sure everyone in the group is aware of their biases and assumptions. Additionally, before making a decision, take the time to review all available evidence and change your mind if new evidence emerges.

9.9.6 Ceiling Effect

The ceiling effect makes us more likely to accept the highest possible score than to objectively evaluate the evidence. For example, you are more likely to accept the highest possible estimate for a particular outcome than consider another estimate. To reduce the ceiling effect, it is important to consider multiple perspectives and evidence, and recognize your biases and assumptions. Additionally, before making a decision, it is important to take the time to review all available evidence and change your mind if new evidence emerges. To reduce ceiling effects, ensure that information is presented objectively without bias or spin, consider multiple perspectives and evidence, and be aware of your biases and assumptions. Before making a decision, take the time to review all available evidence and be prepared to change your mind if new evidence emerges.

9.9.7 Recency Bias

In recency bias people are more likely to accept recently presented information than to objectively evaluate evidence. This can lead to distorted thinking and inaccurate conclusions. For example, you are more likely to accept the opinion of a recent speaker or article than to consider another point of view. To mitigate recency bias, it is important to consider multiple perspectives and evidence and recognize your biases and assumptions. Additionally, before making a decision, it is important to take the time to review all available evidence and change your mind if new evidence emerges. Recency bias can affect decision-making several ways. For example, you are more likely to accept the opinion of a recent speaker or article than to consider another point of view. In addition, they tend to recall more recent events and experiences more vividly than past events and experiences. To mitigate recency bias, it is important to consider multiple perspectives and evidence and recognize your biases and assumptions. Before making a decision, take the time to review all available evidence and change your mind if new evidence emerges.

9.9.8 Primacy Bias

In primacy bias, people are more likely to accept the first information they are presented with than to objectively evaluate the evidence. For example, someone is more likely to accept the opinion of the first speaker or article they read than consider another point of view. To reduce dominance bias, it is important to consider multiple perspectives and evidence and recognize your biases and assumptions. Before making a decision, it is important to take the time to review all available evidence and change your mind if new evidence emerges. To become more aware of your biases and assumptions, it is important to take the time to reflect on your beliefs and opinions.

9.9.9 Perception Bias

Perception bias is a type of bias in which people's perception of a situation influences their judgments and decisions. For example, we are more likely to perceive a situation in a particular way than objectively assess the evidence. To reduce perceptual bias, consider multiple perspectives and evidence, and be aware of your biases and assumptions. Also, evaluate all available evidence before making a decision and be prepared to change your mind if new evidence emerges.

9.9.10 Outgroup Bias

Outgroup bias, also known as outgroup discrimination, is when people discriminate between members of their social group ("ingroup") and members of other social groups ("outgroup"). Refers to a phenomenon that tends to be perceived more positively than more negatively.

Out-of-group biases can result from the natural tendency to divide people into groups based on common characteristics such as race, ethnicity, religion, gender, and nationality. When these groups are formed, people can develop a sense of loyalty and connection to the group, which can lead to prejudice against their group and negative attitudes toward other groups. Out-of-group bias can have negative consequences, conflicts, discrimination, and social inequalities between groups. It can also lead to a lack of empathy and understanding for other group members, which can make relationship-building difficult and promote social harmony.

Reducing out-of-group prejudice requires efforts to increase awareness and understanding of different social groups and efforts to promote empathy and positive interactions among members of different groups. This includes education, inter-group outreach, and promoting diversity and inclusion in various settings such as schools, workplaces, and communities.

9.9.11 Optimism Bias

Optimism bias refers to the tendency of people to be overly optimistic about future life events. People estimate that they are less likely to experience negative events and more likely to experience positive events compared to what objective probabilities suggest. For example, we estimate that divorce and unemployment are much less likely. People believe that they are less vulnerable to negative events than others. Consider, for example, that you are less likely to be involved in a car accident than the average driver. Optimistic people tend to make more risky decisions when given objective probabilities. Promotes positive thinking and risk-taking. Optimism is an innate psychological tendency and cannot be easily modified by facts or logic. It persists even when people have optimism and conflicting knowledge. The trend toward optimism has several benefits as it leads to positive expectations, resilience, and motivation. But it can also lead to bad decisions, poor preparation, and undue surprises from negative events. The propensity for optimism varies from person to person but is stronger among young and inexperienced people. However, it does not disappear completely due to age or life experience.

9.9.12 Negativity Bias

Negativity bias refers to people's tendency to pay more attention to negative experiences, information, and aspects of their surroundings. People sometimes tend to pay attention, and remember negative information. For example, we are more likely to remember a rude patient than a friendly one. People perceive negative information as more important, effective, and useful than positive information of equal value. Negative events are seen as more diagnostic of situations and relationships. Negative experiences greatly influence judgment and decision-making. For example, one bad experience at a restaurant can dramatically change your attitude towards that restaurant, while many positive experiences will not affect your opinion much. Negative biases lead to a more pessimistic view of the world, increased unhealthy fears and worries, lower self-esteem, and a tendency to make poorer decisions out of fear of loss or harm. You should manage negativity and cultivate optimism in a balanced and realistic way.

9.9.13 Ingroup Bias

Intragroup bias, also known as an intragroup preference, is a psychological phenomenon in which individuals prefer members of their group to members of other groups. Intragroup biases are ingrained in our evolutionary history, as humans tended to form tight groups for survival. This prejudice can lead to favoritism, discrimination, and even conflict.

Ingroup bias can manifest itself in a variety of ways, including positive rating, allocation of resources, emotional connection, stereotype, and preferred treatment (individuals are more likely to provide support and assistance to in-group members than to members of other groups).

9.9.14 Implicit Bias

Implicit bias refers to attitudes and stereotypes that unconsciously influence our understanding, actions, and decisions. These prejudices, which include both favorable and unfavorable evaluations, are activated unconsciously, without a person's conscious or intentional control. They are everywhere and often contradict stated or stated beliefs. The main characteristics of implicit bias are: They are everywhere and everywhere. They can subconsciously influence our decisions and actions beyond our control. The implicit associations we develop are influenced by factors such as media and news broadcasts, childhood experiences, cultural stereotypes, and other learned associations. Implicit bias can favor some groups over others, leading to unfair treatment and discrimination. But they can also lead to quicker, habitual responses that make everyday interactions easier. Implicit prejudices are malleable and can be "unlearned," giving way to new mental associations. This requires awareness, moral motivation, and practice. The existence of implicit bias challenges the idea that people's judgments and actions are determined solely by explicit belief systems. Recognizing and understanding implicit bias is critical to reducing discrimination and promoting participation in society. But overcoming implicit bias requires conscious and sustained effort.

9.9.15 Hindsight Bias

Hindsight bias, also known as the "know-it-all effect," is the tendency for people to see an event that has already happened as more predictable than it was before it happened. It can also lead to false learning from past experiences. The main characteristics of hindsight errors are: It makes people believe that the consequences they know were inevitable or should have come from the beginning. This makes events look more predictable than they are. People reconstruct the past and reconcile it with what they know to be true in the present. It leads to the statement "I knew a long time ago." People overestimate how well they could have predicted the event. It prevents people from learning from experience effectively. By attributing consequences to what was inevitable or obvious, people fail to understand the real reason an event occurred and miss an opportunity for improvement that is nearly impossible to completely avoid. Even with retroactive recognition of bias, it continues to have a powerful influence on judgments about past events. People often think someone or something should be blamed when a bad outcome seems to have been predicted from the beginning. Hindsight bias poses significant challenges to effective decision-making and learning. Effective strategies for reducing hindsight bias include recognizing it, how it affects your thinking, considering alternative outcomes, and understanding the information available at the time, recording predictions in advance, avoiding blame, and considering multiple players.

9.9.16 Explicit Bias

Explicit bias is a type of cognitive bias in which people are more likely to accept information that is consistent with their preconceived notions than to objectively evaluate the evidence. For example, someone is more likely to accept information that confirms their existing beliefs than to consider alternative points of view. Additionally, before making a decision, it is important to take the time to review all available evidence and change your mind if new evidence emerges. Several strategies are for objectively evaluating evidence. Take your time and review all the evidence. Look for information from multiple sources and consider different perspectives. Ask yourself if you are interpreting the evidence in a way that is influenced by your beliefs. Ask questions and ask for clarification. If anything is unclear, feel free to ask questions and ask for clarification. It is important to consider the circumstances under which the evidence was collected and how it might be interpreted in different circumstances. Look for patterns in the evidence and consider how they are related. Consider alternative explanations of the evidence and how they affect interpretation.

9.9.17 Ideological Bias

Ideological bias refers to a preference or inclination towards a particular political or social belief or value. It can come in many forms, such as the way information is presented or interpreted, and the choice of sources used to support an argument or position. In journalism, ideological bias can lead to selective reporting and shaping of articles that align with particular political or social agendas. In academia, this can lead to the marginalization of certain perspectives and the promotion of certain ideologies. In politics, ideological bias can lead to the adoption of policies that reflect a particular worldview or set of values. It is important to be aware of ideological biases and to strive for objectivity and balance when presenting information and ideas. It also requires a willingness to acknowledge and address your biases and to seek out different sources and opinions. Ideological bias can also arise in biomedical research and can seriously affect the accuracy and objectivity of research results. For example, ideological bias can arise in the choice of research questions and hypotheses. Rather than objectively consider all possibilities, researchers sometimes choose questions and hypotheses that are consistent with their beliefs and the prevailing ideologies in their field. To mitigate ideological bias in biomedical investigation, researchers need to be aware of their biases and to strive for objectivity and transparency in their research. Additionally, peer review and replication of studies can help to minimize the effects of ideological bias by providing independent critiques and validation of research findings.

9.9.18 Partisan Bias

Partisan bias refers to the tendency to favor one political party, ideology, or candidate over another, often leading to the distortion of information and opinions. In politics, partisan bias can lead to a lack of cooperation and compromise, and it can also lead to the promotion of policies that benefit one party or ideology at the expense of others. Partisan bias in the media can cause news and information to be presented in a way that favors one political party or ideology over another. This can occur in both traditional and social media, where news sources and commentary can be selected based on their alignment with a particular partisan point of view. In order to reduce partisan bias, it is important to seek out a variety of sources and critically evaluate the information presented. Additionally, news outlets can seek objectivity in their reporting and commentary, and social media platforms can take steps to reduce the spread of partisan misinformation and propaganda. Biomedical research is also susceptible to bias, which can seriously affect the accuracy and objectivity of research results. Research aligned with particular political party or ideological priorities may be prioritized over other research areas, resulting in less diversity in the types of research conducted. Partisan bias can also influence the interpretation of research results. Researchers may interpret results to support their partisan views or those of political allies, rather than objectively considering all possible interpretations. This can lead to information bias and a lack of consensus on important biomedical issues may foster a culture of scientific rigor and objectivity, and seek to fund and resource a wide variety of research areas and perspectives.

9.9.19 Institutional Bias

Institutional bias refers to practices or policies within an organization that systematically favor certain groups over others, perpetuating inequalities. A key aspect of institutional bias is the lack of diversity in leadership and key decision-making roles. An institutional policy, procedure, or standard that explicitly or implicitly favors one group over another. For example, the clean appearance requirement that some groups prefer. If an institution's culture, language, or values largely reflect one of its groups, while other groups feel like outsiders, they may feel marginalized or have limited access/opportunities. It can lead to a lack of awareness and sensitivity. Institutional leaders and staff may be unaware of their biases and negative impacts on particular groups, or their lack of sensitivity to the issues most important to different groups. Policies that directly or indirectly exclude or disadvantage members of a particular group in areas such as admission, recruitment, promotion, discipline, or resource allocation. Fear of validating negative stereotypes about one's group can undermine performance and access to opportunities. Something that feels exclusive in a secret way. This dynamic, accountability, inclusive policy, diversity initiatives, implicit bias training, continuous reflection, and feedback to reduce institutional bias. Institutional bias can affect the medical field and medical research in many ways. Some examples are the lack of diversity in leadership and key roles. Stereotype threats in healthcare facilities. Lack of sensitivity or awareness. Addressing institutional bias in medicine requires policy review, staff training, attitude reform, data analysis, patient voice, and an inclusive and equitable view of practices, priorities, and cultural norms. Continuous review is required. It is an ongoing process of awareness building, willingness to tackle difficult problems, and real change.

9.9.20 Actor–Observer Bias

This bias refers to situations where respondents attribute internal factors (e.g., bad character) to justify others' behavior and external factors (difficult circumstances) to justify the same behavior in themselves. Actor-observer bias is the psychological phenomenon of attributing one's behavior to external factors while attributing the behavior of other internal factors. In other words, when we observe the behavior of others, we tend to assume that behavior is the result of that person's character and temperament, whereas when evaluating our behavior, we tend to attribute it to situational factors.

For example, if someone is late for a meeting, the delay may be due to traffic jams or other external factors, but if they are late, we can infer that the person is lazy or disorganized.

Actor-observer bias can have important implications for many areas of life, including interpersonal relationships, workplace dynamics, and social interactions.

9.9.21 Perdana (Information)

Perdana bias occurs when the results obtained from a trial are systematically confounded by the knowledge of the intervention that each participant receives. The perception approach may be applied by the person who prescribes the interventions, the person who receives the interventions (participants), the investigator who evaluates and analyzes the results, and even the person who analyzes the results or writes the trial report. The second step after collecting information is when analyzing the data and reporting the results. For example, the people implementing the interventions can create biases in the trial by purposefully (biased) changing the interventions provided to the participants. In addition, if the people responsible for evaluating and reporting the results know which research group the patients are in, they may consciously or unconsciously report the outcomes of the patients receiving the new drug more favorably than the patients in the placebo group. In ideal conditions, detection bias should be reduced by blinding the people implementing the interventions, the recipients of the interventions, and the people responsible for evaluating and reporting the results. In most cases, if the people who are responsible for analyzing or reporting the results of the trial are informed about the treatment groups, the effects of the new intervention will increase. For example, the person responsible for analyzing the trial data can choose the outcomes or time points that show the maximum benefit of the new intervention and ignore the outcomes or time points that show the ineffectiveness or harmfulness of the new intervention. This source of bias can be controlled by keeping the data analysts and those responsible for reporting the trial results unaware of the identity of the study groups.

9.9.22 Bias Accountability

Memory bias and other information biases are usually associated with exposure measurement in case-control studies. But bias in the diagnosis and reporting of the desired outcome or disease usually occurs during the follow-up of the subjects under study (for example, a cohort study). In addition to the possibility of observer bias, there is a possibility of another bias caused by the response of the subjects under study. For example, when collecting data based on the answers given by the subjects under study, such as the frequency of epileptic attacks, response bias is very important. If possible, the information stated by the subjects under study should be controlled using documentary tools such as hospital records. Whenever such a possibility is not available, such as when it is not possible to collect information about events that occur at times other than when the patient is hospitalized, or when it is possible to evaluate it in a laboratory, one of the methods to reduce the burden of responsibility is to collect accurate and detailed information about signs, symptoms, and possible side effects are the desired outcome. This information is an effective help in evaluating the accuracy of the stated information. For example, in a study that measured the occurrence of migraine headaches, apart from the question about the presence of very severe headaches, questions about the presence of dizziness, lightheadedness, and nausea along with headaches were also asked of the people under study [5]. Evaluation of the occurrence of some complications such as angina pectoris and chronic meningitis have standardized questionnaires.

9.9.23 Monitoring (or Diagnosis) of Patients

This bias occurs when subgroups of society are more concerned by the medical team due to the presence of a specific symptom or prognosis. For this reason, they are examined and subjected to paraclinical tests more than other people in society, or their follow-up is long and more accurate. This issue causes a faster and more accurate diagnosis of some complications in these subgroups. This approach is very significant in the case of diseases or exposures such as diabetes, blood pressure, and the use of oral contraceptive pills (OCP), which leads to the continuous and accurate performance of some examinations and tests. For example, since one of the side effects of OCP use is kidney failure, if women who use OCP are examined repeatedly and their creatinine is measured, the risk of OCP use in developing kidney diseases is much more exaggerated than the actual value.

Conducting similar tests and examinations in all subgroups of society, regardless of the exposure status, minimizes this bias in the studies. For this reason, the same, continuous, and planned examinations are performed in large cohort studies for all subjects under study. Another way to minimize this bias in cohort studies is to hide the exposure situation from the team responsible for diagnosing the outcome under investigation. When this method is not applicable, for example, when the study is retrospective (such as case-control studies) using old cases, in the case of subgroups without exposure or prognosis, quality and continuous information about medical records, results of previous tests and examinations, and medical follow-ups should be obtained. For example, when researchers intend to evaluate the effect of hormone therapy in a disease with specific clinical symptoms such as type II diabetes using a case-control study, paying attention to things such as whether all patients have medical insurance or their medical examinations in the past was similar in terms of quality and frequency is very important and necessary. Another noteworthy point is the status of education, education, and social and economic class of the patients as these factors usually have a high relationship with the availability and use of medical care. In general, the surveillance network makes the disease or outcome in some subgroups of society that have a specific exposure or prognosis be diagnosed faster and more often. For this reason, the complication ratio in cohort studies and the chance ratio in case-control studies are higher in these subgroups than in other investigated groups.

9.9.24 Researcher Bias

For instance, a researcher who believes that driver error is the primary cause of road traffic injuries may design a study that focuses solely on driver behavior and may neglect other factors that could contribute to the occurrence of road traffic accidents, such as road design, vehicle safety features, or environmental factors.

This can lead to a biased study design and may limit the scope of the study, leading to incomplete or inaccurate conclusions about the causes of road traffic injuries.

9.9.25 Bankbook Bias

"Bankbook bias" is a term that describes the tendency to judge others based on their financial status rather than their personal qualities and achievements. It refers to the belief that a person's worth is determined by their income and wealth rather than by their character, abilities, and contributions to society. Medical research is often subject to funding sources and financial interests that can affect research planning, conduct, and dissemination.

Bankbook bias can affect the allocation of research funding and resources. More profitable research or research that is in line with the financial interests of funders may be prioritized over other research areas, and diversity in the types of research conducted may be lost. This can limit the scope of research and divert attention to important but less profitable areas.

Bankbook bias can also affect the interpretation and dissemination of research results. Researchers may interpret results to support the financial interests of funders rather than objectively consider all possible interpretations. This can lead to information distortion and a lack of transparency when reporting research results.

To mitigate the effects of bankbook bias in medical research, researchers need to be aware of the potential impact of funding sources and financial interests in research. For example, a study might recruit participants who have been injured in a road traffic accident from a private hospital that primarily serves individuals with higher levels of income or education. This can lead to a biased sample that does not accurately reflect the broader population of individuals who have been injured in road traffic accidents.

9.9.26 Omitted Variable Bias

Omitted variable bias is a statistical phenomenon that occurs when the variable of interest is not included in a statistical model, resulting in distorted estimates of the relationships between variables in the model. In medical research, omitted variable bias can occur when relevant variables are not included in the analysis, leading to inaccurate or incomplete conclusions about the relationship between two or more variables. For example, studies investigating the relationship between a particular drug and health outcomes may experience omitted variable bias when there are associated variables. This may lead to a biased assessment of drug effects on health outcomes, as pre-existing conditions may be confounding factors influencing the relationship between medication and outcome. To mitigate the effects of omitted variable bias in medical research, it is important to carefully consider all relevant variables that may influence the relationships between variables under study. These steps enable researchers to ensure that their results are accurate and reliable and provide a complete picture of the relationships between the variables under investigation.

9.9.27 "I Am an Expert Bias" (Expertise Bias)

"I am expert bias" or "expert bias" means that experts in a particular field of the study compare the accuracy or appropriateness of their judgments or decisions with those of other experts. A potential source of bias in research studies occurs when there is a tendency to overestimate, leading to over-reliance on expert opinion, which can affect the conclusions of the study.

Expert bias should be minimized by implementing rigorous study designs and analytical methods. This includes blinding experts from investigating hypotheses and other information that might influence their judgment. In addition, multiple experts can be consulted to reduce the potential for bias and increase confidence in the research results. For example, in a study investigating the effectiveness of new traffic injury prevention measures, several traffic safety experts were asked during the design stage of the study to ensure that the study was comprehensive and that all relevant factors were considered. You may consult an expert. Additionally, study design can include expert blinding to intervention groups and careful selection of objective, non-interpretable outcome measures.

9.9.28 Monitoring Bias

Bias in monitoring can result from the tendency to make decisions or act based on preconceived notions or stereotypes. In medical research, it is important to be aware of bias to ensure the reliability and accuracy of research results. This can be achieved by designing unbiased experiments and monitoring the data collection process to ensure data are collected in an unbiased manner. Additionally, researchers should be aware of potential sources of bias when interpreting results. Finally, it is important that organizations provide training and resources so that researchers understand the importance of monitoring bias in research. An example of monitoring bias in healthcare is selection bias. Selection bias occurs when researchers select participants who are not representative of the population being studied. To reduce selection bias, researchers should use random sampling methods to ensure that participants are representative of the study population. Furthermore, when selecting participants, researchers should be aware of potential sources of bias and ensure that the criteria used to select participants are not biased.

9.9.29 Berkson Bias

Berkson bias, also known as Berkson's paradox, is a statistical phenomenon that occurs when a study's sample selection process creates an artificial association between two variables. In particular, bias arises when samples are selected from a population based on the absence of one or more variables associated with the outcome of interest.

A hospital accepts patients with diabetes or cancer, but not both. If the researchers looked at the relationship between diabetes and cancer using only this hospital's data, they found that diabetes may actually increase the risk of cancer, but there is a negative correlation between the two diseases. There is a relationship. Named after the statistician Joseph Berkson (1899–1982), who first described it in his 1946 paper, we find a correlation between these biases. It is important to be aware of this bias, especially in observational studies, as it can lead to erroneous conclusions about the true relationship between variables.

A medical researcher is interested in studying the relationship between high blood pressure (hypertension) and diabetes. The researchers decided to recruit study participants from hospitals, but only those admitted with either hypertension or diabetes, not both.

In this case, the researcher inadvertently introduced Burkson's bias into the study. Despite the fact that hypertension and diabetes are known to be closely related in the general population, the researchers excluded patients with both conditions by including only those with hypertension or diabetes. As a result, this study may find that the association between hypertension and diabetes is weaker than it actually is in the general population, or even absent. Can be derived, jeopardizing clinical decision-making and patient care. To avoid Burkson's bias in this setting, researchers were able to include patients with hypertension and diabetes, and those with both conditions, in the study sample.

9.9.30 Language Bias

One type of publication bias is language bias, which indicates that manuscripts are published and published in journals in different languages, depending on the direction of the results obtained. Most studies with positive results are published in English. Researchers in some countries are known to report only positive results. For example, randomized clinical trials evaluating the efficacy of acupuncture were conducted in China, Japan, Hong Kong, and Taiwan. For example, a systematic review can assess the effectiveness of different interventions to reduce the incidence of road traffic injuries. However, if the review includes only studies published in English, studies conducted in other languages that may contain important results or finding relevant to the review may be excluded.

9.9.31 Bias Caused by Time Delay

This bias caused by time lags can occur when the variable under investigation changes between the time of data collection and analysis. For example, in a longitudinal study tracking disease progression, changes in the health status of participants may occur between the time data is collected and analyzed. These changes can introduce bias into the study, as data collected at different time points may no longer represent the true relationship between the variables studied. In general, it seems that the publication of trials with negative results takes twice as long as positive results. Also, the studies conducted on this bias show that the trial after completion may take years to be presented and published. So that the time spent on completing the trial is equal to the time spent on publication.

9.9.32 Lead-Time Bias

Lead-time bias is a type of bias that occurs in medical research, especially in screening and early detection programs. This occurs when the disease is detected earlier than without a screening program and increases survival without improving a patient's overall survival.

For example, screening programs for certain types of cancer may detect some cancers earlier than they would without the screening program. These cases can be treated earlier and survive longer than those detected later due to treatment. Lead-time bias may be of concern in health screenings as it may overestimate the benefits of screening or early detection programs. To mitigate the impact of her bias, researchers should carefully consider the timing of disease detection and patient overall survival, given the impact of early detection and treatment on overall survival. Furthermore, when analyzing research results, it is important to use appropriate statistical techniques to correct the effects of lead-time bias.

Overall, lead time is an important consideration in medical research, especially in screening and early detection programs, and researchers should seek to minimize its impact to ensure results are accurate and reliable. Measures must be taken.

Several statistical methods that can be used to correct lead-time bias in medical examinations. Some of them are:

Use the "date of diagnosis" as the starting point for survival analysis, using compare groups, use of modeling techniques, and using time-to-event analysis such as Cox proportional hazards regression. For example, a study might compare the survival rates of individuals who have been injured in road traffic accidents before and after the implementation of a new emergency response system that reduces response times. The study may find that the survival rate has increased after the implementation of the system.

However, this apparent increase in survival time may be since the individuals are being treated earlier in the course of their injury, rather than to any actual improvement in the treatment or cure of the injury. This can result in a biased conclusion about the effectiveness of the new emergency response system.

9.9.33 Time Lag Bias

Time-lag bias is a type of bias that occurs in medical or epidemiological studies when there is a time lag between exposure to a risk factor and the onset of the associated disease or outcome. This can lead to inaccurate or incomplete conclusions about the relationship between risk factors and disease or outcome.

Time-lag bias can occur if the time from exposure to outcome is not taken into account or is not sufficiently considered in the study design or analysis. For example, in studies examining the association between smoking and lung cancer, it may take years or decades for the effects of smoking to become apparent, but time-lag bias exists when results are measured soon after quitting. There is a possibility. Smoking.

To mitigate the effects of lag bias in medical research, it is important to carefully consider the timing and outcome of exposures when planning studies. This can be achieved through longitudinal study designs that follow exposures and outcomes over time, and through the use of appropriate statistical methods to account for the effects of time lags.

In addition, it is important to consider potential confounding factors that may be associated with exposure and outcome and control for these factors in study design and analysis. In this way, researchers can ensure that their results are accurate and reliable, and gain a clear understanding of the true relationship between risk factors and disease or outcome.

Several statistical methods can be used to describe the effects of time delays in health examinations. These include time-lagged exposure analysis, time-dependent covariate analysis, propensity score matching, and structural equation modeling. The choice of statistical method depends on the specific study design and the type of data to be analyzed. It is important to carefully consider the timing and outcome of exposures and use appropriate statistical techniques to account for the effects of time lags to ensure that research results are accurate and reliable.

9.9.34 Extraordinary Power Draw

This bias occurs in journalists (and an increasing number of Internet publishers) who deliberately (and biasedly) select, amplify, and publish studies based on biased results. This problem can arise, for example, when journalists try to draw public attention to research that claims the beneficial effects of new interventions for terminal illnesses. Abnormal power consumption can be a problem in medical examinations, especially when using electrical equipment such as imaging equipment and surgical instruments. These devices can consume abnormal amounts of power for short or long periods, which can cause problems such as equipment failure, power surges, or electrical disturbances.

To mitigate the effects of abnormal power consumption during health checks, it is important to properly maintain and inspect all electrical equipment to ensure that it is used within recommended power limits. This may include regular calibration of imaging equipment, replacement of worn or damaged components, and ensuring electrical equipment is properly grounded and connected. The bias of prestigious journal occurs when the results of studies published in a well-known magazine are magnified.

9.9.35 The Bias of the Unpopular Journals

Unpopular journal bias is a type of publication bias that occurs when research studies with negative or zero results are unlikely to be published in academic journals. This may lead to an over-representation of positive results in the published literature and may distort our overall understanding of the relationships between the variables under investigation.

Less popular journals are journals that are less well-known or have a lower impact factor than popular journals in a particular field. Because these journals may have a lower readership and reach, authors are more likely to submit negative results or you are less likely to submit zero results.

To mitigate the bias of unpopular journals, it is important to encourage the publication of all research regardless of the direction or strength of the findings. This can be achieved by implementing policies and initiatives that encourage open-access publication, pre-registration of research protocols, and publication of negative or invalid results.

9.9.36 Famous (Prominent) Author Bias

This bias occurs when the results of studies published by famous authors are magnified. Prominent author bias means that research written by prominent researchers or prominent researchers is more likely to be published in journals or cited in subsequent research, regardless of the quality or relevance of the study. It is a type of publication bias that occurs in some cases.

Famous author bias can arise for a variety of reasons, including the author's standing and influence in academia, the perceived importance of the research topic, or the perceived novelty or innovation of the research results. This bias can lead to over-emphasis on particular researchers or findings, distorting our overall understanding of the relationships between the variables studied.

To mitigate the effects of well-known author bias, it is important to evaluate research studies based on their quality, relevance, and academic merit rather than on the author's reputation or influence. This can be achieved by conducting a rigorous peer review process, evaluating research studies using transparent and objective criteria, and publishing negative or zero results. Additionally, it is important to encourage and support the publication of research researchers from diverse backgrounds, with varying levels of experience and influence.

9.9.37 Famous Institute Bias

Similar to prominent (famous) author bias, this occurs when the results of research published by a well-known institution are magnified. It can also refer to the tendency of researchers associated with a particular institution or organization to prefer findings or results that are relevant to that institution's interests or agenda. This undermines the objectivity of the study and can unwittingly introduce subtle biases. To combat institutional bias, research must be conducted and evaluated by stakeholders who have no personal interest in the results. Truly independent peer review, repetition of studies, and consideration of conflicting results and evidence also help limit the impact of these trends toward subtly biased results. However, institutional biases are likely to persist, at least to some extent, so a critical analysis of the incentives and assumptions behind the research is always warranted. A classic example of institute bias is the tobacco industry researchers in the mid-twentieth century finding that smoking does not cause cancer or other health issues. The researchers had a clear incentive to produce findings favorable to the industry that employed them.[1]

[1]World Health Organization. (2008). WHO Report on the Global Tobacco Epidemic, 2008: The MPOWER Package. Geneva: World Health Organization.

9.9.38 Unknown Institute Bias

Sometimes the important findings of an unknown or famous institution may be ignored and considered unimportant or unimportant by a source or scientific journal. This bias causes the scientific community to be deprived of the important results of a study. It also happens when the results of published studies from unknown or unreputable institutions are purposefully (biased) underestimated. Unknown institute bias can be difficult to identify because it involves biases that are not commonly known or acknowledged.

9.9.39 Small Trial Bias

Sometimes the results of trials with small samples are underestimated, especially when it contradicts the reader's opinion. For example, attributing the possibility of any meaningful or clinical effect found in a small trial to chance, or considering the lack of meaningful results to be due to a reduction in study power. This bias is a kind of publication bias. Small research biases can be caused by a variety of factors, including the preference of journal editors and reviewers for studies with statistically significant results, or the tendency of researchers to selectively report only positive results. This bias can have serious implications for clinical decision-making, as it can lead to the adoption of ineffective or even harmful treatments and interventions. To address small study biases, researchers and clinicians can use systematic reviews and meta-analyses to summarize findings from multiple studies on a given topic. This allows a more comprehensive and accurate estimate of the effect size of a particular intervention or treatment and serves as a guide for evidence-based practice.

9.9.40 Geographical Bias

Geographical bias occurs when research is exaggerated or underestimated according to the country or region in which it was conducted. Geographic bias can seriously affect the generalizability and validity of research results and the fairness and effectiveness of decision-making processes. To counteract geographic bias, consider the diversity of the subject populations studied or affected, and ensure that research and decision-making processes incorporate and are representative of a wide range of perspectives and experiences. is important. An example of geographic bias is a study of the effectiveness of a particular medical treatment conducted in an affluent urban area and only included participants from that area. The results of this study may not be generalizable to other populations such as individuals living in rural or low-income areas who have different access to healthcare and may have different health outcomes.

9.9.41 Unconscious Bias

Unconscious prejudices refer to prejudices that we do not know about or that we have consciously about certain groups of people or certain traits. These prejudices are often rooted and ingrained in stereotypes formed through our experiences, upbringing, and cultural background.

Unconscious bias manifests itself in many ways. How we respect and interact with others, the choices we make, the assumptions we make. For example, people may unconsciously associate certain traits with certain genders or races, leading to biased evaluations of people based on those traits. Unconscious bias can have serious consequences in many areas of life, including education, healthcare, employment, and the criminal justice system. This can lead to discrimination, prejudice, and inequality, as well as missed opportunities and a lack of diversity and inclusion.

To reduce the impact of unconscious bias, it is important to raise awareness of the problem and proactively identify and challenge your bias. This can be achieved through education, training, reflection, and the implementation of policies and initiatives that promote diversity, equity, and inclusion. Additionally, it is important to foster a culture of openness, respect, and empathy, and to actively seek out diverse perspectives and experiences in all areas.

Oversampling technique collects more data than is needed for the study and uses statistical techniques to identify and remove data bias. To reduce bias, it is important to consider multiple perspectives and evidence and recognize your biases and assumptions. Additionally, before making a decision, it is important to take the time to review all available evidence and change your mind if new evidence emerges. Oversampling is a useful tool for reducing the effects of bias in data collection but could be expensive and take more time. To ensure that the data are representative of the population under study, it is important to collect data from a variety of sources and use statistical techniques to identify and remove bias. Finally, it is important to take the time to review all available evidence before making a decision and be prepared to change your mind if new evidence emerges.

9.10 Common Biases Associated with Case-Control and Cohort Studies

In general, almost all the biases that we deal with in the studies are classified into two categories: selection bias and information bias.

9.10.1 Selection Bias

This bias occurs when the people under study have different selection probabilities according to the parameter under study. For example, as seen in Fig. 9.1, cases with exposure have a higher probability of being selected. One of the clear examples of this type of deviation is monitoring bias. For example, when a case-control study is designed to evaluate the relationship between the use of oral contraceptive pills (OCP) and any disease with significant clinical symptoms, such as diabetes, any clinical symptoms caused by the disease in women using OCPs are faster and on

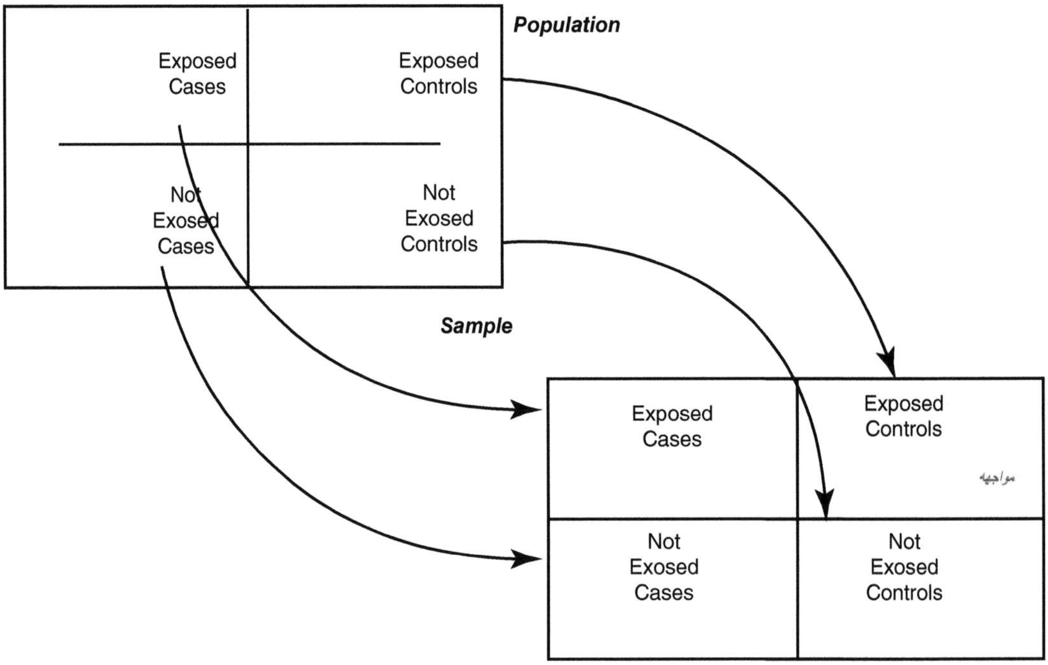

Fig. 9.1 Selection bias: One of the groups investigated in the study (in this case, exposed cases) has a higher probability of being selected and included in the study

average more frequent than the rest because these people are more often under medical examination. This makes it possible that there is a strong relationship between OCP consumption and diabetes.

Selection bias occurs when the diagnosis of the people under study is in a way that systematic errors (estimates less or more than reality) the relationship between the exposure and the event under investigation. In case-control studies, the way cases and controls are identified, and in cohort studies, the presence or absence of exposure are the sources of this bias. Especially in case-control studies related to the selection of hospitalized patients, selection bias is Berkson bias. Tables 9.3, 9.4, 9.5 and 9.6 are devoted to the study of the effect of this theory in a hypothetical case-control study.

Conclusion: The exposure chance and the exposure odds ratio are biasless.

Conclusion: The chance of exposure is in the cases with bias and in the controls without bias. In total, the chances of exposure are the ratio of the chances of having a bias.

Table 9.3 Hypothetical case-control study where all eligible cases and controls have been investigated (there is no information bias and confounding factor in this study)

Population	Risk factor	Cases	Controls
	Yes	500	1800
	No	500	7200
	Total	1000	9000
	Odds of exposure	$\frac{500}{500}=1$	$\frac{1800}{7200}=1.4$
	Odds ratio	$\frac{\left(\frac{500}{500}\right)}{\left(\frac{1800}{7200}\right)}=4$	

Conclusion: The chances of exposure of cases and controls have its bias, but the odds ratio remains the same without its bias.

In Table 9.3, all the real cases and controls in the reference population of 10,000 people have been examined in the case-control study. For this reason, Table 9.3 presents the actual results that can be used as a standard reference.

In Table 9.4, a sample without selection bias is taken from the reference table. The sample taken

Table 9.4 Hypothetical case-control study that was selected based on a random sample of 50% of cases and 10% of community controls introduced in Table 9.3

Sample	Risk factor	Cases 50%	Controls 10%
	Yes	250	180
	No	250	720
	Total	$1000 \times 0.5 = 500$	$9000 \times 0.1 = 900$
	Odds of exposure	$\frac{250}{250} = 1$	$\frac{180}{720} = 0.25$
	Odds ratio	$\frac{\left(\frac{250}{250}\right)}{\left(\frac{180}{720}\right)} = 4$	

Table 9.5 Case-control study despite selection bias. In this study, 50% of cases and 10% of community controls were sampled

Sample	Risk factor	Cases	Controls
	Yes	$500 \times 0.6 = 300$	180
	No	$500 \times 0.4 = 200$	720
	Total	$1000 \times 0.5 = 500$	$9000 \times 0.1 = 900$
	Odds of exposure	$\frac{300}{200} = 1.5$	$\frac{180}{720} = 0.25$
	Odds ratio	$\frac{\left(\frac{300}{200}\right)}{\left(\frac{180}{720}\right)} = 6$	

is a combination of 50% of the cases and 10% of the controls of the whole society. Unscreened sampling allows the exposure probability and calculated odds ratio to evaluate the disease risk factor without screening. Tables 9.5 and 9.6 show the effect of selection bias on the relationship between risk factors and disease.

In Table 9.5, due to the researcher's carelessness in selecting the cases, the study has bias. In this example, as in the example in Table 9.4, the researcher has selected a sample containing 50% of the cases; But the proportion of cases with exposure is more than cases without exposure. In the example in Table 9.6, selection bias exists equally in cases and controls. For this reason, the chances of exposure in cases and controls have nets, but the odds ratio remains without nets.

One of the ways to remove the bias effect caused by differences between groups is to try to spread the bias equally among the groups under study. For example, in retrospective case-control studies, the selection conditions of cases and controls should be completely similar. In case-control studies, the best way to select a control group is to use controls who have participated in a screening program. For example, if women who participated in the breast cancer screening program and were diagnosed (cases) are compared with those who were diagnosed as healthy (controls), because the controls are as exposed to risk factors as the cases, such as a positive family history, old age, and other risk factors, there is less bias than if we choose the control group from the normal people of society. The hypothetical example shin Table 9.6 shows this. In this example as well, bias is the same in both case and control groups. For this reason, even though the chances of encountering a net, the odds ratio remains the same without a net. In this example, the selection bias is the same in cases and controls. This issue compensates for bias.

Table 9.6 Case-control study despite the selection bias, a sample of 50% of the cases and 10% of the controls of the population introduced in Table 9.3 was taken. In this study, cases and controls have the same selection bias

Sample	Risk factor	Cases	Controls
	Yes	$500 \times 0.6 = 300$	$1800 \times 0.136 = 245$
	No	$500 \times 0.4 = 200$	$7200 \times 0.091 = 655$
	Total	$1000 \times 0.5 = 500$	$9000 \times 0.1 = 900$
	Odds of exposure	$\frac{300}{200} = 1.5$	$\frac{245}{655} = 0.374$
	Odds ratio	$\frac{\left(\frac{300}{200}\right)}{\left(\frac{245}{655}\right)} = 4$	

$$\text{Bias} = \frac{\text{Chance to choose cases}}{\text{Real chance to choose cases}} = \frac{\frac{1.5}{1}}{\frac{1}{1}} = \frac{\text{Chance to choose controls}}{\text{Real chance to choose controls}} = \frac{(1/2.67)}{(1/4)} = 1.5$$

To compensate for the balanced bias, there must be the same sources of bias in both groups under comparison. In this case, it can be argued as follows:

$$\text{Real odds ratio}\left(\text{without bias}\right) = \frac{\text{Odds for Cases} \times \text{Bias}}{\text{Odds for Controls} \times \text{Bias}} = \frac{\text{Odds for Cases}}{\text{Odds for Controls}} = \text{Real Odds ratio witout bias}$$

In the example of Table 9.6:

$$\text{Odds ratio} = \frac{\left(\frac{1}{1}\right) \times 1.5}{\left(\frac{1}{4}\right) \times 1.5} = \frac{\left(\frac{1.5}{1}\right)}{\left(\frac{1}{2.67}\right)} = 4$$

In practice, it is very difficult to ensure the compensation of bias in the compared groups. For example, in a study that was conducted to evaluate the relationship between coffee consumption and pancreatic cancer, to adjust the bias in the group of cases (pancreatic cancer patients) and controls (other patients of the same hospital), the same medical team asked them about the level of exposure, i.e., coffee consumption. However, a very important point in this study was not paying attention to the fact that pancreatic cancer patients usually suffer from indigestion, and the treating doctors recommend they consume less coffee. For this reason, the efforts of the researchers to compensate for the bias led to a control group that consumed much less coffee than the real average of society [6]. This issue led to the observation of a positive and strong relationship between coffee consumption and pancreatic cancer. The relationship observed in subsequent studies was not confirmed.

All the examples mentioned in this section were related to case-control studies because the results of this type of study and cross-sectional study are very sensitive to selection bias. In cohort studies, the outcome is created after selecting the subjects under study, i.e., exposed and non-exposed groups, and in clinical trials, the outcome is created after the randomization of patients [7, 8]. For this reason, it does not seem that the method of selecting the sample members has many effects on the observed relationships.

In these studies, the important point is the creation of bias caused by missing cases or those with short-term follow-up in some groups under study [9].

9.10.2 Observer Bias

In cohort studies, it is possible to decide the occurrence of the investigated outcome under the influence of awareness of the exposure status of the people under study. This problem is much more serious when the diagnosis of the intended outcome is somewhat ambiguous, such as migraine attacks, hearing loss or mental illness. However, the occurrence of observer bias is also possible in different stages of outcome diagnosis, which includes pathological and clinical diagnoses. For example, to diagnose cirrhosis of the liver due to alcohol consumption with the help of histological examination of samples, if the pathologist is aware of the addiction or lack of addiction of the subjects under study to alcohol, this issue is considered as one of the potential sources of observer bias. One of the documented examples in this field is a study in which the size of the observer's bias was investigated due to knowing the race of the patients in the diagnosis of advanced renal disease caused by high blood pressure (HSRD). In this study, the medical history of seven patients was referred to a group of kidney specialists. In these cases, the race of the patients was randomly mentioned as black or white. Finally, the chance of diagnosing the disease in black people was twice the chance of being diagnosed in white patients [10]. As mentioned in this section, when the diagnosis of the disease and the knowledge of the exposure situation are not independent, the bias of the observer occurs. For this reason, from a theoretical point of view, if the observer is unaware of the history of exposure (blind), the observer bias will not be created. In cases where blinding is not possible, using two or more observers for diagnosis is one of the appropriate strategies to reduce this bias.

9.11 Common Biases Associated with Cross-sectional Studies

The biases related to cross-sectional studies are divided into two groups: the bias of using incidence instead of prevalence, and the bias of priority of consequence overexposure. One of the common biases in cross-sectional studies is the use of prevalence estimates from these studies to calculate the relative risk. The following relationship exists between the prevalence, occurrence, and duration of the disease.

$$\text{Duration of disease} \times \text{Incidence} = \frac{\text{Prevalence}}{1 - \text{Prevalence}}$$

This relationship can also be shown in this way:

$$(\text{Prevalence} - 1) \times \text{Duration of disease} \times \text{Incidence} = \text{prevalence}$$

In this way, apart from the incidence and duration of the disease, the prevalence is also related to the term (prevalence − 1). This issue in cross-sectional studies causes the relative prevalence, a function of the ratio of the incidence in the exposure group (indicated by the + sign) to the incidence in the non-exposure group (indicated by the − sign) and the ratio of the duration of the disease in the exposure group to the group without exposure and the ratio of the expression (prevalence −1) in the groups with exposure and without exposure means:

$$\text{Prevalence ratio} = \frac{\text{Incidence}+}{\text{Incidence}-} \times \frac{\text{Duration of disease}+}{\text{Duration of disease}-} \times \frac{(1 - \text{Prevalence}+)}{(1 - \text{Prevalence}-)}$$

Ratios 2 and 3 cause the creation of two types of correlation with the names of the correlation coefficient of disease period and correlation coefficient of prevalence.

9.11.1 The Bias of the Disease Period

This bias is a special type of bias. When the relative prevalence obtained from a cross-sectional study is used as an index to show the degree of dependence between exposure and disease, while the course of the disease is not the same in two groups with exposure and without exposure, bias of the course of the disease occurs. Because the length of the disease period in chronic diseases is often related to the survival time of the patients, this bias is sometimes called the bias of survival. When the disease under investigation is rare and the duration of the disease is the same in both groups, the relative prevalence is an almost unbiased estimate of the relative incidence rate; but when the exposure changes the duration of the disease, the results are distorted.

9.11.2 The Bias of the Complementary Ratio of Prevalence

When the length of the disease period is independent of the exposure, the relative prevalence rate causes an estimate to be lower than the actual value of the relationship between the exposure and the outcome under investigation (it causes the estimate of the relative prevalence rate to lean towards 1). The size of this bias depends on the relative prevalence and prevalence in two groups with exposure and without exposure. When the prevalence is higher in the exposure group, the complementary ratio of prevalence is less than 1. This ratio becomes close to 1 when the prevalence is rare in both groups. For example, if the prevalence of a disease in the group with exposure is 0.04 and in the group without exposure is 0.01, the relative prevalence is equal to $\frac{0.04}{0.01} = 4$ and the bias caused by the complementary ratio of prevalence can be neglected ($\frac{0.96}{0.99} = 0.97$). On the other hand, when the prevalence in the exposed group is relatively high, the complementary ratio of the prevalence and the swelling caused by it will be important. For example, if the prevalence of the disease in the exposed group is 0.4 and in the non-exposed group is 0.1, the relative prevalence is the same as the previous example, but the complementary ratio of the prevalence is equal to $\frac{0/6}{0/9} = 0/67$. In this case, estimating the relative incidence using relative prevalence causes the relative incidence to be estimated at 33% less than the actual value.

9.11.3 Precedence of Consequences Overexposure

This type of bias occurs when the time sequence necessary to establish a causal relationship is not considered in the study. This type of bias occurs more in studies that collected exposure and outcome at the same time. For example, from observing an artificial relationship between high blood pressure and high creatinine, it is possible to infer that high blood pressure causes an increase in creatinine or vice versa; however, conducting a prospective study on people with high blood pressure with normal creatinine levels showed that high blood pressure is one of the predictors of creatinine levels and ultimately kidney disease [11].

9.12 Common Biases Associated with Clinical Trials

The design of a trial can happen in the stages of planning, selecting participants, implementing interventions, measuring outcomes and analyzing data, interpreting and reporting results, and publishing study results. Bias may occur even when one is reading the report of a trial [12].

The main reason for investigating, revealing, measuring, and controlling the bias is the fact that the real effects of any intervention are unknown. The overall goal is to provide results in a way that can be generalized to the entire target population. It is impossible to be sure of the presence or absence of bias in the results of a research because it is impossible to prove the systematic deviation of the research results from the unreality.

A large number of potential sources of bias have been identified over the years. The discussion of bias is traditionally focused on biases that can occur at any stage of the implementation of a trial, from the selection of participants in research groups to the implementation of interventions, outcome measurement, interpretation, and reporting of results.

Imagine that a new drug to treat MS has achieved promising results in animal studies and phase I trials. These results have that the drug is capable of delaying the onset of severe movement disorder in the patient, and it has been widely advertised in the media over the past 3 months. As a result of these findings, patient groups have put pressure on the government to make the new medicine available to patients as soon as possible. Considering that MS is a debilitating disease that affects millions of people in the world and considering that there is no secure for it, the investigators (all doctors who have been in contact with MS patients for years), the company making the new drug (which has spent a lot of resources perfecting the drug) and the media (which is interested in confirming the widely advertised drug) are all interested in finding effective results in new combinations. After holding discussion sessions on the treatment course, the government formed a multicenter working group including consumer representatives and agreed to conduct the next stage in the form of a randomized clinical trial. A research agreement is prepared by another special group of reviewers and consumers, and a well-research group at a large healthcare center is selected to conduct the study.

The elements of this hypothetical scenario will be explained in the following sections according to the biases that may be created during the trial.

9.12.1 Other Biases in Clinical Trials

9.12.1.1 Placebo Effect

The placebo effect is the phenomenon in which patients perceive improvement in their symptoms and well-being after receiving a treatment that has no positive therapeutic effect. The placebo effect is often attributed to the patient's belief in the effectiveness of the treatment rather than to the actual biological or physiological effects of the treatment itself.

Placebo effects can occur in a variety of settings, such as clinical trials, where patients perceive improvement in symptoms after administering a placebo instead of an active drug. The placebo effect can also occur in clinical settings, patient experiences symptomatic improvement after receiving non-aggressive treatments such as sugar pills or saline injections.

The placebo effect is a complex phenomenon, not fully understood, but thought to involve a combination of psychological, neurological, and social factors. For example, the patient's expectations, beliefs, and emotions can influence the placebo effect, as can the patient's relationship with the provider and the social and cultural context in which the treatment is provided.

To mitigate the impact of placebo effects in medical research, it is important to use appropriate control groups and study designs that help isolate the specific effects of the treatment under study. Additionally, researchers can use blinding and randomization techniques to minimize the impact of patient expectations and beliefs on study outcomes. These steps ensure that researchers have accurate, reliable results and a clear understanding of the true effects of the treatment being studied.

9.12.1.2 Tarmac bias

Tarmac bias is a term used to describe a potential source of bias in clinical research studies that arise when patients who are sicker or have more severe medical conditions are more likely to be hospitalized and enrolled in the study during their wait in the emergency room (i.e., while waiting on the tarmac). This can lead to an over-representation of patients with more severe diseases in the study sample and impair the generalizability of the study results. For example, in a study examining the effectiveness of a new intervention to treat traffic injuries, patients who are more severely injured might be more likely to be hospitalized and enrolled in the study while waiting on the tarmac rather than being treated on the tarmac accident site or in outpatient treatment. This can lead to an over-representation of patients with more severe injuries in the study sample and impair the generalizability of the study results.

9.12.1.3 Bias Caused by Insufficient Reviews of Withdrawals and Proposal Rejections

Ideally, all participants in a trial should complete the study, follow the research protocol, and provide information on desired outcomes at all time points; But in practice, trials have missing data. The lack of data may be due to the withdrawal of participants before the end of the trial or failure to follow the research protocol consciously or accidentally, and incorrect measurement of some outcomes at one or more time points. Regardless of the cause, improper handling of missing data can lead to bias. For example, if in the MS trial, patients for whom the new drug was not useful due to harmful side effects, often withdraw from the study, due to their absence, the beneficial effects of the new drug will increase and its side effect will be to be less than the actual value.

9.12.1.4 Publication Bias

Some evidence shows the tendency of the reviewers, those responsible for compiling and presenting the article, the group of critics, and editors to accept manuscripts for publication in which trials with positive results have been reported [13]. What is publication bias in meta-analysis? Many studies are conducted in different parts of the world, but their results are not published for various reasons, or at least they may be published in non-indexed journals. The existence of significant differences increases the possibility of publishing the article. The non-printing of articles without meaningful results is called a file-drawer. The meta-analysis results of these articles have a systematic error called publication bias. So, publication bias means that a meta-analysis does not include all studies. In case of publication bias, meta-analysis results will be overestimated.

9.13 Common Biases Associated with Ecological Studies

Ecological studies have limitations and potential biases that must be carefully considered when interpreting research results. Researchers should carefully select study populations, consider confounding variables, and use appropriate statistical techniques to minimize the effects of bias on study results.

Ecological studies are a type of observational study that examines exposure-outcome relationships at the group or population level rather than at the individual level. Some common prejudices associated with ecological research include the following ones.

Ecological fallacy This happens when inferences are made about individuals based on group-level data. For example, if environmental studies found that populations with higher levels of air pollution had higher rates of respiratory disease, it would not be reasonable to assume that all individuals within those populations are at higher risk.

An example of an ecological fallacy in studies of traffic injuries is when ecological studies find that populations living in high-traffic areas have a higher incidence of traffic injuries. It is a mistake to assume that all individuals living in these areas are at increased risk of road traffic injuries, because the relationships observed at the group level do not necessarily apply to all individuals [14].

To minimize ecological bias in road traffic injury studies, researchers sometimes use individual-level data whenever possible, rather than relying solely on group-level data. Individual-level data allow more accurate and accurate estimates of exposure-outcome relationships and help minimize the potential for bias and error associated with group-level data. For example, studies examining the effectiveness of new interventions to prevent injuries from road traffic accidents use individual-level data to estimate the impact of the intervention on each participant, rather than relying solely on aggregated group-level data. May be evaluated. This helps minimize the potential for ecological fallacy and ensures that research results accurately reflect the target population.

Confounding Confounding is a potential source of bias in ecological studies that can occur when exposure-outcome associations are influenced by a third variable that relates to both exposures and outcomes. Confusion can arise in ecological studies when different populations have different underlying traits that influence both exposures and study outcomes.

For example, ecological studies examining the relationship between traffic density and traffic injuries find that people living in densely populated urban areas have a higher incidence of traffic injuries. However, this relationship can be confounded by other factors related to both traffic density and road injuries, such as age, gender, socioeconomic status, and access to healthcare.

To control for confounding in ecological studies, researchers can use statistical techniques such as multivariable regression analysis to adjust for the effects of potential confounding variables. Additionally, researchers can carefully select study populations to ensure they are comparable concerning potential confounding variables.

Temporal bias Temporal bias is a potential source of bias in ecological studies that occurs when exposure timing and outcomes are not adequately accounted for. In ecological studies, this can occur when data on both exposure and outcome are aggregated over time, making it difficult to establish a temporal relationship between the two.

For example, ecological studies examining the link between air pollution and respiratory disease find that people living in areas with high levels of air pollution are more likely to suffer from respiratory disease. However, this relationship can be disrupted by transient factors such as changes in air pollution over time, changes in respiratory disease diagnoses or reports, and demographic changes.

To control for temporal bias in ecological studies, researchers can use time series analysis to examine the relationship between exposure and outcome over time. This helps establish temporal relationships between exposures and outcomes and controls for temporal factors that may be related to both.

For example, in a study examining the relationship between air pollution and respiratory disease, researchers used time-series analysis to account for temporal factors such as changes in air pollution, and changes in air pollution over time. Relationships between levels and incidence of respiratory disease can be examined.

Measurement bias In ecological studies, this can occur when data are aggregated or averaged across groups, which can obscure within-group variability. Measurement bias is a potential source of bias in ecological research that occurs when exposure or outcome measurements are subject to error or misclassification. In ecological studies, this can occur when data are aggregated or averaged across groups, which can obscure within-group variability.

For example, in ecological studies investigating associations between air pollution and respiratory disease, air pollution can be measured at several fixed measurement stations in a city and averaged across the population. This approach may not take into account differences in air pollution levels within cities, such as differences in air pollution in different parts of a city or differences in exposure due to proximity to major roads or industrial sites.

To control measurement bias in ecological studies, researchers can use more detailed and accurate exposure and outcome measures. For example, in the air pollution and respiratory disease example, researchers can use more advanced air pollution monitoring techniques such as satellite remote sensing and mobile surveillance to understand spatial and temporal variations in air pollution.

Additionally, researchers can use individual-level data whenever possible, rather than relying solely on group-level data. Individual-level data allow more accurate and accurate estimates of exposure-outcome relationships and help minimize the potential for bias and error associated with group-level data.

Selection bias Selection bias occurs when the study population selection is not representative of the wider population of interest. In ecological studies, this can occur when populations are selected for convenience or availability rather than being representative of the wider population.

For example, in ecological studies investigating the relationship between traffic density and road injury, researchers can choose easily accessible study populations, such as road injury risk.

To control selection bias in ecological studies, researchers can use sampling techniques to ensure that the study population is representative of the broader target population. In the traffic density and road traffic injuries, for example, researchers used random sampling to select study participants from different neighborhoods or regions within a city, ensuring that the study population is representative of the wider population. In addition, researchers can use statistical techniques such as propensity score matching to control for potential confounding variables and allow study groups to compare important traits.

9.14 Bias in Qualitative Investigations

Bias is an important consideration in qualitative investigations. Qualitative research typically involves the collection and analysis of non-numerical data such as interviews, focus groups, and observations.

Qualitative research has some limitations that should be considered when interpreting the findings. These limits include limited generalizability, subjectivity, limited quantitative data, time and resource intensive, and limited control over variables.

Qualitative studies, like other studies, are prone to error. Here are some common sources of bias in qualitative research:

Researcher bias Researcher bias occurs when the researcher's personal beliefs, values, or experiences influence the research process and analysis. Researcher bias can affect all aspects of qualitative research, from study design and data collection to data analysis and interpretation.

There are several strategies researchers can employ to minimize researcher bias in qualitative research. One approach is reflexivity, which reflects the researcher's biases and assumptions and their impact on the research process. Researchers can keep a journal or record their thoughts and feelings throughout the research process. This helps identify areas of potential bias. Another approach is to use a team-based approach to data analysis and interpretation. This requires multiple researchers to independently analyze the same data and compare their results to identify areas of concordance and discordance. This approach helps identify potential biases and ensure that the data are interpreted unbiased and rigorously.

Researchers can also use coding frameworks and analytical tools to ensure data is analyzed systematically and consistently. This minimizes the potential for researcher bias in data analysis.

Participant bias This bias occurs when research participants provide biased or inaccurate information. It can occur in some ways, including social desirability bias, recall bias, and response bias. To minimize participant bias in qualitative research, researchers can employ several strategies. One approach is to build rapport and trust with participants. This helps create a safe and value-free environment for participants to share their experiences and perspectives. Researchers can also use open-ended questions and prompts to allow participants to freely express their thoughts and feelings without being restricted to open-ended answer options.

Another approach is to use multiple methods of data collection such as interviews, focus groups, and observations. This helps triangulate the data and check the consistency and accuracy of participant responses. Researchers can also share research results with participants, using member reviews to ensure that participants accurately reflect their perspectives and experiences.

Sample bias This bias occurs when the sample of participants is not representative of the population being studied. Self-selection bias, convenient sampling, and sampling from limited populations can lead to sample bias.

To minimize sample bias in qualitative research, researchers can employ several strategies. One approach is targeted sampling, where participants are selected based on certain characteristics or criteria relevant to the research question. Another approach is to use the Snowball-Her pattern to recruit participants through referrals from other participants. This allows you to identify hard-to-reach or marginalized populations and ensure your samples are diverse and representative. Researchers can also use the member's review. This involves reviewing research results with participants to ensure that they accurately reflect their perspectives and experiences [14].

9.15 How to Avoid Bias in Research

Avoiding bias in research requires careful attention to study design, data collection, and analysis methods [15–17].

Researchers should use rigorous study designs, develop comprehensive study protocols, use appropriate sampling techniques, minimize measurement errors, use appropriate statistical techniques, and perform sensitivity analyses. This will minimize the impact of bias on research results.

Bias is a potential source of error in research, and several strategies can be used to minimize its impact on research results. Use a rigorous study design, a well-designed and rigorous study design helps minimize bias. Comprehensive research protocols help ensure that research is conducted in a systematic and standardized manner. The protocol should include details of the study design, data collection, data analysis, and quality control measures. A representative and unbiased sampling method helps to make research results generalizable to a wider population. Researchers must use reliable and valid means to minimize sources of variability in data collection. Statistical techniques can be used to control for confounders and other sources of bias. Sensitivity analysis can be used to examine the impact of potential sources of bias on study results. Sensitivity analysis is a statistical technique used to assess the robustness of research results to various assumptions and sources of bias. Sensitivity analysis involves changing one or more key parameters or assumptions in a statistical model and examining the impact on research results.

References

1. Willett WC, Sampson L, Stampfer MJ, Rosner B, Bain C, Witschi J, et al. The Nurses' Health Study: a cohort study of factors affecting women's health. N Engl J Med. 1984;311(9):508–15. https://doi.org/10.1056/NEJM198408303110901.
2. Alavi SS, Mohammadi MR, Soori H, Kalhori SM, Jannatifard F, Sepahbodi G. Personality, driving behavior and mental disorders factors as predictors of road traffic injuries based on logistic regression. Iran J Med Sci. 2017;42(1):24–31. https://doi.org/10.30476/ijms.2017.40647.
3. Barnett AG, van der Pols JC, Dobson AJ. Regression to the mean: what it is and how to deal with it. Int J Epidemiol. 2005;34(1):215–20. https://doi.org/10.1093/ije/dyh299.
4. Pepe MS. The statistical evaluation of medical tests for classification and prediction. Oxford: Oxford University Press; 2003.
5. Stovner LJ, Hagen K, Jensen R, Katsarava Z, Lipton RB, Scher AI, et al. The global burden of headache: a documentation of headache prevalence and disability worldwide. Cephalalgia. 2007;27(3):193–210. https://doi.org/10.1111/j.1468-2982.2007.01288.x.
6. Barr EL, Pike MC, Beral V, Green J, Reeves GK. Coffee and cardiovascular disease: a review of the current research. J R Soc Med. 2018;111(11):424–32. https://doi.org/10.1177/0141076818806298.
7. Higgins JPT, Altman DG, Gøtzsche PC, et al. The Cochrane Collaboration's tool for assessing risk of bias in randomized trials. BMJ. 2011;343:d5928. https://doi.org/10.1136/bmj.d5928.
8. Sterne JAC, Savović J, Page MJ, et al. RoB 2: a revised tool for assessing risk of bias in randomized trials. BMJ. 2019;366:l4898. https://doi.org/10.1136/bmj.l4898.
9. Kinner AC, Slifkin RT. Trends in disparities in diagnosis of overweight and obesity using objectively measured weight and height data from primary care clinics, 1997 to 2016. Ann Intern Med. 2019;171(9):637–8. https://doi.org/10.7326/L19-0378.

10. Hsu CY, McCulloch CE, Iribarren C, Darbinian J, Go AS. Risk factors for end-stage renal disease: 25-year follow-up. Arch Intern Med. 2009;169(4):342–50. https://doi.org/10.1001/archinternmed.2008.605.
11. Schulz KF, Grimes DA. Sample size slippages in randomized trials: exclusions and the lost and wayward. Lancet. 2002;359(9308):781–5. https://doi.org/10.1016/S0140-6736(02)07882-0.
12. Altman DG, Schulz KF, Moher D, et al. The revised CONSORT statement for reporting randomized trials: explanation and elaboration. Ann Intern Med. 2001;134(8):663–94. https://doi.org/10.7326/0003-4819-134-8-200104170-00012.
13. Deeks JJ, Higgins JPT, Altman DG. Analysing data and undertaking meta-analyses. In: Higgins JPT, Green S, editors. Cochrane handbook for systematic reviews of interventions. Version 5.1.0. The Cochrane Collaboration. 2011. www.handbook.cochrane.org.
14. Salkind NJ, editor. Hawthorne effect. Encyclopedia of research design. New York: SAGE Publications; 2010.
15. Rothman KJ, Greenland S, Lash TL. Modern epidemiology. 3rd ed. Philadelphia: Lippincott Williams & Wilkins; 2008.
16. Carroll R, Ruppert D, Stefanski L, Crainiceanu C. Measurement error in nonlinear models: a modern perspective. 2nd ed. Boca Raton: Chapman and Hall/CRC Press; 2006.
17. Spertus JA, Winder JA, Dewhurst TA, Deyo RA, Prodzinski J, McDonell M, et al. Development and evaluation of the Seattle Angina Questionnaire: a new functional status measure for coronary artery disease. J Am Coll Cardiol. 1995;25(2):333–41. https://doi.org/10.1016/0735-1097(94)00397-9.

Study Guide: Pilot, Pre-test, Quality Assurance, Quality Control, and Protocol Modifications

10

Quality is not an act, it is a habit. In research studies, a commitment to quality is essential for ensuring the validity and reliability of study results. This requires a systematic approach to study design, implementation, and analysis, including the use of quality assurance and quality control measures to minimize errors and bias.

—Aristotle (384–322 BC)

10.1 Introduction

The previous topics were related to study design. This part includes the contents related to the left side of Fig. 10.1 (that is, the gray part). In this chapter, the issues related to the implementation of the study, study guide, pre-test, quality control, violation of the protocol, and modification of the protocol are discussed.

First, we will review the study guide. Even the best thought-out designs may change in practice. The number of responses obtained or the follow-up rate may be much less than the predicted value and the measurements may lead to impractical results. The best way to reveal these problems is to study the guide. By conducting a pilot study before starting the main study, appropriate changes can be made to the protocol. The next step is quality control. Many researchers do not pay much attention to the implementation of the study because this issue is boring and less attention is paid to it than the analysis and design stage. The results of a well-designed study can be misleading as a result of low accuracy in implementation and the occurrence of errors at this stage. The solution to this problem is to improve the system and increase the quality of data at the time of conducting the study.

H. Soori, *Errors in Medical Science Investigations*, https://doi.org/10.1007/978-981-99-8521-0_10

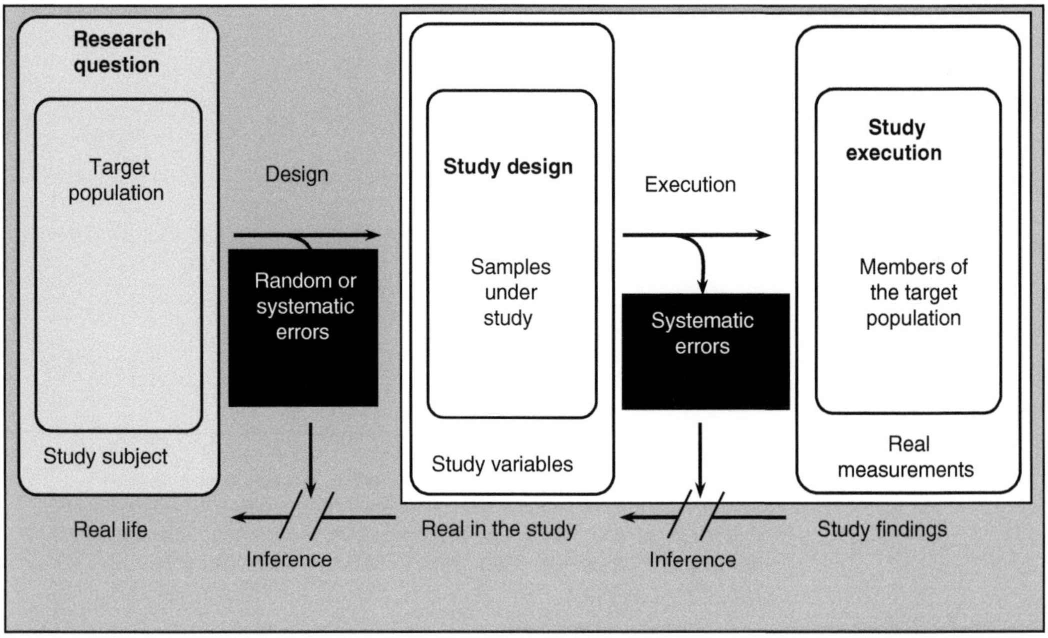

Fig. 10.1 How to conduct the study

10.2 The Importance of Pilot Studies

The term "guide or pilot studies" refers to a small version of a full-scale study as well as a specific pre-test of a specific research tool, such as a questionnaire or an interview program. Guided studies are an important component of a good study plan. Conducting a pilot study does not guarantee the success of the main study, but it increases the probability of success. The term "pilot study" is used in two ways in applied research. On the one hand, this term refers to the feasibility of the study, which consists of small-scale studies or trials that are conducted to prepare the main study. On the other hand, it is possible to pre-test or evaluate a specific research tool in the study guide. One of the advantages of conducting a pilot study is that before conducting the main study, you can find out which part of the research project may fail, stop, or that the proposed methods or tools are inappropriate or too complicated. Other reasons such as persuading the funders that the research proposal is worth investing in are one of the other reasons for conducting the pilot study. Therefore, there are various reasons for conducting guideline studies. Table 10.1 is dedicated to the study of the reasons for conducting the pilot study. Guidance studies are conducted based on quantitative or qualitative methods. Large-scale studies need to conduct multiple pilot studies before conducting the main study.

For example, to conduct the 1385 Population and Housing Census, which is the largest 10-year survey in the country, methodological changes and other changes compared to the 1375 census questionnaire were tested. These test censuses provided basic information on people's reactions to the questions and new writing styles of the questionnaire, how to conduct field operations and the method of reducing non-responses, and the success rate of management, implementation, collection, and processing methods was evaluated.

In pilot studies, an attempt is made to identify potential practical problems for conducting research. Other problems such as the incompleteness of the documents, the low response rate of the missing cases, and the violation of the proposal can also be identified by reading the guide

Table 10.1 Reasons for conducting guideline studies

Reasons for a pilot study
• Preparing research tools and testing the adequacy of these tools • Evaluating the feasibility of a study or investigating the possibility of its implementation on a large scale • Research protocol design • A realistic assessment of the practicality of the research protocol • Ensuring the effectiveness of the framework and sampling technique • Evaluating the success rate of the proposed methods for entering people into the study • Identification of legal or ethical problems that may occur while using the proposed methods • Estimating the variability of outcomes to determine the sample size • Collecting primary data • Determining the required resources such as personnel or financial resources for the designed study • Arranging research questions and plans • Teaching the research process to researchers • Convincing the funders that the research team has the necessary competence and knowledge • Convincing funders that the original study is feasible and worth investing • Convincing other interested groups that the original study is worth supporting

and taking precautionary and reassuring measures. The steps of the pre-test for a questionnaire on a small group of volunteers who are as similar as possible to the target population of the study have been reviewed in Table 10.2. Pilot studies can reveal policies or local problems and issues that may affect the research process.

10.2.1 Problems of Guidance Studies

Guideline studies also have limitations, which include: the possibility of predictions or incorrect perceptions based on the data of the guidebook study, problems caused by contamination, and budget-related issues. In this section, each of these topics is discussed.

Successful completion of the pilot study is not a guarantee for the success of the main study in large dimensions. Although the results of the pilot study indicate the possible response rate in the main study; it does not guarantee it, because it has no statistical basis and in almost all cases it

Table 10.2 The methods of conducting a pilot study to improve the internal validity of a questionnaire

How to do a pilot study questionnaire
• Present the questionnaire to the subjects of the pilot study exactly as it is presented in the main study • Ask the people under study to identify ambiguous items and difficult questions • Record the time taken to complete the questionnaire and decide on its reasonableness • Eliminate all unnecessary, difficult, or ambiguous questions • Evaluate the adequacy of the available options for each question • Make sure that the answers can be interpreted according to the required information • Check that the subjects have answered all the questions • Rephrase any question that is not answered as expected or replace it in the questionnaire • Summarize and revise the questionnaire and, if possible, read another guide

was obtained based on insufficient sample size. In addition, other problems may not be identified until a larger-scale study is conducted. The next issue to consider is pollution. Pollution can be created in two ways:

- *When the data of the pilot study are included in the results of the main study.*
- *When the participants in the pilot study also participate in the main study, new data is collected from them.*

One of the main features of the pilot study in quantitative studies is that when reporting the results, its data is not used for hypothesis testing and is not analyzed in the real study. It is clear that if the results of the study guide show that there are problems related to the research tool and it is necessary to make changes to it, these data may be incomplete or incorrect; But when a standard and valid research tool is used and the study guide determines other methodological aspects such as the rate of people entering the study, the resulting data are valuable.

A more common problem is deciding whether participants or study sites in a pilot study should be included in the main study. The important issue is that these people have already faced the intervention and as a result, their response may be different compared to people who have not faced this intervention before. For example, the participants get to know how to use the instrument or the measurement method, but on the other hand, repeating the research steps may harm them, and we may encounter many cases of violation of the protocol by the people under research study because this protocol is no longer attractive to them.

Therefore, the presence of the participants in the pilot study in the main study because only the people examined in the pilot study gain more experience (which does not apply to all the people under the study) causes a kind of distortion in the study; But in some cases, it is not possible to easily remove the participants of the pilot study from the main study, because in this case, the sample size of the main study will be very small. This issue is more evident in cases where the sampling plan is clustered. In these cases, sensitivity analysis or sub-group analysis can be performed to evaluate how much the pre-test process or pilot study affects the size of the intervention effect.

In qualitative studies, the issue of contamination is less important, and researchers often use part of the data from the pilot study or all of it in the main study. The collection and analysis of data resulting from qualitative research are often gradual and continuous, and the second interview or subsequent interviews are usually more effective than the previous interview because the interviewer uses the insight and information obtained from the previous interviews, the interview plans, and questions. It corrects some of it. For this reason, some people argue that in qualitative approaches, it is not necessary to conduct pilot studies separately.

Other problems may arise when the study of the guide requires a large investment, as a result, it is difficult for the research group to stop the research if the study of the guide is unsuccessful. Instead of concluding that their proposed study is unfeasible due to available resources, time, population, and other available factors, researchers may be encouraged to make many changes to the original study. On the other hand, if the guideline study is large and comprehensive, the funders lose their desire to invest more in this study, because they no longer see it as a new (original) study, especially if the results of the guideline study are published.

10.2.2 Pilot Study Report

A pilot study report is a document that summarizes the findings and results of a small study conducted before a larger study. The purpose of a pilot study is to test the feasibility and validity of the study design and methodology and to identify any potential problems or issues that may arise during the larger study. A pilot study report is a valuable tool for researchers to evaluate the feasibility and validity of their study design and methodology, and to identify potential problems or problems that may arise during the larger study. This helps ensure that the larger study is being conducted rigorously and validly and that the results are reliable and accurate. Pilot studies are conducted to test the feasibility and validity of a research study before conducting a larger study. One of the main goals of a pilot study is to identify and fix any potential errors or issues that may arise during the larger study.

A pilot study report usually contains an introduction, methods, results, discussion, conclusion, and references. The pilot study could include a small sample of participants, e.g., 10–20 people who have recently been in a car accident. Participants would be asked to use the smartphone application to capture information about the location and severity of their injuries, as well as any other relevant information such as the time and location of the accident. The pilot study would evaluate the feasibility and validity of the smartphone application as a tool for collecting road accident data. It would also identify any potential issues or issues with the application such as technical malfunctions or difficulties with data entry. The pilot study report would include a description of the study design and methodology, including sampling strategy and data collection methods. It would also present the results of the pilot study, including all data collected and analyzed. The report would discuss the feasibility and validity of the smartphone application as a data collection tool and identify any limitations or potential sources of bias in the study design.

10.2.3 Conclusion

Pilot studies are less discussed and used and less reported. It is rare to find a complete report of the guideline studies in the research literature. If these studies are reported, they often confirm only specific research methods or research tools. In many cases, in research articles, only one component of the pilot study is mentioned, such as "pre-testing" or examining a questionnaire. These articles simply state: "The validity and reliability of the questionnaire were tested."

When details of pilot studies are presented in articles and reports, researchers often acknowledge that they learned from the pilot study and made necessary changes, without providing the reader with the details of what exactly they learned. Some of these processes and results obtained from successful and unsuccessful pilot studies can be useful for those who start similar projects. This is very important because guideline studies are "time-consuming, frustrating, and associated with unpredictable problems." However, it is better to conduct a pilot study before spending a lot of time, money, and effort on the main study.

Pilot studies that are well designed and implemented can inform researchers about the best way to conduct research and sometimes its possible consequences. Therefore, researchers should be encouraged to report the guideline studies more fully and especially to state the real reforms that have been made in the study design and research process accurately and in detail.

10.2.4 Finalizing the Protocol

The final goal of studying the guide is to decide how to design intervention methods and measure and manage human resources. Guideline studies to investigate human resources management methods, an estimate of the number of available people who are willing to cooperate, and the effectiveness of different management methods are used in the study.

The guide studies provide the researcher with a perspective of the structure of the society from which the sample was taken, and the distribution of age, sex, race, and other indicators that are important in the study are estimated. Study guides are important in improving methods of measuring variables. Small comparative pre-tests are used to test different methods in the initial stages.

In the pre-test stage, it is possible to check sub-reactions, comprehensibility of questionnaire questions, and study improvement methods. It is possible to conduct extensive pre-tests on people who are members of the main community in the planning stage. This work is done to check the validity and ensure the correctness of the implementation methods. If the samples in the study include people of different ages, sexes, races, and cultures and the measurements are sensitive to this variety, in the pre-test, suitable representatives should be selected from each main subgroup.

If a new intervention is used in studies, pre-tests are very useful. Interventions designed to change behavior, such as AIDS prevention programs in schools, are questionable.

10.3 Quality Assurance

Quality assurance and errors are closely related concepts, as quality assurance aims to minimize defects and ensure that a product or service meets defined quality standards [1, 2]. Quality assurance is a set of activities and processes designed to ensure that a product or service meets or exceeds defined quality standards. In healthcare, quality assurance aims to ensure patient care is delivered in a safe, effective, and efficient manner. Quality assurance activities may include developing and implementing policies and procedures, monitoring and evaluating performance, identifying areas for improvement, and implementing corrective actions as needed. These activities can help healthcare organizations improve the quality of patient care, reduce errors, and increase patient safety by providing ongoing education and training to healthcare providers.

Quality assurance may also include working with patients and their families to gather feedback and identify opportunities for improvement. Overall, quality assurance is an important aspect of healthcare that can help ensure patients receive quality care that is safe, effective, and efficient. For example, when a study examines the effectiveness of a new intervention to prevent road traffic injuries, researchers can collect data on various outcomes such as the number and severity of injuries, length of hospital stay, and patient satisfaction. To ensure the quality of the data collected, researchers could develop a standardized data collection form and protocol that includes clear definitions and instructions for each variable. The quality assurance measures might include training all data collectors on the data collection protocol, conducting regular checks of the collected data for completeness and accuracy, and implementing procedures for resolving any discrepancies or errors in the data. Additionally, the study may include a data monitoring committee that reviews the data regularly to ensure that the study is being conducted according to the protocol and that any issues are identified and addressed on time.

Quality assurance in clinical practice is essential to ensure patients receive quality care that is safe, effective, and efficient. By implementing a systematic approach to quality assurance, healthcare providers can continuously improve the quality of care and improve patient outcomes. Quality assurance in clinical practice is a systematic approach to ensure patient care is delivered in a safe, effective, and efficient manner. It includes a range of activities aimed at improving the quality of care, reducing errors, and improving patient safety. Some key components of quality assurance in clinical practice include: implementing corrective actions and providing ongoing education and training. Quality assurance in medical research involves a systematic approach to ensuring that research studies are conducted in a manner that produces accurate and reliable results. It includes a range of activities aimed at improving the quality of research and reducing errors. Some key components of quality assurance in medical investigations include study design, data collection, data analysis, quality control, and reporting.

10.4 Quality Control

Quality control and errors are also closely related concepts, as quality control aims to prevent defects from occurring during the production process and to ensure that the final product meets desired quality standards [3]. Quality control includes a set of activities aimed at monitoring and improving the quality of a product or service and plays an important role in minimizing errors. One of the most important topics in clinical research that are usually neglected is the assurance of data quality and consistency because the data collection process is usually repetitive and boring, and the measurements often seem more accurate than they are. If there are no proper quality control methods to provide reliable data, the presence of incorrect and missing data will cause problems.

Quality control in clinical practice is essential to ensure patients receive quality care that is safe, effective, and efficient. By implementing a systematic approach to quality control, healthcare providers can continually improve the quality of care and patient outcomes. Some key components of quality control in clinical practice are: establishing clinical guidelines and protocols, monitoring and evaluating performance, identifying implementation of corrective actions, and providing ongoing education and training. Quality control in medical science research involves a systematic approach to ensure that research studies are conducted in a manner that produces accurate and reliable results. It includes a set of activities aimed at monitoring and improving the quality of the study, and it plays an important role in minimizing errors and improving the validity and generalizability of the results. Standardized data collection, data analysis, quality control measures, and reporting. For example, when a study examines the effectiveness of a new intervention to prevent road traffic injuries, researchers can collect data on various outcomes such as the number and severity of injuries, length of hospital stay, and patient satisfaction. To ensure the quality of the collected data, researchers could develop a standardized data collection form and protocol that includes clear definitions and instructions for each variable of the collected data on completeness and accuracy and implementation of procedures to fix any discrepancies or errors in the data. In addition, the study may include a data monitoring committee that regularly reviews the data to ensure that the study is being conducted according to protocol and that any issues are identified and addressed on time.

10.4.1 Missing Data

If a large proportion of the measurements are missing data or even multiple measurements are missing from the study, the results will be misleading and biased. For example, consider a long-term follow-up study of surgery that has a 5% mortality rate if 10% of patients in follow-up are dropped (lost) from the study, and death among them is common is folks, this complication is seriously underestimated. Misleading results related to missing data can sometimes be corrected during the analysis phase.

There are various statistical methods, especially in multivariate analysis where the presence of missing data in front of many independent variables makes a lot of information available, to replace the missing response based on the available information. However, the only proper solution is to design and conduct the study in such a way that the missing data is minimized. Although these methods are useful, there is no guarantee that the responses will be unbiased if there are a significant number of missing observations.

10.4.2 Incorrect Data with Low Accuracy

Incorrect data with low accuracy causes problems that often remain unknown. This problem occurs especially when more than one person collects data (when a researcher designs a study and leaves data collection to his colleagues). In the data analysis stage, some of these measurements, along with the continuous use of an inappropriate analysis method, seriously distort the results. When the errors related to data entry are not revealed after conducting the study, a more serious problem arises.

10.4.3 Misleading Data

Clinical researchers leading a research system must consider that research team colleagues may not cooperate closely. These people have found entering wrong information as the easiest way to do their job. The ways to ensure that such big errors do not occur are careful selection of colleagues and project members, communicating with the research team and making them understand the importance of the research topic, being aware of the possibility of intentional errors and random evaluation of data when conducting the study [1].

10.4.4 Quality Control of Clinical Stages of Research

The quality control of the clinical stages of the research starts from the implementation stage and continues throughout the study (Table 10.3)—Research operational instructions. The operational instruction is a supplementary part of the study protocol. The operational instruction pre-

Table 10.3 Quality control steps in clinical research

Quality control
Study design
• Preparation of instructions about entry and exit criteria and measurements • Standardization of measurement methods and tools • Determining the methods of data management and analysis • Compilation of quality control system • The necessity and possibility of blinding • Research team training • Confirming the skills of the research team
Execution
• Continuous guidance and leadership • Periodic work sessions • Reconfirming the skills of the research team • Periodic reports

cisely defines the subjects of the study, how to measure the variables and the method of conducting the study. Operational guidelines are very necessary when research is conducted by multiple people, especially when several researchers collaborate in several different centers. Even when a researcher does all the work alone. Operational instructions help him in reducing random changes and changes in measurement techniques over time.

The important topics of operational instruction are stated in Table 10.3. These tables include all the tools and forms used in the study, which include how to contact the subjects, conduct interviews, fill out questionnaires, code and modify forms, collect samples, analyze data, and quality control methods.

- ***Training and confirmation of skills***

  In group studies, people who perform important measurements are trained and their competence is tested and confirmed.
- ***Leadership and guidance***

  In the studies that are done in a group, the task of quality control is the responsibility of the main executive. He cannot see all the measurements of his colleagues, but if he has doubts about the correctness of the data, he can test the accuracy of the measurements, observe and record the information, or control the performance of the research team members.
- ***Working meetings***

  From the beginning of the design phase, the researcher should have regular meetings with all members of the research team. In the meetings, instructions for the next steps should be distributed and the people who were responsible for each step of the study should present a work report. These meetings provide an opportunity to discover and solve problems and make everyone fulfill their responsibilities according to the progress of the study program and schedule. Regular meetings are a good reference for evaluating the realization of study objectives.
- ***Reviewing***

  All team members should participate in a review system, in which the methods used by each member of the research team are reviewed. After obtaining permission from the subjects, the main project manager can give at least one complete example of the interviews or show the technical process of each member of the research team. It is useful to use a standard checklist during the observation (prepared in advance). The communication between the project lead and each member of the research team is facilitated by reviewing the checklist. The drafts are used to record the actual results of the inspection and analyze the results of the quality control unit.

  Exploratory looks at the research team as a reviewer, encouraging, attracting cooperation, and making sure to use the same standardized methods among the members of the research team are very useful. Another advantage of exploratory views of the system is that all members of the research team feel that they are contributing to the quality control process.
- ***Periodic reports***

  Data tabulation is important for checking the technical quality of clinical stages of research and measurements at regular intervals. With this method, it is possible to determine missing, incorrect, and inaccurate measurements. For example, if in a blood pressure screening team, the average blood pressure level measured in two consecutive months is different, it can be concluded that different measurement methods were used, and similarly, there are wide changes in the standard deviation of the measurements. In consecutive months, it indicates the inappropriateness of the measurement technique.

  Quality control often includes tests to measure the reliability and repeatability of study measurements. For example, collecting two sets of data from a series of people to test the existence of an agreement between the measurements, checking the internal consistency between the related data, and using the reference standard to validate the measurements in a sample of Subjects are the steps that are taken to ensure the quality of the research (refer to Chap. 4).

10.4.5 Special Methods for Drug Interventions

In clinical trials related to the use of drugs, especially for those that are blind, it is necessary to careful monitoring of compliance with the medication order [2–4]. This issue is achieved through careful planning with the drug manufacturing company, controlling the way the drug is distributed, and monitoring the health of the drug and the dosage.

10.4.6 Coordination for Quality Control

In large studies, one of the members of the research team should be responsible for the proper implementation of quality control methods. The purpose of this work is to identify potential problems before they occur and prevent them from occurring.

10.4.7 Quality Control of Laboratory Processes

By using the described methods to control the quality of clinical procedures, the quality of laboratory processes can also be controlled (Table 10.4).

The displacement of laboratory samples of individuals and the error-prone nature of laboratory methods lead to the adoption of special strategies in this field [4].

- *Attention to labeling*

  When a person's blood test sample is mistakenly labeled with the name of another person, it is almost impossible to correct or detect the mistakes made. The only solution is to prevent and avoid displacement errors by carefully checking the name and identification code of the people under study when pasting the laboratory samples. Using a computer, you can print a set of labels for laboratory tubes containing blood and record them. This method speeds up the labeling process and prevents the displacement of figures. When the separated serum is transferred from one test tube to another, it is better to label the new test tube in advance and keep the two tubes close together. In this method, it is checked by reading one of the others, and you can also use automatic barcodes.
- *Blinding*

  If the researcher does not know the study group or the values of other key variables when measuring the samples taken from the patients, blinding is done. Even in processes like automatic blood glucose determination, this method reduces bias and prevents the use of personal judgments when reporting results. When samples, laboratory results, or medical images are sent to a central laboratory in a multicenter study, it is better to have double-blind labels. This standard method is suitable for evaluating the accuracy of laboratory methods and can be designed in a way that tests both the consistency of a single observation and the consistency between observations.

Table 10.4 Quality control of laboratory procedures

Quality control
Design
• Solutions available in Table 10.1 • Accurate and appropriate labeling
Execution
• Solutions available in Table 10.1 • Periodic control of equipment • The possibility of blinding

10.4.8 Data Quality Control

The researcher should pre-test the data management system before starting the study. This process includes designing forms to record measurements, selecting a database for data editing and management, and designing blank tables to ensure that all research variables are collected. Table 10.5 lists the steps in data quality control.

- *Form design*

  The design of data collection forms has a great impact on the quality of data. Designing the data entry system before starting the data entry phase allows the researcher to standard-

Table 10.5 Data quality control in the design stage

Data quality control (study design stage)
• Solutions available in Table 10.1 • Only required variables should be collected • Preparation of empty tables for designing the data analysis stage • Preparation of information forms that have the following features: • Understandable • Compatible • Clear and orderly • Proper printing • Validated • Labeled on every page • Preparing a data bank that is sensitive to out-of-range, missing, and inconsistent observations

Table 10.6 Data quality control during the study implementation phase

Data quality control (study execution stage)
• Investigating major errors in uncompleted forms and when completing the form when the subjects are still available • Ensuring that the name, identification number, and date of examination are correct on each page • Ensuring that the forms are completed for each part of the examinations • Ensuring that different parts of the questionnaire do not fit • Checking the correctness of entered data employing random review • Preparation of periodic frequency tables to detect possible errors

ize responses during the design phase and reduce errors during the data entry phase. It also makes the researcher avoid using questions that are difficult to code or interpret. Subjective measurements (such as clinical diagnoses) need a clear operational definition. These definitions should be accurately stated in operational instructions and forms related to measurement registration [5]. The options must have a connection and a logical sequence. Readable and motivating forms make the people under study pay more attention to completing the forms. The pre-test ensures the clarity of the questions and the ease of the instructions for completing the form. Labeling each page with the date, name, and ID number of people's files prevents the information from being lost.

– ***Data collection and management***

Consistent and structured management is an important part of quality control, increasing the efficiency and accuracy of data. In clinical measurements, quality control and consistency of data should be done when the person is still available [5, 6]. One member of the research team should edit the forms and another should review the completeness and correctness of the information (Table 10.6). If the editor does not participate in data collection, the probability of discovering missing values and other errors increases. Another method is computer editing. In this method, the computer is programmed in such a way that missing data, inconsistent information, and out-of-range values are automatically identified. This method is not suitable for small studies. An alternative method is to select a random sample from the original forms and re-prepare the original data table and compare the two together.

– ***Periodic tables***

Examining the frequency distribution of important variables at regular time intervals allows the researcher to check the completeness and quality of the data. This makes it possible to correct previous errors and prevent possible errors in the continuation of the study.

10.4.9 Quality Control in Multicenter Studies

In many types of research, the sample size is very high and is more than the number of samples available in one center. This issue leads to multicenter studies. These studies are carried out by research teams in different centers. Sometimes these centers are in one city or one region and one researcher can supervise all research teams [7]. However, most multicenter studies are conducted by several researchers in different cities. In this type of study, certain steps are necessary so that all centers conduct the study in the same way and provide comparable and integrable data for analyzing and publishing the results. A coordinating center should facilitate communication between different centers, coordinate guidelines, and handle other aspects of quality control, training of each center's staff, review, data management, analysis, and dissemination. A common mistake is a tendency to collect too much data. Considering that the initial clinical examination stage when patients enter the study is the only time when the researchers have the chance to measure the background variables, it makes it difficult for the researchers to record any interesting variables (for example, recording routine data from the physical examination that has little relation to the research question) to register. Usually, researchers collect much more data than what is analyzed or published. The problem with this method is wasting time to measure unimportant parameters. Subjects get tired and upset and more important data loses its quality. Another problem is the large volume and complexity of data, which makes quality control and data analysis more difficult. It is better to examine the need to collect the variables and remove many of the variables that are arbitrarily considered. The reduction of additional variables increases the validity and accuracy of important variables.

10.5 Improvement of the Protocol When Conducting the Study

When conducting research, it is important to consider how protocols can be improved so that research is conducted in an ethical and effective manner. This may include reviewing the protocol to ensure they are clear and comprehensive and making any necessary changes or additions to the logs. Additionally, it is important to ensure that protocols are consistent across sites and that logs are regularly monitored and updated as needed. Regardless of the results of the pre-test, the problems of designing, implementing, and measuring the parameters appear when the study started. The general rule is to apply fewer changes after the beginning of the study. However, sometimes improving the protocol can give validity to the study.

10.5.1 Minor Changes

Deciding whether small changes will improve the study or not is often a balance between the methodological advantages of the improved protocol and changing the uniformity of the study, spending time and money to change the system. Decisions that make an operational definition more precise are relatively simple. For example, in "a study where smoking is one of the exit criteria, what decision should be made for people who quit smoking?". This decision should be made uniformly for all people and in all centers.

10.5.2 Basic Improvement

Major changes in the study protocol, such as changes in the entry and exit criteria of patients or changes in the intervention, lead to more serious problems. Although there may be good reasons for applying these changes, if these changes lead to a different interpretation of the findings, the analysis and reporting of the data should be examined separately. When improving medical research protocols, it is important to consider how to ensure that research is conducted in an ethical and effective manner. This may include reviewing the logs to ensure they are clear and making any necessary changes or additions to the logs. Ensure that logs are consistent across sites and that protocols are regularly monitored and updated as needed. Finally, it is important to ensure that the protocol is communicated to all research staff and participants in a clear and understandable manner.

References

1. Sánchez-Jerónimo P, Silva-Cerón M, López-López M, Hernández-Morales V, Gochicoa-Rangel L. Implementation of an integrated total quality management system in a pulmonary function laboratory. Qual Manag Health Care. 2022;31(2):74–9. https://doi.org/10.1097/QMH.0000000000000333. PMID: 35132004.
2. Szklo M, Nieto FJ. Epidemiology beyond the basics. 4th ed. Burlington: Jones & Bartlett Learning; 2019.

3. Badrick T. Integrating quality control and external quality assurance. Clin Biochem. 2021;95:15–27. https://doi.org/10.1016/j.clinbiochem.2021.05.003. Epub 2021 May 7. PMID: 33965412.
4. Brownson RC, Petitti DB, Bao S. Applied epidemiology: theory to practice. 3rd ed. Oxford: Oxford University Press; 2019.
5. Salkind NJ, editor. Encyclopedia of research design. New York: SAGE Publications; 2008.
6. Roberts MS, Korn DS, editors. The fundamentals of clinical research: a universal guide for implementing good clinical practice. Berlin: Springer; 2018.
7. Smith J, editor. Multicenter research: design, challenges and solutions. Berlin: Springer; 2020.

11 Errors in Medical Procedures

11.1 Introduction

Medical errors refer to mistakes or errors made by healthcare professionals, which can occur due to errors of omission, errors in planning, and errors in the execution of a planned healthcare action, whether it causes harm to the patient. Such errors can increase morbidity and mortality rates, decrease patient satisfaction, and reduce hospital productivity. The objective of this study is to determine the prevalence of medical errors in Iranian hospitals.

There are two main types of medical errors:

1. Omission errors happen when important actions are left undone. Examples include failing to secure a patient in a wheelchair or stabilize a gurney before moving a patient.
2. Commission errors involve taking an incorrect action. Examples include giving a patient a medication they are allergic to or failing to label a lab sample, leading it to be attributed to the wrong patient.

Both types can lead to serious consequences for patients. Preventing either type requires consistent protocols, checklists, and staff training to reduce opportunities for human error.

The key is building systems that make it hard for errors to occur in the first place, rather than relying solely on individuals to avoid mistakes.

Healthcare workers are reluctant to report errors due to fear of punishment and job loss. They want to ensure patient safety but dread disciplinary action. Underreporting contributes to serious patient harm. Rigid policies create an adversarial environment, making staff hesitant to report, minimize or document issues. This allows errors to multiply.

The term "error" is seen as overly negative and blame oriented. It can damage workers' confidence and performance or cause them to leave the profession. Neutral terms are preferred. However, adverse outcomes do occur due to errors, ignoring this obscures goals like prevention. Most errors result from multiple factors, not just individual actions. Intolerance for errors reflects a lack of understanding that some may be unavoidable.

Punishing individuals for systemic errors does not address the causes or prevent recurrence. The focus should be on improving safety systems, not blaming individuals.

Institutions need to remove blame while retaining accountability. With this approach, all errors, even those causing adverse outcomes, can be measured as targets for improvement. Neutral, non-punitive reporting and analysis can reduce future risk. The key takeaways are that a blame-free culture is needed to encourage reporting and learning from errors, while still holding institutions accountable for patient safety and quality improvement [1].

H. Soori, *Errors in Medical Science Investigations*, https://doi.org/10.1007/978-981-99-8521-0_11

Patient safety incidents (PSIs) are defined as any unintended or unexpected event that could have or did lead to harm for one or more patients receiving healthcare [2]. Medical error is defined as a preventable adverse effect of medical care, whether it is evident or harmful to the patient. It can result from an action taken or not taken by a healthcare professional, equipment failure or malfunction, whether communication or coordination among healthcare providers, or from a system issue. Medical errors can range from minor errors with no harm to the patient to serious adverse events that result in disability, prolonged hospitalization, or even death [3].

Medical errors are different from malpractice, because the error is an accident or mistake despite good intentions, but in malpractice, blameworthy negligence and ignorance occurred with or without criminal intent.

11.2 Some Definitions in Errors in Medical Procedures Setting

Active Errors Occurring at the point of contact between a caregiver and the larger system. Examples include operating on the wrong body part or providing an incorrect medication dose. Active errors are committed by people carrying out operational tasks and include slips, lapses, mistakes, and procedural violations. Examples include administering an incorrect dosage of medication or operating on the wrong patient.[1]

Adverse Events Injuries caused by medical errors versus underlying conditions. They can be prevented through better practice. Examples include prolonged hospitalization or disability caused by poor management. Common types of adverse events include surgical injuries, medication errors, healthcare-associated infections, falls, blood clots, and procedure-related complications. An adverse event is an injury caused by medical management, rather than the patient's underlying condition. It may result in prolonged hospitalization, permanent disability, or death. Not all adverse outcomes are due to errors; some can be unavoidable complications of necessary treatments. However, many adverse events are preventable and result from errors or system flaws.

Latent Errors Issues in system design, equipment installation, or management structures. They remain hidden until triggered by an active error, resulting in an adverse event. These are "time bombs" waiting to happen. They are often more difficult to identify because they do not immediately result in any noticeable effects. Latent errors within processes, equipment, and environments increase risk by creating weaknesses that active human errors can then expose.

Medical Error Failing to achieve intended goals through wrong or omitted actions. These deviations from best practice may or may not cause harm. Medical errors encompass a wide range of issues, from misdiagnoses and medication mistakes to surgical mishaps and unsafe discharge planning. Errors can happen at any stage of a patient's care, from admission to follow-up.

Negligence Failure to meet the reasonable standard of care expected of an average qualified caregiver in similar circumstances. Negligence arises when an individual caregiver's failure to meet the standard of care results in harm. However, errors are more often attributable to systemic factors outside an individual's control. A systems approach focused on process improvements, rather than blame, is most effective at reducing patient harm. Examples include failure to review test results leading to a missed diagnosis or injuring a nerve during surgery.

[1] To reduce active errors, healthcare systems implement measures to: enhance training and verify staff competence to ensure proper knowledge and skills, formalize procedures using checklists and guidelines to standardize care and minimize variations that lead to mistakes, automate tasks through technology like electronic health records, computerized order entry, and barcoding to reduce the potential for human mistakes. Implement verification steps like patient wristbands and ID bracelets to confirm patient identity before procedures and medications to avoid wrong-patient errors.

Near Miss Events that could have caused harm but did not either by chance or intervention. Near misses offer opportunities to develop preventative strategies. Near misses are sometimes called "close calls" because harm was narrowly avoided. They typically involve deviations from best practices or standard procedures that introduce risk to the patient. Encouraging the reporting and analysis of near misses can reveal system weaknesses that can then be fortified to enhance overall patient safety.

Never Events Errors that should never happen, like pressure ulcers or wrong-site surgery. Never events are serious, largely preventable patient **safety events that should never occur in healthcare.**[2] **The term "never event" signifies that these errors should nev**er happen even with reasonable diligence. They indicate vulnerabilities within the system that require immediate intervention and process changes to prevent recurrences.

Patient Safety Methods to prevent or minimize harms from healthcare processes. The World Health Organization (WHO) defines patient safety as: "The prevention of errors and adverse effects to patients associated with health care. An approach to improving the safety of patient care aims to prevent and reduce risks and hazards, with a focus on systems and processes rather than individual performance."[3]

Root Cause Fundamental deficiencies or decisions that, if corrected, would eliminate undesirable consequences. Common root causes include lack of training/expertise, poor communication, inadequate policies/procedures, insufficient staffing, technical failures, no audits, and lack of accountability.

Clinical Malpractice Failure to provide a reasonable standard of care expected of an average practitioner in that situation. Not all medical mistakes constitute malpractice, but some clear deviations from the standard of care may meet the criteria. Most malpractice claims in hospitals are related to surgical errors, whereas most claims for outpatient care are related to missed or late diagnosis.

11.3 Magnitude of the Problem of Errors in Medical Procedures

Clinical procedure errors pose a significant issue in healthcare systems worldwide. As per the Institute of Medicine report, medical errors result in around 98,000 deaths per year in the USA, ranking them among the leading causes of death in the country [3]. According to an analysis by the World Health Organization (WHO), published in 2017, the global costs associated with medication errors are approximately 42 billion USD per year.[4]

Various studies have demonstrated that clinical procedure errors can occur at any stage of healthcare, including diagnosis, treatment, and follow-up care. These errors can arise due to several factors, such as inadequate training, fatigue, communication breakdowns, and equipment malfunctions [4, 5].

Moreover, medical errors significantly affect patient safety, healthcare providers, and institutions. They can result in legal action, loss of trust in healthcare providers, and harm to the reputation of healthcare institutions [6]. Therefore, comprehending the extent of clinical procedure errors is crucial in devising effective strategies to prevent them.

While most research does not show conclusive differences in error rates between provider types, factors like workload, stress, fatigue, experience,

[2]Common interventions aimed at never events include standardized procedures, checklists, safety briefings, unique patient identifiers, and color coding of equipment. Computerized physician order entry and bar-coded medications can help eliminate some transcription errors.

[3]Patient safety. https://www.who.int/news-room/fact-sheets/detail/patient-safety. Accessed May 2023.

[4]https://www.who.int/initiatives/medication-without-harm#:~:text=Medication%20Without%20Harm%20aims%20to,Germany%20on%2029%20March%202017. Accessed May 2023.

and the quality of oversight/protocols likely interact in complex ways to influence patient safety risks for various groups.

Clinical errors can happen to patients of any age or background, but some populations, such as elderly, critically ill, or those with multiple chronic conditions, may be more vulnerable due to the complexity of their care. Patients with limited health literacy or language barriers may also be at increased risk of clinical errors. Healthcare providers may also be at risk of clinical errors when they are fatigued, overworked, or stressed. Examples of clinical errors may include incorrect medication dosage, misdiagnosis, or failure to recognize important patient information.

Patients with certain characteristics may be more vulnerable to medical errors, such as children, older adults, and those with multiple chronic conditions. Moreover, certain healthcare settings, like emergency departments and intensive care units, may be more prone to medical errors.

Errors in clinical procedures are a significant problem in low and middle-income countries (LMICs) as well. According to a systematic review of studies on medical errors in LMICs, the overall incidence of adverse events in these countries is estimated to be 8.2%, with a mortality rate of 2.1% [7]. Another study conducted in India found that medical errors were responsible for 5.2% of hospital admissions, with an associated mortality rate of 0.8% [8]. A systematic review in Iran showed that the prevalence of medical errors among Iranian physicians ranged from 38.1% to 65%. The most common errors were prescription error with 17.3% [9].

Research has identified various factors contributing to clinical procedure errors in LMICs, including inadequate resources, limited access to training and education, and a lack of regulation and oversight [10]. In addition, communication breakdowns and cultural factors can also contribute to medical errors in these settings [11].

The impact of medical errors in LMICs is not limited to patient harm but also has significant economic consequences. A study conducted in Ghana estimated that the cost of medical errors was $1.5 million annually, which accounts for 9% of the country's healthcare budget [12].

Clinical errors in low- and middle-income countries (LMICs) occur due to various reasons. One of the primary challenges is the lack of resources, such as equipment, medication, and qualified healthcare providers. Another critical factor contributing to clinical errors is the limited access to training and education for healthcare workers in LMICs. Moreover, inadequate regulation and oversight of healthcare systems in these countries also play a significant role in clinical errors [11].

Communication breakdowns between healthcare providers, patients, and their families can also lead to clinical errors in LMICs. Additionally, cultural factors, such as beliefs and practices that may contradict evidence-based medical practices, can contribute to clinical errors in these settings. Furthermore, the combination of high patient load and the need for healthcare providers to work extended hours in LMICs can lead to fatigue and burnout, which can increase the likelihood of clinical errors [13].

11.4 Perceptions of Medical Errors by Physicians

Despite clinical services being provided to people with the aim of returning and improving their health, errors in clinical environments can even lead to severe illness and death. Since ancient times until now, healthcare providers and physicians have been striving to minimize clinical errors. Some studies have shown that the risk of death in a healthcare setting is even higher than driving, chemical industry accidents, and air travel [12] (See Fig. 11.1). Health care professionals experience profound psychological effects such as anger, guilt, inadequacy, depression, and suicide due to real or perceived errors.

Physicians' views on medical errors can vary depending on their training, experience, and personal beliefs. While some may consider errors an inevitable part of healthcare, others may regard them as preventable and unacceptable.

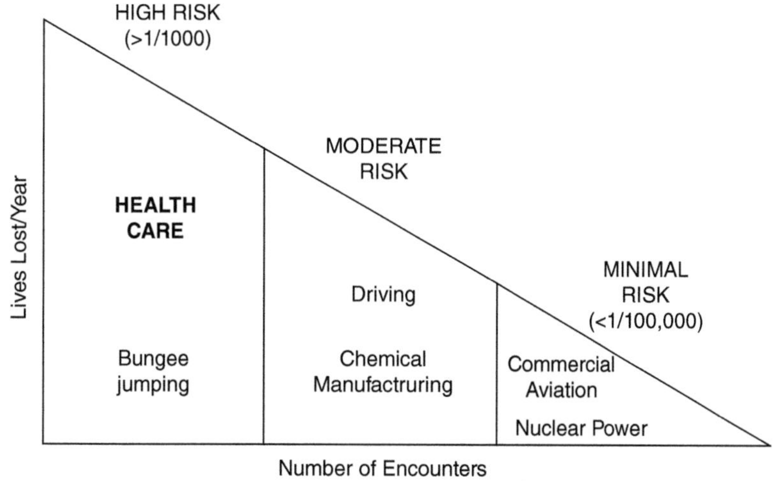

Fig. 11.1 Comparison of risk in health care and other industries. (Source: Kalra [12])

Medical errors can be a source of stress and anxiety for some physicians who fear disciplinary action or legal consequences. Nevertheless, others see errors as an opportunity to learn and improve patient outcomes by implementing changes in practice.

Although some physicians may feel guilty or ashamed when an error occurs, it is important to understand that errors often result from complex systems and processes. Blaming individuals can be counterproductive, and it is more beneficial to identify and address underlying systemic issues contributing to errors.

Physicians' perceptions of medical errors can significantly affect their response to and learning from errors. Establishing a culture of openness, transparency, and continuous improvement can reduce the stigma associated with errors and promote a proactive approach to patient safety.

The possibility of legal action can intensify negative emotions and undermine the confidence of healthcare professionals. They associate errors with failure, breaching public trust, and causing harm to patients, despite their mandate to prioritize patient safety. Medical errors can have serious consequences for physicians and may face disciplinary or legal action. Punishments may include license suspension or revocation, fines, civil lawsuits, criminal charges, or loss of reputation. Severe errors that result in patient harm are more likely to lead to consequences for physicians. However, there are several healthcare institutions that have implemented programs to support physicians and learn from errors to prevent future occurrences. While not all medical errors result in punishment, many healthcare institutions have programs to support physicians and learn from errors to prevent future occurrences. The goal is to promote a culture of transparency, accountability, and continuous improvement to enhance patient safety and prevent medical errors.

Consequently, healthcare workers may be hesitant to report errors due to fear of disciplinary action, which can contribute to a cycle of medical errors and harm patients. Some experts argue that the term "error" perpetuates a culture of blame and negative connotations, which can damage the morale and effectiveness of healthcare professionals. However, identifying errors can lead to constructive changes and improvements in healthcare delivery. It is crucial to improve healthcare systems' safety and accountability while avoiding a culture of blame to reduce medical error rates and associated costs and injuries. Healthcare professionals must work together to achieve this goal.

11.5 Healthcare Providers Workload and Medical Errors

Medical errors can be influenced by physician workload, as overworked healthcare providers may be more prone to making mistakes, including prescribing incorrect medication or dosage, misinterpreting test results, or overlooking important patient information. Studies have linked high physician workload to an increased risk of medical errors, particularly in emergency departments and intensive care units. Additionally, physician burnout, which is often caused by workload and stress, can further increase the risk of medical errors. To mitigate the risk of medical errors caused by physician workload, healthcare organizations can implement various strategies such as reducing workload by hiring more providers or implementing balanced staffing models, providing tools and resources to help manage workload such as electronic health records and decision support systems, supporting physician well-being and addressing burnout through wellness programs and counseling services, and offering ongoing training and education on topics such as medication safety, communication, and teamwork. By addressing physician workload and providing support to healthcare providers, healthcare organizations can improve patient safety and reduce the risk of medical errors. The workload, fatigue and drowsing are strongly associated with medical errors. Research has shown that healthcare providers who work long hours or have irregular schedules are at an increased risk of making medical errors. In addition, fatigue and sleep deprivation can impair cognitive function, including attention, memory, and decision-making, which can further increase the risk of medical errors [14].

Monitoring symptoms of burnout and its associated factors in the workplace and proposing an alternative organizational and behavioral system and sharing it with relevant authorities may help prevent or reduce job burnout and medical errors. Restricting successive shifts, reducing workload, increasing training and supervision, and implementing smart clinical decision support systems may help reduce prescription errors.

The key strategies are ensuring adequate staffing, reducing administrative burdens, utilizing support staff, limiting work hours, implementing protocols, fostering teamwork, providing training, identifying, and removing system error risks, and encouraging error reporting in a non-punitive manner.

Specifically, healthcare organizations should:

- Hire enough providers, nurses, and technicians for the patient load and monitor workload indicators.
- Offer flexible scheduling, part-time options and share work among teams to accommodate staff needs.
- Streamline paperwork through electronic health records and limit non-clinical duties to save time.
- Have medical assistants and nurse practitioners take on some routine tasks to free up higher-level providers.
- Enforce regular meal and rest breaks for staff and allow time off as needed.
- Limit the maximum number of hours worked per shift and week to reduce burnout.
- Standardize tasks through checklists and automate functions to make work more efficient.
- Foster communication among care teams so tasks can be shared, and handoffs done properly.
- Ensure staff are fully trained and feel competent through simulations and skill verification.
- Identify and fix underlying systems issues that contribute to workload pressures and errors.
- Implement a "just culture" approach where errors are reported and analyzed to improve systems, rather than to blame individuals.

A systems-level solutions that complement efforts to directly support overburdened staff can help control workload pressures and reduce medical mistakes. Ongoing monitoring and adjustments are also part of an effective workload management strategy.

11.6 Common Errors in Clinical Procedures

11.6.1 Infection Control Errors and Failure to Follow Proper Hand Hygiene Protocols

The World Health Organization defines hand hygiene as "Washing hands with plain or antimicrobial soap and water".[5] In healthcare settings, hand hygiene is a critical measure to prevent and control the spread of pathogens and reduce the risk of infection transmission to patients. It is a crucial practice that all healthcare workers, including physicians, midwives, nurses, pharmacists, dentists, and other care providers, such as community health workers and family members, must follow to ensure the safety of patients and themselves. By implementing proper hand hygiene protocols, healthcare workers can minimize the risks of patients acquiring infections and promote patient safety.

Maintaining clean hands is the most crucial measure in preventing the spread of pathogens and antibiotic resistance in healthcare environments. Proper hand hygiene reduces the occurrence of healthcare-associated infections. Numerous studies have shown that hand hygiene is an effective measure in reducing the incidence of infections. For instance, Semmelweis [14] conducted a study at the first obstetrics clinic in Vienna's General Hospital, which revealed that the mortality rate among mothers who delivered there was significantly lower when hospital staff cleaned their hands with an antiseptic agent than when they washed their hands with plain soap and water. This study provides compelling evidence that proper hand hygiene can have a significant impact on reducing the spread of infections. According to CDC estimates, almost 2 million patients in the USA develop hospital-acquired infections each year, leading to approximately 90,000 deaths. The utilization of hand hygiene products that improve adherence to recommended hand hygiene practices can significantly enhance patient safety and prevent infections. By implementing these measures, healthcare providers can promote patient safety and reduce the risk of harm [14].

Hand hygiene is a critical issue in healthcare settings such as nosocomial infections worldwide. According to the World Health Organization (WHO), healthcare-associated infections (HAIs) affect hundreds of millions of patients worldwide each year, and hand hygiene is the most effective way to prevent the spread of HAIs [15].

In the USA, HAIs are a significant problem, with the Centers for Disease Control and Prevention (CDC) estimating that approximately 1 in 31 hospitalized patients develops an HAI [14]. Hand hygiene is one of the most critical measures in preventing these infections, and failure to follow proper hand hygiene protocols can have severe consequences for patients, including prolonged hospital stays, increased healthcare costs, and even death.

Moreover, failure to follow proper hand hygiene protocols can contribute to the emergence and spread of antibiotic-resistant bacteria, which pose a significant threat to global public health. The overuse and misuse of antibiotics have contributed to the emergence and spread of antibiotic-resistant infections, and hand hygiene is one of the critical strategies to prevent the spread of these infections.

There is extensive scientific evidence to support the effectiveness of hand hygiene in reducing the incidence of infections. A landmark study conducted by Semmelweis at the First Obstetrics Clinic in Vienna's General Hospital demonstrated that the mortality rate among mothers who delivered there was significantly lower when hospital staff cleaned their hands with an antiseptic agent than when they washed their hands with plain soap and water [15]. This study provides compelling evidence that proper hand hygiene can have a significant impact on reducing the spread of infections.

Additionally, numerous other studies have confirmed the importance of hand hygiene in preventing the spread of infections in healthcare settings. For example, a systematic review and meta-analysis of 77 studies found that hand

[5] https://www.ncbi.nlm.nih.gov/books/NBK144013/pdf/Bookshelf_NBK144013.pdf. Accessed June 15, 2023.

hygiene interventions significantly reduced the risk of healthcare-associated infections [16].

There are multiple factors that can lead to healthcare workers failing to comply with proper hand hygiene protocols, including insufficient knowledge or training, heavy workload and time constraints, forgetfulness, skin irritation, perception of low risk, lack of accountability, and prioritizing patient care.

Controlling the failure to follow proper hand hygiene protocols requires a multifaceted approach that includes education and training, adequate resources, monitoring and feedback, accountability measures, and improving the culture of patient safety.

11.7 Administering the Wrong Medication or Dosage

The administration of incorrect medication or dosage is a prevalent medication error that can result in severe harm to patients. It happens when healthcare providers administer the wrong medication or an inappropriate dose, which can occur due to various reasons, such as misinterpretation of prescriptions, confusion between drugs with similar names, or miscalculation of doses. Such errors can lead to adverse drug reactions, allergic reactions, or other complications.

The wrong medication or dosage can be life-threatening for patients and its effects depend on various factors such as the medication involved, dosage, age, weight, and medical history of the patient. It can cause adverse drug reactions or severe complications such as organ damage, seizures, respiratory failure, or cardiac arrest. Children are particularly vulnerable as they require different dosages than adults. Administering the wrong medication or dosage can also result in chronic health conditions, disability, or increased healthcare costs. Healthcare providers can prevent medication errors by using technology, double-checking medications before administration, and verifying patient identity to ensure safe and effective care.

To prevent this type of medication error, healthcare providers must take measures to confirm the accuracy of the medication and dosage, such as cross-checking the medication label and verifying the patient's identity. Furthermore, healthcare facilities can implement strategies that can minimize the risk of medication errors, such as computerized order entry systems, bar coding, and automated dispensing machines.

The National Coordinating Council for Medication Error Reporting and Prevention offers a definition of medication errors, but there is no universally accepted definition.[6] According to the Council, a medication error is a preventable event that may lead to inappropriate medication use or patient harm while the medication is within the control of healthcare professionals, patients, or consumers. This includes errors related to various aspects of healthcare, such as prescribing, order communication, product labeling, compounding, dispensing, distribution, administration, education, monitoring, and use. However, despite efforts to define and prevent medication errors, they continue to occur and are often underreported, resulting in significant morbidity and mortality.

Mistakes with medications are common in healthcare, from prescribing to administering. Giving the wrong drug or wrong amount is a serious issue, potentially causing harm and even death.

Many reasons exist for these errors: illegible writing, similar drug names, copying errors, poor communication, and lack of training. Children are especially at risk due to their size and dosing needs.

To prevent errors, providers must verify the patient's identity, check the drug and amount, and ensure the medication fits their condition. Healthcare systems can also implement strategies like electronic prescribing, barcodes, and automated dispensing to:

- Reduce transcription mistakes.
- Catch potential drug interactions and allergies.

[6] https://www.nccmerp.org/about-medication-errors. Accessed May 2023.

- Ensure the correct drug and amount reach the patient.

This improves medication safety by lowering the chances for errors.

11.8 Miscommunication Between Healthcare Providers

Miscommunication between health providers is common due to differences and barriers but can be mitigated through strategies to improve interactions, information exchange, and shared understanding.

It refers to breakdowns, errors, and ambiguities in how information is exchanged between providers involved in patient care. This can lead to medical mistakes, delays in care, inappropriate treatments, and threatened patient safety.

Common causes of miscommunication include differences in experience levels and roles (for example, a resident physician fails to communicate a new treatment plan to the nursing staff because he/she assumes they already know his role and responsibilities), incomplete knowledge of patient histories (e.g., a nurse handing off to the next shift neglects to mention that a patient had an unexpected reaction to medication the previous day), use of assumptions (e.g., a resident assumes the attending physician is aware of a change in a patient's status when they have not spoken yet), medical jargon and abbreviations (e.g., a pharmacist interprets an order for "SL" insulin differently from the physician who meant "subcutaneous" insulin), focus on technology over face-to-face discussions (Misunderstandings occur more often in email communications versus face-to-face discussions), external distractions (e.g., a telephone ringing during handoff interrupts the exchange of critical patient information), and lack of assertiveness (e.g., a medical assistant fails to speak up when they think a resident physician misunderstood a caregiver's report, leading to an error).

The consequences of miscommunication can be severe.

To minimize miscommunication interventions such as standardizing processes and communication techniques, limiting distractions during handoffs, fostering trust and teamwork, promoting transparency, and speaking up, using technology to support—not replace—interactions, and standardizing terms and definitions could be effective.

11.8.1 Language Barrier Errors in Clinical Practice

In clinical practice, a language barrier between healthcare providers and patients or their families can lead to errors. Effective communication can be challenging when patients and healthcare providers speak different languages, and this can result in misunderstandings, misdiagnoses, and inappropriate treatments. Common errors that can arise due to language barriers include patients having difficulty expressing their symptoms accurately, not understanding the healthcare provider's instructions or recommended treatment options, not receiving adequate information to provide informed consent, and delayed or missed diagnoses due to incomplete medical histories or ineffective communication. To overcome language barriers, healthcare providers can use trained medical interpreters, bilingual staff members, or translation services to facilitate communication with patients who speak different languages. It is crucial to provide patients with information in a language they understand to ensure they receive appropriate care and treatment and can make informed decisions about their healthcare.

In countries with large numbers of immigrants or refugees who speak different languages, language barrier errors can be a significant issue in clinical practice. For instance, in Canada, the USA, and Australia, where there are substantial immigrant populations, healthcare providers often encounter patients who do not speak the official languages of the country, leading to misunderstandings and miscommunications that can result in inadequate care or treatment. In Canada, for example, there are over 200 languages spoken, which poses challenges for healthcare providers. To overcome these language barriers, healthcare providers often use trained medical interpreters or language translation services to facilitate communication with patients who speak different languages.

11.9 Inadequate Patient Identification

Inadequate patient identification refers to healthcare providers not being able to correctly identify the patient they are treating. This can result in serious medical errors like giving the wrong medication, performing procedures on the wrong patient, and misinterpreting test results for the wrong patient.

Inadequate identification can occur due to incomplete medical records, communication issues, language barriers, and lack of standardized patient ID protocols.

Errors in patient identification continue to be a significant problem in the healthcare industry, leading to medication errors, testing errors, transfusion errors, and other serious mistakes such as performing procedures on the wrong person or discharging infants to the wrong families. The United Kingdom National Patient Safety Agency reported 236 incidents and near misses related to missing or incorrect wristbands between November 2003 and July 2005, while the United States Department of Veterans Affairs cited patient misidentification as a root cause for over 100 incidents from January 2000 to March 2003.[7] However, there are interventions and strategies available that can significantly reduce the risk of patient misidentification.

Patient misidentification can occur in critical areas, such as drug administration, phlebotomy, blood transfusions, and surgical interventions. The trend toward limiting working hours for clinical team members can lead to an increased number of team members caring for each patient, increasing the likelihood of communication problems during handovers. Patient misidentification is a root cause of many errors, leading the Joint Commission in the USA to prioritize improving patient identification accuracy as the first of its National Patient Safety Goals in 2003. While wristbands are traditionally used to identify hospitalized patients, missing bands or incorrect information can limit their efficacy. The color-coding of wristbands can facilitate quick visual recognition of specific issues, but the lack of a standardized coding system has led to errors by staff who provide care at multiple facilities. Newer technologies, such as barcoding, have proven to be cost-effective in improving patient identification. Regardless of the technology used, careful planning for the care processes can ensure proper patient identification before any medical intervention and provide safer care with significantly fewer errors.

1. The World Health Organization (WHO) recommends the following strategies for its member states to improve patient identification in healthcare organizations:
2. Implement systems that prioritize the responsibility of healthcare workers to verify patient identity before administering care, using at least two identifiers such as name and date of birth.
3. Standardize patient identification approaches across different facilities within the healthcare system, such as using white ID bands with standardized patterns or markers, or biometric technologies.
4. Develop clear protocols for identifying patients without identification or those with the same name, including non-verbal methods for identifying comatose or confused patients.
5. Encourage patient participation in all stages of the process, including labeling of containers used for blood and other specimens.
6. Provide clear protocols for maintaining patient sample identities throughout pre-analytical, analytical, and post-analytical processes, and for questioning laboratory

[7] Wristbands for hospital inpatients improves safety. National Patient Safety Agency, safer practice notice 11, 22 November 2005. http://www.npsa.nhs.uk/site/media/documents/1440_Safer_Patient_Identification_SPN.pdf. Accessed June 2023.

results or other test findings that are inconsistent with the patient's clinical history.
7. Incorporate training on patient identification procedures into the orientation and continuing professional development of healthcare workers.

Educate patients about the importance of correct patient identification in a positive manner that respects privacy concerns.[8]

11.10 Inadequate Monitoring of Patients

Poor monitoring and processes are responsible for some medical errors. Inadequate monitoring of patients in clinical settings can lead to serious adverse events and complications, highlighting the importance of regular and thorough monitoring of patients in healthcare settings. Patients monitoring systems are collections of machines or equipment used to constantly monitor patients through various vital signs and warning systems to detect and record changes in patient well-being.

Patient monitoring systems allow for constant surveillance of patients' vital signs and condition through measuring devices, data capture, trend tracking, alerts, and alarms. Collecting this information in close to real time helps clinicians optimize care delivery and outcomes.

Patient surveillance technologies provide constant monitoring of patients' condition by tracking vital signs like heart rate, blood pressure, oxygen levels, respiratory rate, and temperature. These systems detect changes in physiological functions, conscious state and movement that can indicate deterioration or improvement in a patient's status as well as adverse developments requiring clinical intervention.

They typically consist of sensors that measure physiological variables, transducers that convert signals into readable data, monitors that display measurements and trends, and alarms that notify staff of critical developments. Data obtained from patient monitoring systems enable clinicians to guide care management, determine bedside interventions, evaluate treatment responses, identify issues promptly, and prevent further health declines. In summary, automated monitoring of patients' vital signs and activities over time provides information that helps clinicians optimize patient care and outcomes through more timely detection of changes and alerts.

Patients in clinical settings may experience inadequate monitoring due to a variety of factors, such as:

Insufficient monitoring of vital signs: Regularly monitoring vital signs, including blood pressure, heart rate, respiratory rate, and temperature, is crucial in assessing a patient's health status. Neglecting these indicators can result in delayed recognition of changes in a patient's condition, leading to life-threatening situations.

Inadequate monitoring during anesthesia: Patients undergoing surgery are often under general anesthesia, which can cause changes in vital signs and other physiological parameters. Inadequate monitoring during anesthesia can lead to severe complications, such as hypoxemia, hypotension, and cardiac arrest.

Absence of monitoring for medication side effects: Many medications have potential side effects that can be fatal if not promptly identified and treated. Failure to monitor patients for medication side effects can result in severe adverse events, including organ failure, seizures, or anaphylaxis.

Lack of monitoring for patients with chronic conditions: Patients with chronic conditions, such as diabetes, heart disease, or kidney disease, require regular monitoring to ensure their conditions are well-managed. Neglecting to monitor these patients can lead to complications such as diabetic ketoacidosis, heart failure, or kidney failure.

Healthcare providers can reduce inadequate monitoring of patients by standardizing monitoring protocols based on evidence, utilizing auto-

[8] World Health Organization. Patient Identification. WHO Collaborating Centre for Patient Safety Solutions. 2007.

mated monitoring systems to supplement manual monitoring, increasing staff awareness of risks and protocols, improving staffing levels to meet patient acuity needs, streamlining communication between shifts and teams through checklists and rounding procedures while limiting distractions, reducing non-monitoring tasks through automation, fostering assertiveness to speak up about patient concerns, establishing standardized monitoring workflows with reminders and checklists, ensuring all staff can accurately assess patients through training and competency verification, requiring rapid response times to monitor alarms, and thoroughly investigating incidents to identify systems issues needing process or policy changes. Together, these strategies can help address inadequate patient monitoring by minimizing protocol variability, catching more subtle changes in patient conditions earlier, improving staff competence and communication, reducing non-essential tasks, fostering a culture of transparency, routinizing monitoring activities, enforcing monitoring policies, and identifying and correcting underlying systems issues that contribute to the problem.

11.11 Inadequate Informed Consent

Doctors are required to provide patients with an informed consent form that outlines the treatment, risks, and financial obligations prior to performing any medical procedure or treatment. Failure to obtain informed consent can leave doctors vulnerable to medical malpractice lawsuits if the patient experiences harm as a result. Lack of informed consent medical is a malpractice.

Informed consent is both a legal and ethical necessity for any medical or surgical procedure, as it ensures that patients comprehend the nature, risks, benefits, and alternatives of the proposed treatment. It aims to respect patient autonomy by supplying individuals with the information necessary to make voluntary decisions about their own care, thus promoting patient-centered care. The basic elements of informed consent include a thorough explanation of the advised procedure or treatment, identification of material risks and side effects, description of viable alternatives, and clarification that the patient can refuse treatment without repercussions. Informed consent must be given freely, without coercion, and patients must possess the mental capacity to comprehend the provided information and make an informed choice. Legally, informed consent demands disclosure of information a reasonable person would want to know to make an informed decision, though the patient's personal values and wishes ultimately would determine what is "material" information. Informed consent is an ongoing process, not a single event, and clinicians should check for patient comprehension and re-obtain consent if aspects of care change significantly. The ethics principles of autonomy, beneficence, nonmaleficence and justice underlie the legal requirements for informed consent, upholding trust in the patient–provider relationship. The lack of informed consent violates patients' rights and autonomy and can constitute negligence or battery in malpractice cases.

Inadequate informed consent can contribute to clinical errors. Inadequate informed consent characterized by failures like incomplete disclosure of risks, not discussing viable alternatives, not ensuring patient comprehension, pressuring patients to consent, having language and cultural barriers, neglecting to reconfirm consent when plans change, and lack of verification of patient understanding can contribute to various clinical errors. When providers do not fully explain potential risks, side effects and complications of treatment, patients may experience preventable adverse events due to lack of information, leading to harm, distress, and complaints. When providers do not discuss alternative treatments, patients may undergo unnecessary interventions. When providers do not make sure patients comprehend what was discussed by avoiding jargon and speaking slowly, patients may consent without truly understanding. When providers pressure hesitant patients to accept treatment, it can breed mistrust interfering with the relationship. When informed consent discussions are not tailored for those with limited health literacy and English proficiency, it can result in confusion, misunderstanding, and suboptimal care. When providers fail to reconfirm consent when aspects of treatment plans change, it can violate trust and autonomy. And when providers do not verify patient comprehension, they cannot ensure treatment reflects patients' informed choices. All these breakdowns in the informed consent process can set the stage for errors stemming from misunderstanding, confusion, reluctant consent, and a threatened patient–provider relationship.

This is an example of inadequate informed consent and its consequences:

During a knee replacement surgery consultation with a 75-year-old Persian-speaking patient, the surgeon communicates through an interpreter. However, the surgeon only emphasizes the benefits of the procedure, neglecting to fully disclose the potential risks and complications involved. Despite the patient signing the consent form and agreeing to the surgery, the language barriers, rushed discussion, and lack of clarity around risks prevent the patient from fully comprehending the possibility of complications such as blood clots, infections, and cardiovascular issues. Following the surgery, the patient experiences a postoperative infection that requires prolonged antibiotic treatment and physical therapy. The patient feels upset about the unforeseen complications and expenses, believing that the risks were not adequately explained before the surgery. The inadequate informed consent process is characterized by incomplete disclosure of risks and complications, possible language and cultural barriers, and a failure to assess patient comprehension. As a result, clinical errors occur, including the development of an avoidable postoperative infection due to a lack of awareness about potential risks. Furthermore, the inadequate informed consent process causes distress, dissatisfaction, and erosion of trust due to unmet expectations.

11.12 Inadequate Training of Healthcare Providers

Insufficient or inadequate healthcare training can lead to numerous issues, such as an increased likelihood of patient harm, legal complications, and difficulties in maintaining a positive doctor–patient relationship. Some believe that if a person can only answer less than 80% of the questions related to her field or has the skills to do it, she is known as a person with insufficient training.

A 1995 British Medical Association report[9] criticized the way British medical schools and hospitals train doctors, stating they fail to provide the necessary training and supervision. It recommended less rote memorization and more continuous assessment in medical schools. Hospitals needed to properly oversee junior doctors and abandon the philosophy of "education through humiliation." The report noted that medical mishaps in hospitals often involve unsupervised junior doctors.

The report pointed out that British doctors are not trained in important areas like how to communicate with patients, avoid errors, and deal with complaints—increasing the risk of repeated errors and serious malpractice suits.

The key issues highlighted were:

- Medical schools relied too much on rote learning and not enough on continuous assessment.
- Hospitals did not adequately supervise junior doctors, who were often left unsupervised even for critical tasks.
- Doctors lacked training in soft skills like communication, error avoidance, and handling complaints—undermining quality and safety.
- This training gap contributed to the risk of repeated medical errors and malpractice suits.
- The report recommended reforms to how medical schools and hospitals educate doctors, calling for less emphasis on memorization, more supervision of junior doctors, and training in competencies beyond medical knowledge alone. These changes, the report argued, were needed to improve doctor performance, reduce medical errors and strengthen the healthcare system.

[9] British Medical Association. Training the doctors of tomorrow: undergraduate medical education. London: British Medical Association; 1995.

Insufficient or incomplete training of healthcare providers concerning medical knowledge, clinical skills, communication, error prevention, change recognition and supervision can contribute to medical errors in several ways. For example, a resident physician who is undertrained in diagnosing rare conditions fails to properly identify a patient's disorder. This occurs because the resident lacks sufficient knowledge about the various signs, symptoms, and testing for this uncommon disease. The patient suffers delays and unnecessary tests before finally receiving the correct diagnosis from a more experienced physician. More comprehensive training during residency may have avoided this misdiagnosis.

Providers who do not receive thorough training in medical sciences, clinical skills and treatment guidelines may lack the knowledge base needed to properly diagnose conditions, interpret tests, and prescribe appropriate treatments, potentially resulting in misdiagnoses, inappropriate treatments, and medication errors. Providers who lack training in practical skills like taking patient histories, performing physical exams, using medical devices, and executing procedures competently may struggle to perform these tasks correctly, leading to errors during assessments, procedures, and interventions. Providers who are not trained in how to effectively communicate with patients explain diagnoses and treatments or work in interprofessional teams may have issues accurately conveying and receiving important information, causing errors stemming from miscommunication, failure to clarify and misinterpretation. Providers who lack training in techniques to reduce medical errors like double-checking orders and recognizing warning signs may fail to catch errors before they cause harm, meaning more errors will go unnoticed until adverse outcomes occur. Delays in identifying and responding to clinical deterioration may also result from insufficient change recognition training. And when training programs inadequately prepare new providers to supervise less experienced staff, there is an increased risk that providers will make errors due to a lack of appropriate oversight and guidance.

Inadequate training contributed directly to errors that caused harm due to lacking knowledge, safety practices, diagnostic skills, or procedural competencies. With proper training that addressed these deficiencies, these errors may have been avoided.

11.13 Equipment Errors and Malfunction

Health professionals commonly believe that technology can significantly improve healthcare, resulting in increased efficiency, quality, safety, and lower costs. However, it is also true that these same technologies can introduce errors and adverse events, which can be a significant challenge. Since there are around 5000 types of medical devices used by millions of healthcare providers worldwide, device-related errors are inevitable. Unfortunately, the benefits of technology may not be fully realized due to the prevalence of four common pitfalls: inadequate maintenance, insufficient plans for implementing technology into practice, poor technology design that neglects human factors and ergonomic principles, and inadequate technology interface with the environment and patient [1].

Medical and equipment flaws in design, mishandling, user error, and malfunction are the most common causes of medical errors. User errors are often due to differences in device functions between manufacturers, inadequate testing, lack of standardization, poor design, and poor maintenance.

Medical errors can arise from equipment errors and malfunctions in several ways. These include misdiagnoses due to inaccurate results from imaging machines, laboratory equipment, and monitoring devices. Treatment delays can occur when equipment fails or malfunctions, leading to delays in diagnosis and treatment. Improper treatment may also result from malfunctioning medical devices. Adverse events can occur when malfunctioning equipment directly causes patient injuries. Equipment errors can increase the length of hospital stays and lead to medication errors and missed changes.

Procedural errors can occur during surgery due to malfunctioning procedural devices. Proper maintenance and use of medical equipment is crucial for ensuring patient safety, as medical device errors and malfunctions can have severe consequences. To guarantee the safety of patients and users, it is crucial to maintain medical equipment in accordance with the manufacturer's specifications. This ensures that the machine is functioning correctly.

Due to the utilization of a vast array of medical equipment and multiple functions in healthcare institutions, it is crucial to monitor and maintain the equipment to ensure optimal performance and safety levels. However, maintenance management may prove to be challenging for healthcare providers who encounter issues such as insufficient competent personnel and limited resources, including replacement parts and funds. The World Health Organization (WHO) has identified initial expenses and operating expenditures as two categories of necessary financial resources for maintaining medical equipment. The proper maintenance of medical equipment is critical for ensuring optimal functionality and safety. To prevent equipment failure, which can lead to medical errors, patient harm, and increased costs, healthcare providers must regularly monitor and maintain their equipment. Regular maintenance and calibration of medical equipment also help ensure that it meets the manufacturer's specifications and regulatory requirements.

However, healthcare providers may face challenges in maintaining their medical equipment. One of the most significant challenges is the lack of competent personnel with the necessary skills and knowledge to service and repair the equipment. The shortage of replacement parts and funding can further compound this issue.

To overcome these challenges, organizations such as the World Health Organization (WHO) have identified two critical categories of financial resources necessary for maintaining medical equipment: initial expenses and operating expenditures. The initial expenses cover the cost of purchasing the equipment, installation, and training personnel on its use. Operating expenditures include the cost of maintenance, calibration, repair, and replacement of parts.

Proper maintenance management of medical equipment is crucial for ensuring patient safety and optimal healthcare outcomes. It is essential to allocate sufficient resources and investments for maintenance programs to address the challenges and ensure that healthcare providers have the necessary competencies and resources to maintain medical equipment correctly [16, 17].

A systematic review on medical equipment reliability assessment suggests the development of a comprehensive strategic maintenance management system that covers PM, CM, and RP activities, as well as the application of machine learning techniques to anticipate and prevent equipment failures. The adaptive framework based on the functionality of healthcare providers can also improve maintenance prioritization. The use of appropriate techniques can help comply with national standards and statutory requirements and improve healthcare services [16].

11.14 Diagnostic Errors

According to the Joint Commission, diagnostic errors lead to the death or injury of 40,000–80,000 patients annually.[10] Primary care solo practices are most susceptible to diagnostic errors due to heavy workload and the inability to cross-reference with colleagues. However, healthcare institutions, where patients are seen by multiple healthcare providers, have a lower chance of diagnostic error. A significant number of these deaths are preventable, and better safety measures are necessary. One in every six patients is affected, and 1 in every 1000 primary care visits causes preventable harm. Diagnostic errors can occur with clinicians, radiologists, and pathologists, with the most common errors being the failure to order appropriate tests, faulty interpretation, failure to follow-up, and failure to refer. Prematurely ending the diagnostic process

[10] "The Joint Commission. Improving America's Diagnosis: Rebuilding After COVID-19. September 2020."

is a cognitive error that can lead to misdiagnosis. Delaying treatment after diagnosis is the third most common error and leads to increased costs for readmission and further treatment. Various diagnoses are commonly missed, including acute renal failure, appendicitis, metastatic cancer, and urinary tract infection. Diagnostic errors affect virtually all medical specialties, with an overall misdiagnosis rate of 10–15% [18].

Cardiac diagnoses often result in diagnostic errors, with coronary atherosclerosis being frequently missed, and aortic disease like an aneurysm and dissection being misdiagnosed. Procedures like angioplasty and cardiac catheterization are significant sources of medical cardiovascular liability. Diagnosing pulmonary embolism (PE) is also challenging due to nonspecific symptoms, and it can be an incidental finding in approximately 3% of chest CTs. Failure to diagnose and treat cancer early can result in difficult therapy and lower cure rates, with tissue diagnosis error rates as high as 15%. Making an initial neurologic diagnosis can be challenging, particularly in young patients, psychiatric patients, and those with other diseases that may cause stroke-like symptoms. Clinicians can prevent diagnostic errors by being aware of commonly misdiagnosed conditions and taking extra precautions to seek and confirm the diagnosis. They should also be aware of common "high-risk" diagnoses [2].

Diagnostic errors can occur for several reasons, and it is not always the fault of the physician. Diagnostic errors can occur due to various factors. These include the complexity of the diagnostic process, which involves multiple variables like a patient's medical history, symptoms, physical exam, and test results. The presence of conflicting information or a lack of clarity can also lead to errors. Additionally, physicians' cognitive biases, such as confirmation bias, anchoring bias, or availability bias, can lead to assumptions or erroneous conclusions based on limited information. Limited access to information, including a patient's complete medical history or test results, can also contribute to diagnostic errors. Time pressure in a fast-paced healthcare environment may cause physicians to make quick diagnoses without considering all available information. Furthermore, poor communication between healthcare providers or between providers and patients can lead to errors, such as delayed test results or unclear instructions for treatment. A comprehensive approach to reducing diagnostic errors includes improving communication, providing complete patient information, and addressing cognitive biases.

Preventing diagnostic errors in medicine requires a comprehensive approach that includes several strategies. One effective approach is to improve communication between healthcare providers and patients by ensuring that providers listen actively and communicate clearly. Communication among healthcare providers can also be improved by promptly sharing test results and consulting specialists. Diagnostic decision-making tools such as clinical decision support systems can help providers make more accurate diagnoses by providing real-time information and evidence-based recommendations. Enhancing training and education for physicians and healthcare providers on diagnostic reasoning, cognitive biases, and effective communication can minimize diagnostic errors. A culture of safety within healthcare organizations can promote reporting of errors and near misses, leading to the implementation of strategies to prevent future errors. Providers should have access to complete patient information, including past medical history, previous test results, and medications, to ensure accurate diagnosis. Encouraging teamwork and collaboration among healthcare providers can ensure that all necessary information is shared, and all perspectives are considered during the diagnostic process.

11.15 Common Surgical Errors

Most malpractice claims in hospitals are related to surgical errors, whereas most claims for outpatient care are related to missed or late diagnosis. Globally, more than 200 million surgical procedures are performed annually, yet surgical errors continue to occur at a high rate despite awareness of their adverse effects.[11] Surgical errors contribute significantly to adverse events, with at least 4000 occurring annually in the United States alone. Operating on the wrong body part is a common source of surgical error, and robotic surgery has been found to increase accidental hemorrhage due to lacerations and injury to surrounding tissues. Interestingly, surgical errors tend to occur more frequently before and after the surgical procedure rather than during the operation.

Although all patients who undergo surgery are at risk of surgical errors, certain factors can increase this risk. These factors include complex surgeries that involve multiple procedures or surgeons, emergency surgeries without sufficient preparation time, patient-related factors such as obesity, age, or underlying medical conditions, poor communication between members of the surgical team, inadequate training for inexperienced or poorly trained surgeons or other team members, lack of standardization in surgical protocols or procedures, and systemic factors such as poor staffing levels or inadequate resources within the healthcare system. It is important for healthcare providers to be aware of these risk factors and take appropriate measures to minimize the risk of surgical errors.

Some of the common surgical errors that can occur during surgery include:

Wrong-site surgery: This happens when the surgeon operates on the incorrect body part or the wrong side of the body, which can result in severe harm to the patient, such as amputations or paralysis.

Retention of surgical instruments or other foreign objects inside the patient: This type of error can cause infections, pain, and other complications.

Anesthesia errors: Administering too much or too little anesthesia can cause severe harm to the patient, including brain damage or death.

Infection: Surgical site infections are a common complication of surgery and can result in severe harm to the patient.

Bleeding: Uncontrolled bleeding during surgery can lead to severe complications, such as shock, organ damage, or death.

Nerve damage: Nerve damage can occur during surgery, leading to pain, numbness, or paralysis.

Postoperative complications: Complications that occur after surgery, such as blood clots, pneumonia, or wound infections, can result in severe harm to the patient.

Causes of surgical errors include inadequate surgeon training and education, the absence of standardized rules and regulations, communication gaps between surgeons, anesthesiologists, and other staff, communication gaps between surgeons and patients, use of unreliable systems or protocols, rushing to complete cases, and human factors.

To reduce surgical errors, it is crucial to understand when and where errors can occur during surgery. Key risk factors that providers need to be aware of include surgeons' attitude of not accepting questioning, distraction, incomplete or missing imaging information, incomplete preoperative assessments, multiple surgeons performing more than one procedure, poor staffing, time pressures, and wrong-site surgery.

To prevent surgical errors and improve patient safety, hospitals have adopted guidelines such as using a checklist to confirm the patient's identity, site of surgery, and type of procedure, and performing a timeout before surgery to ensure the correct site, procedure, and patient. Engagement of patients, family members, and healthcare providers in minimizing risks and increasing communication is essential to avoid grave mistakes. The most crucial surgical safety measure is a timeout, a preoperative pause involving all members of the surgical team to minimize costly mistakes, which must follow a defined protocol.

[11] Christensen, J. N. (2015). Surgical errors and risks. Surgery, 33(9), 397–401.

11.16 Causes of Medical Errors

Medical errors can arise from various root causes, which include changes in mental acumen such as not seeking advice from peers, misapplying expertise, not formulating a plan, not considering the most obvious diagnosis, or conducting healthcare in an automatic fashion. Communication issues can also lead to medical errors, including having no insight into the hierarchy, no solid leadership, not knowing whom to report the problem to, failing to disclose the issues, or having a disjointed system with no problem-solving ability. Other causes of medical errors include deficiencies in education, training, orientation, and experience, inadequate methods of identifying patients, incomplete assessment on admission, failing to obtain consent, and failing to provide education to patients. Inadequate policies to guide healthcare workers, lack of consistency in procedures, inadequate staffing and/or poor supervision, technical failures associated with medical equipment, no audits in the system, and no one prepared to accept blame or change the system can also contribute to medical errors. It is essential to identify the root causes of medical errors to develop effective strategies to prevent them and improve patient safety.

11.17 Strategies for Preventing Medical Errors

Providing ongoing education and training to healthcare providers on best practices, safety protocols, new technology and error prevention techniques including communication skills, teamwork, and professionalism can help minimize errors. Developing evidence-based standardized protocols for procedures, treatments, and medications and ensuring consistent use through checklists, order sets, and physician order entry systems can also reduce errors. Utilizing automation and technologies like computerized physician order entry, barcode medication administration, electronic health records, and clinical decision support systems can minimize human error. Implementing medication safety measures such as automated dispensing cabinets, double checks, tall man lettering, and allergy verification in addition to limiting dangerous abbreviations can improve medication safety. Using checklists, timeouts and reminders can verify the correct patient, procedure, and consent while checklists for high-risk procedures are particularly helpful. Educating patients to be active members of the healthcare team and encouraging them to speak up if they notice potential errors can also intercept mistakes. Establishing a non-punitive error reporting system to identify root causes, implement solutions, and share lessons learned across the organization in a culture of safety and transparency where all staff feel empowered to speak up can minimize recurrence of the same errors. Public reporting of quality and safety metrics, tying executive compensation and accreditation to patient safety measures, performing root cause analyses of serious errors, and conducting failure mode analyses to anticipate where errors could occur can all complement strategies for a comprehensive approach to error prevention.

The WHO has created a strategy to prevent medical errors, consisting of several key elements.[12] These include establishing a culture of safety that values error reporting and learning from mistakes, improving communication between healthcare providers and patients, providing education and training to healthcare providers on safety and effective communication, developing and implementing safety systems, strengthening healthcare systems, conducting research to identify root causes of errors and prevention strategies, and involving patients and families in their care. By following these components, healthcare providers and organizations can take practical measures to prevent medical errors, enhance patient safety, and improve healthcare quality.

Furthermore, there are some global strategies for preventing clinical errors as follows:

[12] World Health Organization. Patient safety: making health care safer. https://www.who.int/teams/integrated-health-services/patient-safety. Accessed June 2023.

The High5s initiative: A global patient safety program by the WHO (launched in 2018), aims to reduce harm in health facilities by implementing five evidence-based interventions: hand hygiene, patient identification, a surgical checklist, maximum barrier precautions during high-risk procedures, and safe IV medication administration. The program seeks to halve rates of adverse events related to these five areas within 5 years, improving millions of patients' safety worldwide. The WHO provides tools, training, and monitoring to help countries promote High 5s and achieve this goal. The interventions require health facilities to improve compliance with safety practices and adopt safe practices for IV medication administration using technology when available. Implementing these actions can significantly reduce the most common causes of harm in healthcare settings and result in meaningful reductions in preventable patient harm.

The Medication Safety Challenge: This strategy (launched in 2017) aims to reduce severe, avoidable medication-related errors globally by 50% over the next 5 years. The WHO identifies five strategic areas of focus, including adherence to guidelines, infrastructure, education, and training, reporting, and learning, and smart technology. The WHO helps countries develop national action plans, implement targeted interventions, and provides tools and resources to track progress. Countries that have severe avoidable medication-related errors will receive public recognition from the WHO.

Joint Commission International (JCI): JCI accredits healthcare organizations based on their compliance with international healthcare quality and safety standards, including a focus on patient safety and the prevention of medical errors. JCI requires healthcare organizations to implement strategies to prevent medical errors, such as evidence-based practices, performance measurement, and continuous quality improvement. The accreditation process helps healthcare organizations identify areas for improvement and provides assurance to patients and their families that the organization meets international standards for quality and safety.

National Patient Safety Goals: Many countries have adopted their own national strategies and goals for clinical error reduction based on WHO guidance and tailored to the needs of their health systems. For example, Iran has established several national patient safety goals and initiatives to help reduce medical errors and improve patient safety. Iran has implemented a multifaceted approach to patient safety, which includes developing national standards, conducting an annual patient safety culture survey, establishing an adverse event reporting system, designating a National Patient Safety Day, providing patient safety training programs, supporting research and evaluation, and engaging patients and families through educational initiatives. These efforts aim to reduce medical errors and improve outcomes in the country's healthcare system by driving a systematic, data-informed approach to patient safety.

References

1. Rodziewicz TL, Houseman B, Hipskind JE. Medical error reduction and prevention. In: StatPearls. Treasure Island, FL: StatPearls Publishing; 2023. PMID: 29763131.
2. NHS England and NHS Improvement. Improving medication error incident reporting and learning. London: NHS; 2023. https://www.england.nhs.uk/2014/03/improving-medication-error-incident-reporting-and-learning/. Accessed Jun 2023.
3. Kohn LT, Corrigan JM, Donaldson MS, editors. To err is human: building a safer health system. Washington, DC: National Academies Press; 1999.
4. Leape LL, Bates DW, Cullen DJ, Cooper J, Demonaco HJ, Gallivan T, et al. Systems analysis of adverse drug events. JAMA. 1995;274(1):35–43.
5. Reason J. Human error: models and management. BMJ. 2000;320(7237):768–70.
6. Wachter RM, Shojania KG. Internal bleeding: the truth behind America's terrifying epidemic of medical mistakes. New York, NY: Rugged Land; 2004.
7. Michel P, Saghatchian M, Hofman P. Medical errors in developing countries. Int J Qual Health Care. 2012;24(6):564–7.
8. Khilnani P, Choudhary A, Dewan P, Singh A, Chawla R. Medical errors in hospitals: a review of literature. J Patient Saf Infect Control. 2018;6(2):40–4.

9. Khammarnia M, Setoodehzadeh F, Ansari Moghaddam A, Rezaei K, Peyvand M. Medical errors, and their effective factors in Iranian physicians: a systematic review. RJMS. 2021;28(10):58–73. http://rjms.iums.ac.ir/article-1-6319-fa.html.
10. Kruk ME, Gage AD, Arsenault C, Jordan K, Leslie HH, Roder-DeWan S, et al. High-quality health systems in the Sustainable Development Goals era: time for a revolution. Lancet Glob Health. 2018;6(11):e1196–252.
11. Ahmed M, Arora S, Tiew S. Medical errors in developing countries: a systematic review of literature. Int J Med Rev. 2017;4(1):25–32.
12. Kalra J. Medical errors and patient safety: strategies to reduce and disclose medical errors and improve patient safety. Berlin: De Gruyter; 2011.
13. Ahmadi A, Soori H, Mehrabi Y, Etemad K. Spatial analysis of myocardial infarction in Iran: national report from the Iranian Myocardial Infarction Registry. J Res Med Sci. 2015;20(5):434–9. https://doi.org/10.4103/1735-1995.163955. PMID: 26487871; PMCID: PMC4590197.
14. Semmelweis I. The etiology, concept, and prophylaxis of childbed fever. Madison: University of Wisconsin Press; 1983.
15. Bazmi E, Alipour A, Yasamy MT, Kheradmand A, Salehpour S, Khodakarim S, Soori H. Job burnout and related factors among health sector employees. Iran J Psychiatry. 2019;14(4):309–16. PMID: 32071605; PMCID: PMC7007511.
16. Zamzam AH, Abdul Wahab AK, Azizan MM, Satapathy SC, Lai KW, Hasikin K. A systematic review of medical equipment reliability assessment in improving the quality of healthcare services. Front Public Health. 2021;9:753951. https://doi.org/10.3389/fpubh.2021.753951. PMID: 34646808; PMCID: PMC8503610.
17. World Health Organization. Medical equipment maintenance programme overview, WHO medical device technical series. Geneva: Department of Essential Health Technologies, World Health Organization; 2011.
18. Singh H, Schiff GD, Graber ML, Onakpoya I, Thompson MJ. The global burden of diagnostic errors in primary care. BMJ Qual Saf. 2017;26(6):484–94.

Appendix A: Setting Up the Proposal and Providing Research Resources

Abstract
This appendix highlights the significance of proposal preparation and allocation of research resources in medical research. It further emphasizes the importance of project monitoring, evaluation, and planning to address potential risks. The abstract provides an overview of the key elements of effective propositions in medical research. Additionally, it discusses the value of providing pertinent background information and research, as well as exploring the potential risks and benefits associated with the proposed solution.

Introduction

A research proposal is the written part of a study, in which writing gives the researcher the ability to organize, clarify and improve all elements of the study. In this way, some practical problems of the project will be improved. In addition, even if financial resources are not needed for the study, the proposal is necessary to guide the implementation. A proposal is a written document to attract financial resources from research centers. The proposal includes the technical parts of the study, the study protocol, the budget, the schedule of the project implementation, and other supplementary information. In this section, the structure of a successful proposal is discussed.

Regulation of Proposals

The difficult part of preparing a proposal is organizing, writing, and revising it, which requires spending several months. Proposal regulation refers to the process of ensuring that a proposed project complies with applicable laws and regulations. This may include reviewing proposed projects to ensure that they are consistent with the mission and goals of the organization and comply with relevant laws and regulations. Additionally, it is important to ensure that the proposed project is reviewed and approved by the appropriate stakeholders and that any necessary changes or modifications are made to the project before approval. Finally, it is important to ensure that the project is monitored throughout its implementation to ensure that it is being executed according to approved protocols. The following steps can help you get off to a good start.

Decide where the proposal will be sent. Each research center has unique methods to attract proposals. Therefore, the researcher should start by deciding where the proposal will be sent, determining the financial limits, and explaining the objectives of the proposal for the desired research centers.

1. Formation of the research team and selection of a supervisor. Most of the proposals are written by a team consisting of several people who have a lot of experience in designing and conducting scientific research. This team may be

H. Soori, *Errors in Medical Science Investigations*, https://doi.org/10.1007/978-981-99-8521-0

small (only the researcher and a consultant) or large (including colleagues, a vital statistics consultant, a financial affairs officer, and a support officer). This team must have the ability and skill needed to design and start the study. One of the team members should be responsible for implementing the plan. Usually, this person is the main researcher. The main researcher of research projects should be an experienced person whose information and wisdom are sufficient and useful for making decisions. Probably, the history and previous studies of the members of the research team increase the chances of funding. In some studies, a project manager is considered. This person is usually a novice researcher whose task is daily management and coordinator of proposal preparation programs. Sometimes the project manager is the main researcher of the study. The duties of the main researcher or project manager include: regularly guiding the study, preparing and organizing the proposal, organizing regular meetings of the research team, and making sure that all the work is done completely and on time.

2. Following instructions to receive financial aid. All research centers have written instructions that the researcher must read carefully before writing the proposal. This information includes the outline of the proposal, the page limit, information about the amount of budget that can be requested, and the principles that must be followed in preparing the proposal; But this instruction does not include all the important information that the researcher needs to know the functions and requirements of receiving financial aid. Research centers have a scientific team that is responsible for evaluating proposals. When preparing the proposal, it is better to discuss the topic with the person who is responsible for coordinating the requests. In this way, the desired points of the institution (such as budget limitations, purpose, and explanations required in the proposal) are well presented and it is ensured that the research plan is within the scope of the institution's requests. Rejecting a proposal due to a lack of attention to detail is a failed and unavoidable experience.
3. Preparing the timetable and establishing regular meetings. Preparing a timetable to complete the tasks makes the members of the research team under pressure to submit their tasks on time. Before the proposal is sent to a research institute, it is better to review its budget again with the financial department of the institute. Failure to pay attention to these details causes a crisis that damages other well-made proposals.
4. Finding a sample proposal. It is better to prepare a copy of the successful proposals of the institution that is going to financially support the project. Successful proposals are a sure way to know how to write and content of a good proposal. The researcher can get the best opinions and design a proposal that is more clear, more logical, and more persuasive. It is also useful to review the written reports that the institute has prepared for all successful and unsuccessful proposals. To search for financial opportunities, you can find interesting proposals using the Internet.
5. Regulation of the structure of the proposal. The stages of setting up the proposal are presented in Table A.1. The structured proposal form is useful in dividing the responsibilities of different parts of the proposal.
6. Review, pre-test, and continuous improvement. Writing a proposal is a gradual process, usually, many versions are prepared, each of which reflects ideas, recommendations, and experiences. Before the final version is written, the proposal should be critically reviewed by colleagues who are familiar with the subject. Special attention should be paid to the quality of the research question, validity of the design, used methods, and editing points. It is better to critically review the proposal before presenting it. Otherwise, the project will be rejected due to haste and writing problems. When the proposal is almost ready, the final step is to carefully review the proposal for its internal consistency, comply with the instructions of the center where the proposal is submitted, and correct the editing (writing) errors.

Table A.1 The main elements of writing a proposal

Title
Summary
Table of Contents
Budgeting form
Introduction of study researchers
Required resources, technical equipment, and required physical space
Specific objectives
The importance of conducting the study
Literature review
Methods
Revision of the study plan
Study time frame
People under study
Selection criteria
Sampling plan
How to reach sample members
Measurements
Main independent variables (intervention in case of experimental study)
Response variables
Potential confounders
Guide study plan
Statistical analysis
Data analyzing method

Elements of a Proposal

The constituent elements of a proposal are presented in Table A.1. Some institutions may need less information or a different structure. The researcher should organize the proposal based on the institution that is responsible for the financial support. These items should be written for all studies even if the financial institution does not require them. Elements of the proposal typically include an introduction, problem description, proposed solution description, implementation timeline, budget, list of required resources, and conclusion. Additionally, the proposal should include all relevant background information and research, as well as a discussion of the potential risks and benefits of the proposed solution. Finally, your proposal should include a summary of your proposal and a call to action.

The Starting Stage

The title should be brief, useful, and clear. A proper title creates a proper first impression and is a constant reminder of the content and plan of the study. A good title summarizes the content of the study. The abstract is a useful summary of the contents of the proposal. It is best to start with a research question. Then the plan and methods are explained and it ends with an important sentence about the basic findings of the study. Most institutes state a word limit for the abstract. Therefore, it is better to use effective and clear expressions. Generally, after the other parts of the proposal are prepared, the abstract is written and then reviewed. The abstract is the only page that is read by most of the judges and it should easily represent the main idea of the proposal so that it can be used by anyone other than the judge. The table of contents is an essential help for the reader. Proposals may include larger, more complex, or unusual sections. In these cases, the table of contents should be mentioned and it should match the chapters or sub-chapters in the text.

Executive Departments and Institutional Review Board

Almost all institutions require an executive department that includes budget, provision of personnel expertise, the institution submitting the proposal, the amount of access to equipment, required space, and skills. The budget section is usually organized according to the guidelines of the financial institution. The budget form should not be prepared in the last part of the proposed design. Many things require the passage of time (for example, the passage of time is important to obtain a proper estimate of costs, space, skills, and personnel).

The role of the Institutional Review Board (IRB) in medical research is to ensure that research is conducted ethically and effectively. IRB reviews proposed research projects to ensure that they comply with applicable laws and regulations and do not pose a risk of harm to participants. In addition, the IRB reviews informed consent forms used in research to ensure that they are clear, and provide participants with all necessary information. IRB also reviews data collection and analysis procedures to ensure they are appropriate and reliable. Finally, the IRB will review the results and recommend any necessary changes or additions to the study protocol. IRBs can also provide researchers with guidance on ethical considerations and the design and conduct of research protocols.

IRBs can support researchers by reviewing research protocols, providing feedback on potential risks and benefits associated with research, and educating and training researchers on ethical considerations and research protocols. Gain. IRBs can support research participants by ensuring that they are well-informed and protected throughout the research process.

The IRB process for evaluating research proposals typically involves several steps. First, ensure that our research protocol is comprehensive and compliant with applicable laws and regulations. The IRB reviews consent forms used in research, reviews data collection and analysis procedures to ensure that they are appropriate and reliable, reviews study results, and reviews the research protocol for any required changes or modifications that can be identified.

After the outline of the proposal is determined, the supervisor can start his work and propose the amount of the budget. The regulations and the time frame for submitting the proposal to each institution must be respected. An experienced supervisor can help the researcher to always overcome administrative rules, unexpected problems, and possible delays. Also, the supervisor can be an effective help in drafting the text of the sections related to the budget and collecting resources, appendices, and other matters.

All expenses should be clearly stated in the budget form. Usually, the salary includes the highest cost of the clinical research project. Therefore, the salary and hours of duty should be specified for all people in the budget list. It should be noted that the description of duties stated for the researcher and other members of the research should not leave any doubts in the minds of the judges and it should be ensured that the work estimated for each person is only for the success of the project.

Most judges pay attention to the percentage of the cost allocated to the main members of the project. Members who have very little responsibility based on the budget form are rarely evaluated. (Because they have many other duties and cannot spend much time studying the proposal.) If the needs of the study change or there are unexpected expenses, the best budget plan may also change. If the researcher wants to change the cost of some cases or increase or decrease the duties of the main researchers, he must obtain permission from the research center to provide the research budget. Institutions usually agree to reasonable requests for budgeting changes as long as the researcher does not want increased financial support. Researchers' specifications are usually mentioned on the second page of the proposal, which includes university education, current and previous jobs, and honors, and should be prepared in the following order: the title of all publications, all articles, and books published in the last 3 years.

Equipment and materials that are necessary for the project, including computers and technical equipment, laboratory materials and equipment, office space, and library, should be fully explained. These are usually available in pre-written proposals.

Sections of Objectives and Review of Sources

The specific objectives are the same as the research questions in terms of content, but they are expressed as expected from the research results. Each goal should be explained in one or two sentences. Most of the proposals have several objectives that should be presented in order and time sequence. The most logical way is to state the descriptive goals first, then the analytical goals.

The special goals section can be used to adjust other sections. It is better to review the sources and methods sections one after the other.

When many aspects are examined in a study, it is better to provide the reader with a complete list of specific objectives. If there are many special goals, it is better to state only the most important and interesting ones. In any case, the number of pages should not be large. The resource review section makes the proposal rich in terms of content. The details of this section should be written as much as possible. In this way, it becomes understandable for a person who is not an expert in that field. Sufficient information should be provided about how this particular study is done and why it is important to do it. The purpose of this section is to inform the researcher about how to conduct research, problems, and needs. Comprehensive or partial review depends on the concentration of special goals, the complexity of the issues, etc. Usually, reviewing 20 or 30 of the latest and best sources is enough. In many proposals, it is very important to conduct a guided study that confirms the validity of the research question and the practicality of the study.

Scientific Methods Section

The scientific method is the process scientists use to study and answer questions about the natural world. It involves making observations, forming hypotheses, designing experiments to test the hypotheses, analyzing data, and drawing conclusions. The scientific method consists of communicating the results of experiments and making them available for peer review, modifying hypotheses, and designing new experiments based on the results of previous experiments.

The referees carefully examine the methods section. A common reason for proposal rejection is weakness in technical methods. The first issue is how to organize this section. Sometimes research centers provide guidelines on how to set up methods; otherwise, we suggest the list in Table A.1. At this stage, a summary table about the content of the methods section is very useful, and a review of the design along with the presentation of diagrams and tables is very useful to inform the reader.

It is better to start the statistical section with data analysis methods. Its logical process can be as follows. First, the descriptive tables, then the method of analyzing the relationships between the variables, and after this stage, the problem of sample size is raised, which is better to start with the null hypothesis and choosing the appropriate statistical test, before determining the sample size, and estimate the effective sample size using and. The executive part of the proposal should include a schedule, that is α, β it should be determined when the main phases of the study will start and when they will end.

Indicators of a Good Proposal

A good proposal in medical sciences should be clear and provide an overview of the proposed project and its goals. Additionally, the proposal should include a detailed description of the proposed solution, implementation timeline, budget, and list of required resources. Additionally, the proposal should include all relevant background information and research, as well as a discussion of the potential risks and benefits of the proposed solution. Finally, your proposal should include a summary of your proposal and a call to action. In addition to the above elements, a good medical research proposal should also include a discussion of ethical considerations and a plan for project monitoring and evaluation. In addition, the proposal should include a plan to manage potential risks associated with the project and a plan to ensure that the project is carried out under applicable laws and regulations. Finally, the proposal should include a plan for communicating project results to stakeholders.

The characteristics of a good proposal are:

1. ***Scientific quality of the research plan:*** The research plan should be prepared based on a suitable research question. The plan and methods of doing it should be precise and practical. The research team has enough experience and skills and is committed to conducting research.
2. ***Technical quality of the proposal:*** proper presentation is one of the most important factors that determine the fate of the proposal. Even if the research question is important and the study design is excellent, the poor presentation will cause the referees to reject the proposal. The proposal should be concise, useful, and attractive, and should not destroy the judges' concentration with vague writings about sub-topics. A well-designed, carefully written, attractively presented, and error-free proposal makes the reader confident about the content of the research.

It is better to pay attention to the personal characteristics of the reviewer when writing the proposal. Most of the judges are involved in a lot of long proposals, so the salient points of the project should be identified so that they are not missed by reading quickly and carelessly. You can provide clear results, short sections with meaningful sub-chapters, accurate and short summaries, and concise and useful tables. And the simple diagrams drew the judge's attention to the very important points of the proposal. It is better to have white and empty spaces on the pages.

Most reviewers are very experienced and do not mind the extra sentences and multiple budget request forms. A proposal that exaggerates the importance of the project causes doubt. It is a good idea to write with enthusiasm, but the researcher should be realistic about the limitations of the project. Most of the judges are experts in determining the small problems of the design or the practicality of the research project design.

Instead of eliminating the basic defects, the researcher can clearly state them and explain the advantages and disadvantages of the selected plan. However, paying too much attention to these business issues is a mistake, because the weak aspects of the proposal may be noticed and the strong points of the proposal may be ignored. The goal is for the judges to make sure that the researcher prevents the occurrence of basic problems and has a thoughtful and realistic method of dealing with them.

Appendix B: Questionnaire Design and Interview Guidance

Abstract

This appendix presents the importance of questionnaire design and interviews in medical scientific research. The elements of a good survey: clear and concise questions, good answer options, and ample space for comments is outlined. Important elements of a proposal are explained.

Introduction

Measurement tools are tools that the researcher can use to gather the necessary information for analysis and investigation of the desired phenomenon and finally to discover the truth.

There are three main methods for collecting data on behaviors, health information, and personal history: observation, questionnaire, and interview. Observation is the most popular and natural tool for gathering information. The questionnaire is a tool that the respondent completes, but the interview is conducted by the interviewer. The use of the observation method becomes more accurate and efficient day by day with the progress of science and the invention of precise devices. One of the most important reasons for using the observation method is that with this method, the phenomenon or behavior under study is examined directly and live. This method is very suitable when the phenomenon under investigation must be investigated in a wide dimension, other methods cannot be used (such as studying the behavior of children), the presence of the researcher or the questioner affects the answers of the subjects under study. One of the problems of this method is that it is highly dependent on the personal perception and inference of the observer. This issue appears especially in the case of human behavior where different motivations can cause similar behaviors. The start and end time of observation can have a profound effect on the results obtained. In the questionnaires, the same method is used to answer simple questions such as age and smoking habit. Questionnaires are cheaper than interviews and do not require much time. Interviews are a better way to collect answers to complex questions that need more explanation, and the interviewer makes sure that the answers are complete. Interviews are better when the participants have different abilities to read and understand the questions. Expensiveness, time-consuming and being influenced by the answers from the relationship between the interviewer and the respondent are among the disadvantages of the interview.

The interview and the questionnaire can be standardized, but the execution of the interview changes a little each time. Both methods are sensitive to memory error and are affected by socially motivated responses to varying degrees.

Interviews may be expensive or impossible. When both methods are applicable, the choice depends on the cost-effectiveness and complexity of the investigated questions.

H. Soori, *Errors in Medical Science Investigations*, https://doi.org/10.1007/978-981-99-8521-0

Interviews and questionnaires are divided into two general categories: standard and non-standard which are invented and introduced by the researcher.

Standard tools have been modified and improved over time due to their many uses in various researches and have good reliability and repeatability. Usually, one of these standardized measurement tools can be found in most researches. Researchers should make a decision about this issue before starting the research and while designing the proposal by searching the sources related to the topic. When there are standardized tools for measurement and measurement, it is not logical to use the tools made by the researcher, and in fact, the use of the tools made by the researcher is only when there is no standard tool for research. However, there are many cases where standard tools (such as questionnaires) need to be modified and adjusted based on parameters such as culture, language, special conditions of the people under study, etc.

Designing a Questionnaire and Data Collection Tool

Many clinical research data are collected using questionnaires or interviews. The questionnaire is a set of predetermined questions to collect information (clinical data, social status, occupational groups, etc.). In many studies, the validity of the results depends on the quality of this tool. In this part, we explain how to properly design the questionnaire.

Designing Open and Closed Questions

The two main types of questions are open and closed questions, which are used for different purposes. Open-ended questions are used when it is important for researchers to hear the answers of the subjects under study. For example, an example of an open question is: "What habits do you think increase the risk of a heart attack?" Open questions make the researcher answer the question with fewer restrictions. These questions are useful in the initial stage of investigation and during design, because it introduces researchers to the attitude and thinking of the people under study. The phrases and words used in the answers are the basis for making better options in the next steps. The methods of coding and analyzing answers to open questions require more time than coding closed questions, which is one of the disadvantages of this type of questions. Closed questions are more common and create more standardized criteria. The answers to these questions are chosen from among several predetermined answers. For example, an example of a closed question is: Which of the following do you think increases the risk of heart attack more? (only one answer is correct) ≤ Smoking ≤ Obesity Worry. Since closed questions provide a list of possible answers, they are answered faster and easier and are easily analyzed. In general, the list of possible answers makes the meaning of the question clearer. Closed questions are useful in designing multiple-choice rating scales. There are many disadvantages of closed questions. These questions lead to directional answers. The answer list may not contain the most appropriate answer. The last problem can be solved by doing a pre-test using the answers given to an open question. However, the set of answers may not include all possible options. It is very important to include options such as "other cases" or "none of the above" in the questionnaire. When a specific answer is desired, the possible answers should not overlap. When a question has more than one answer, it is not appropriate to have the option "all items." For multiple-choice questions, it is better to use "yes, no, I don't know" answers for each option. Example: Which of the following increases the risk of heart attack?

	Yes	No	Do not know
Smoking			
Obesity			
Anxiety			

Continuous Scale Spectrum (VAS)

A continuous scale spectrum is another method of coding answers to closed questions using lines or other shapes. In this method, a continuous scale that includes the worst state to the best state is used. Subjects are asked to mark their answer on this scale. The final words should indicate the final exaggerated values. For ease of measure-

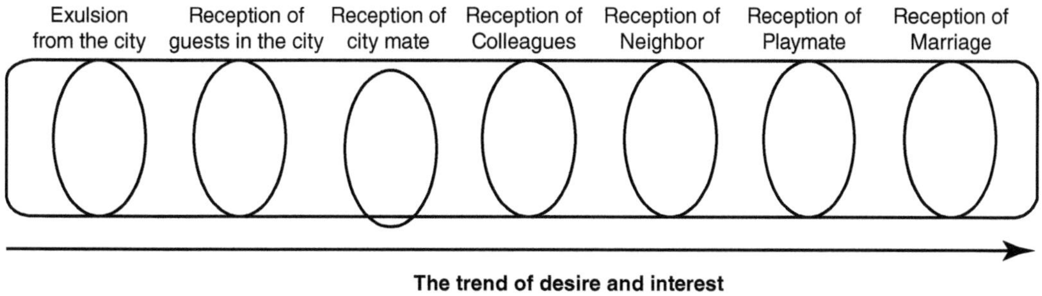

Fig. B.1 Measuring inclination and interest by spectrum

ment, 10 cm lines are often used, and the distance scale is in centimeters. In continuous spectrum scale, because the indicators are estimated on a continuous scale, they are very interesting. This scale is more sensitive to changes. Another method is to make multiple circles instead of a line, which may be easier to rank; But some answers are difficult to understand. Therefore, it is important to explain and provide examples of how to answer the question. For example, in measuring the degree of desire or lack of desire of a person or people from group "A" in relation to other social groups, a spectrum like Fig. B.1 is available to the people under study.

Elements of a Proposal

Questionnaire Structure

It is customary to explain the purpose of the study and the method of data collection in short sentences on the cover of the questionnaire. At the beginning of the interview, similar information is stated. To ensure the correctness and standardization of answers, all measurement tools must have specific instructions to be completed. This issue should be observed not only for the questionnaires that are completed by the people under study, but also for the forms that are asked orally by the interviewer. Sometimes a completed example of a simple question is useful. In order to improve the response, it is better to group the questions according to the topic and explain them with short sentences. It is better to ask neutral questions such as health status at the beginning of the questionnaire. More sensitive questions should be placed in the middle of the questionnaire and questions about personal issues, such as income, should be asked at the end of the questionnaire. The answer method for any question or set of questions that is different from other questions in the questionnaire should be clearly explained. If the questionnaire includes different time frames, it is useful to include the time frame at the top of each new set of questions. For example, questions such as:

- How many times has the doctor visited you during the last year?
- During the last year, how many times have you been examined in the emergency room of a medical center as a patient?
- During the last year, how many times have you been admitted to a hospital? can be summarized as follows:
- Several times during the past year.
  - Has the doctor visited you?
  - Have you been examined as a patient in the emergency department of a medical center?
  - Have you been admitted to a hospital? The external design of the questionnaire should be such that all questions can be answered as easily as possible. If the questionnaire is too complex, respondents or interviewers may miss questions or answer them incorrectly, which causes missing or incorrect data, or even the entire questionnaire may be invalid. A regular questionnaire with enough space is more interesting and easier to use compared to an irregular and crowded questionnaire. Although researchers are often interested in questionnaires

with fewer pages, it becomes problematic when there are too many questions on one page. Answer scales should have enough space to write an integer or draw a mark so that high or low answers are not accidentally marked. An open question should have enough space for the respondent to easily write the answer in that space. Questionnaires designed for people with vision problems should be large and bold. Possible answers to closed questions should be listed below, with boxes to be ticked or numbers circled around them. Example: How many different medicines do you take every day? (only one answer).

Nothing ≤2–1 ≤ 4–3 ≤ 5–6 ≤ 7 or more. Sometimes researchers want to get more detailed information about people who have specific answers to certain questions. One of the appropriate methods to achieve this goal is to use follow-up questions. In this type of questions, researchers screen the people under study according to the initial answers.

Example: Have you ever been told that you have high blood pressure? ≤ Yes ≤ No If yes, at what age were you first told that you have high blood pressure? .... age If yes, go to question 11. Sequential questions save time and make the respondent ignore irrelevant and repetitive questions. Guiding the respondent to the next appropriate question is done by using sentences like "go to question 11."

Sentences

Every word in a question can affect the validity of the answers. The goal is to make the questions simple and unambiguous so that the people under study can answer the questions honestly and correctly and not be afraid of the possible consequences of the answers.

Clarity

Questions should be clear and specific as much as possible. In general, the definition of words should be explained in the list of words. For example, to measure the amount of sports activities in the question "How many hours do you devote to sports during a particular week?," it is better to replace the following question: "How much do you usually do sports?"

Simplicity

Questions should be simple and use common words and avoid using specialized and complicated terms. For example, people easily understand the sentence "Which drugs can you buy without a doctor's prescription?", but they are less familiar with the term "self-administration of drugs." Sentences should be short and have a simple grammatical structure. The use of inductive words and cliché words that cause the desired answer to be induced should be avoided. In the question "How many times did you drink a lot of soft drinks in the last month?", the phrase "a lot" implies the negative effect of sugary soft drinks on health, and it is better to ask the question as follows: "During the last month, how many times during the day did you drink more than five Have you had a glass of soft drink?" [1]. Sometimes it is better to start the sentences with a tone so that the respondent imagines that a habit or action that is against the custom or inappropriate is done by many people and doing it is not unexpected, for example, "many patients sometimes forget the order to take medicine. Have you ever forgotten to take your medicine?." Collecting information in cases such as bad habits or income is difficult. Some people prefer to answer these questions in a questionnaire rather than in an interview; but a very skilled interviewer sometimes gets good answers. In personal interviews, it is better to write the desired answers on cards and the respondent to mark the answers.

Timing

The main questions of the questionnaire are usually designed to measure the frequency of specific behaviors such as eating habits or drug consumption. To measure the frequency of behavior, the respondent must provide the answer in the time scale, such as the number of bottles of soft drink drunk during a day. If this behavior is repeated daily, for example, one pill is taken every morning, a very simple question arises: how many pills do you take in a day? Many daily behaviors change from season to season or year to year. To measure these behaviors, the researcher must first decide what indicators are the important behavioral aspects in the study, mean or Frein states. For example, in the study of the chronic effect of alcohol in increasing the risk of heart attack, it is probably necessary to measure the average consumption of alcohol at a certain time, while the study that is designed to investigate the role of alcohol in the occurrence of injuries caused by falling, probably needs to measure the frequency of times that excessive drinking of alcohol causes Eating the balance of people has been studied. Questions about average behavior are asked in two ways: asking about typical behavior or counting over a period of time. For example, researchers may measure the average consumption of soft drinks with the following question:

Approximately how many glasses of soda do you consume during the week? (Each bottle of soft drink is equivalent to 200 cc) .... soda per week This structure is simple and concise. The respondent expresses the average of his behavior with a simple estimate. Because drinking changes over short periods of time, the respondent may have difficulty deciding which week to talk about. When individuals are asked about their daily behaviors, they frequently provide a report based on their typical activities, often overlooking transient or infrequent states.. Asking about soft drink consumption during the week usually provides a lower estimate of soft drink consumption at the end of the week. Another alternative method is to specify the exact time of exposure. Example: How much soda have you consumed in the last 7 days? .... soft drinks in the last 7 days. Focusing on a specific and short period of time (such as last week) provides the respondent with the ability to remember and make a more accurate estimate. It is possible that the time period defined in the question is not the same as the usual days of the year. If the time interval includes weekends or special occasions, for example, it may cause the average consumption of soft drinks to be overestimated. When asked about a specific behavior, it is difficult for the respondent to remember the performance in a longer period of time, and their answer tends towards more usual behavior. If the behavior under investigation is not regular and common, using a calendar is very useful. In this method, the researcher can calculate the average daily rank.

Two-Sided Questions

Each question should explain only one concept. Sometimes the answers to questions that include words such as "and" and "or" seem incomprehensible. Suppose a question is designed to assess caffeine consumption. "How many cups of coffee or tea do you drink in a day?." The caffeine in coffee is more than the caffeine in tea. For this reason, measuring the amount of caffeine consumed is not accurate. When a question is asked to evaluate two categories at the same time, it is better to turn it into two questions. "How many cups of coffee do you drink in a day?" and "How many cups of tea do you drink in a day?."

Contractual Assumptions

Sometimes the questions include assumptions that do not apply to all members of the study. For example, a standard question about "anxiety" asks the respondent to recount the number of times he has experienced such a feeling. A question like "I feel that even with the help of my family I cannot solve my worries." It is difficult for those who do not have a family or their family does not support them. On unrelated questions and options: The question and the answer options must be related. This is an important point that seems simple but is often not followed properly. For example, for the question "Have you had pain in the last week?" sometimes the answer options are "never, rarely, very often, often" which is grammatically incorrect and may mislead the respondent. The question should be changed as follows: "How many times have you felt pain during the last week?" or that the answers to the first question should be "yes or no." Another problem occurs when the answer options are agreement or disagreement. For example, if a question is asked as follows: "I am sometimes depressed" and the answer options are "I agree, I do not agree," the answer is misleading for those who are often depressed. Not agreeing with this statement means that the person is often depressed or never depressed. In this case, it is better to use clearer questions. For example, "How depressed do you feel?" with the answer options "never, sometimes, often."

Scoring to Measure Qualitative Variables

Quantitative evaluation of subjective concepts such as quality of life by one question is difficult, and summary indicators are usually measured by scoring a series of questions. Using multiple options to evaluate a concept in comparison with a single question or multiple questions has advantages. In comparison with other methods, multiple choice scales increase the range of possible answers. (For example, the score range in a multi-choice scale for evaluating the quality of life is from 1 to 100. In the case of a single question, it may include four or five answers from very inappropriate to completely appropriate.) One of the disadvantages of multi-choice scales is that the results (for example, quality of life = 46.2) are difficult to understand. They usually use the Likert scale for quantities such as attitudes, behaviors, and quality of life. These scales provide a list of questions to the respondent. Then the respondent is asked to choose the option closest to his opinion. Finally, the answers are given points. In each question, circle the number that is the best answer in your opinion.

		Very agree	Agree	No idea	Disagree	Very agree
		1	2	3	4	5
A	Smoking in public facilities should be made illegal					
B	Advertising for cigarettes should be banned					
C	The national income should be spent on the fight against smoking					

A researcher can easily calculate the respondent's total score by adding up the score of each question or the average for the answered questions. For example, the score of the person who strongly agrees with the first and second questions (1 point) but disagrees with the third question (4 points) is 6. The internal consistency of each spectrum can be measured with statistical criteria such as Cronbach's alpha test [2]. This test evaluates the internal consistency of the scale. Cronbach's alpha is calculated using the correlation between the scores of each question. Values above 0.7 are usually acceptable for this criterion, and values of 0.8 or more are excellent. Lower values indicate that each group of questions measures different indicators (there is no internal consistency).

Creating New Scales and Questionnaires

Sometimes the researcher measures an index for which there is no standard questionnaire or interview method. In this case, new questions or scales should be designed. The scope of this activity can range from creating a new question about a sub-variable in the study (for example, how many times a day do you brush your teeth) to developing and testing a multiple-choice scale to measure an outcome (job satisfaction) of the study. It may be necessary to develop a new tool to measure an important concept such as measuring IQ, systematic and long-term methods to convert the initial version to the final result. When the questionnaire or interview is prepared, the next step is critical review by expert and skilled persons.

Stages of Questionnaire Preparation in the Study

There are several steps to collect a set of questionnaires for each study. These steps include preparing a list of variables that may be suitable for the study, collecting existing questionnaires and designing a new questionnaire that is clear, attractive, and easy, conducting a pre-test to estimate the time required to execute the questionnaire and test the repeatability and validity of the answers.

Preparing a List of Variables

Before designing an interview or questionnaire, the researcher must prepare a list of the data to be collected and the concepts measured in the study (e.g., outcomes and confounders).

Collection of Existing Questionnaires

Complete a checklist to measure each variable. A useful method is to create a folder for each variable. Then, optional questions are prepared for the subject. The best questionnaire or interview method should be used to measure the consequences and exposures. There are usually different sources for questionnaires and interviews. First, it is better to collect the questionnaires of other researchers who have studied the desired criteria. Many standard questionnaires are available in books, review articles and electronic resources such as CDs and websites. By using phrases such as "questionnaires related to the study of nutrition patterns" you can find the desired site and collect the questionnaires. Also, the published questionnaires of other studies with similar topics, or contacting other researchers can be useful for collecting the questionnaire. Using questionnaires from other studies saves time and the findings can be compared with the results of other studies. It is possible that the existing questionnaires are not completely suitable for the question or the studied community, or that they are too long; But if some topics are not suitable, some questions can be removed, added, or changed (all these problems occur when a questionnaire prepared and adjusted for a specific culture or topic is used in other situations).

Draft Preparation

Compared to the original questionnaire, the initial draft should include more questions about the topic, but in terms of structure, it should be completely similar to the final questionnaire. On correcting, the researcher should read the initial draft carefully and imagine himself as a respondent. Answer all the questions and check all the possible explanations for each question. The goal is to change words or phrases that may mislead even a small number of respondents or may not be understood correctly. Finding short or incomprehensible words and translating them into simpler and more understandable terms is also one of the goals. Complex questions that include expressions such as "and" and "or" can be converted into two or more simpler questions. It is better to use expert and skilled people to review and design the questionnaire. The purpose of each question must be stated very clearly. In shortening the study questionnaire, usually, more data is collected in studies compared to what needs to be analyzed. Long interviews and questionnaires may tire the respondent and reduce the validity of the answers. When the questionnaire is available to people by post, less attention is paid to long questionnaires. Questions whose answers are not related to the main purpose of the study cause extra time to enter, correct and analyze data and reduce the accuracy of the study. In order to decide whether there is a question in the questionnaire or not, first think about the analysis and reporting of its results in the study. By summarizing the final tables, you will be sure that all the required variables are present in the study. If you have doubts about whether a topic or criteria will be used in the next analysis, it is better to delete it.

Pre-test

In order to clarify, correct, and estimate the time to complete the questionnaire, a pre-test should be done. The role of the pre-test is much more valuable than the latter when examining the validity and repeatability of questionnaires. Validation Like any other criteria, the validity and repeatability of questionnaires and interviews should be checked. The first step is to check the apparent validity of the questions. This stage is a matter of taste and subjects that include the researcher's desired indicators are examined. The validity of the new questionnaires is examined in comparison with the standard reference criteria. When the reference standard is not available, the responses of two groups of patients who are at different levels of the desired conditions are compared. When there is a big difference between two groups, we conclude that the questions are more valid. The predictive validity of a questionnaire is evaluated by the correlation coefficient with future events. For example, in the question "Can you read a newspaper without glasses or contact lenses?", the answers are compared with the answers of the valid questionnaire that was completed for patients with cataracts and people with healthy eyes. By comparing the responses of cataract patients before and after surgery, the validity of the questionnaire is tested.

Sequence of Questions

Most of the time, the best way to start the questions is everyday and normal questions. If the initial questions are very personal, it is possible to induce the feeling of alienation to the participants. The fact that all information related to the subjects of the study, even information such as age, race, etc., remains confidential, must be brought to the notice of all study participants. It is very important to create motivation about the research topic and to prepare interesting questions so that the people under study patiently answer all the questions. Probably the best way to design the sequence of questions is to put important and basic questions in the middle of the questionnaire. It should be noted that the answers that the subjects write for open-ended questions do not affect the subsequent questions.

Response Rate

The response rate to the questionnaires varies depending on the strata of the society that have been examined; But generally, they have reported low response rate. According to the researches, the response rate is about 40% and if the sampling is simple random from the whole community, it will be even lower than this value [3]. Compliance with the following may increase the response rate:

- Using appropriate and high-quality paper, especially if the questionnaire is mailed.
- Use legible and clear lines.
- The coarseness of the line, especially when the people under study have vision problems.
- Consider the empty space to answer the questions.
- Instructions for answering the questions should be prepared with a different and specific font for each part.
- Ensure the correct arrangement of the tables for marking the answers.
- Use the typed version of the questionnaire.
- Number the pages of the questionnaire.
- In postal questionnaires, a stamped envelope with a return address should be given to the people under study.
- An abstract version of the research should be made available to the people under study.
- Specify the date of return of the answers.
- In an attachment letter, describe the objectives of the current research and introduce the researchers.
- Make sure that the people under study complete the questionnaire in the right environment and time.
- Do not give the questionnaires to the sample members when they are very busy. For example, end-of-year holidays, end-of-semester exams, etc. are not suitable times to complete the questionnaire.

Advantages and Disadvantages of the Questionnaire

Advantages

- It saves money and time.
- It becomes possible to reach a large group of people in a relatively easy and cheap way.
- The face-to-face contact between researchers and subjects under study, which causes social and psychological effects on subjects under study, is eliminated.
- Researchers have a lot of time to design questions and can ask more serious questions than interviews.

Disadvantages

- The answers given can be apparent and unreal and the people under study provide researchers with information contrary to reality.
- The lack of face-to-face contact between researchers and subjects may cause confusion

and misunderstanding in answering questions.
- Questionnaires are not suitable for certain members of society such as children or illiterate people.
- The response rate is usually low and the percentage of incomplete or carelessly completed questionnaires is very high.

Interview

Interview is not a research method, but a set of research methods that are common in only one topic. An interview consists of a conversation between two people in which one person plays the role of a researcher [4]. The interview can be very calculated and structured to the extent of an oral questionnaire or completely unstructured and to the extent of a common conversation. Most of the interviews are somewhere between these two extremes [5].

Regular interview; Semi-regular interview; Irregular interview; Structured interview; Semi-structured interview; Unstructured interview.

Regular Interview

In this type of interview, the interviewer has a precise template about the questions to be asked, their order and sequence, and the exact words that should be included in each question, and acts on the issued instructions. In a regular interview, the interviewer usually reads the questions to the study subjects on special forms that have special instructions and codes corresponding to each answer and marks the answers in the form. The only difference between a regular interview and a questionnaire is that the study subjects in a regular interview do not have the form of the questions and answer the questions orally. In this case, factors such as the attractiveness of the questions, the clarity of the instructions for filling out the forms, and the inability to read them accurately are not very effective. The important point is the accuracy of the questioners in the way they express the questions, which should be done in such a way that the people under study are not influenced unconsciously.

Semi-regular Interview

In this type of interview, the interviewer is fully aware of the subject of investigation; But there is freedom of action in the way of phrasing the questions, their sequence and order. It is possible to use special forms; But the questioner is allowed to ask only specific questions from the form. In this type of interview, the interviewers encourage the subjects to give more complete and accurate answers. To see examples of this type, readers can refer to sources [6–9].

Irregular Interview

In this type of interview, there is no predetermined set of questions. The people under study are allowed to express their feelings and opinions without any restrictions, control or guidance from the questioner. In an informal interview, the questioner asks some obscure points from the subject and tries to get more information about more interesting topics. The main use of informal interviews is in psychological studies, counseling sessions and special diseases such as AIDS, special mental diseases, etc.; but in other studies, especially in the early stages of the research, this type of interview is used to collect primary information. References [10–12] are successful examples of this issue.

Advantages and Disadvantages of Regular Interview

- Regular interview is a precise, clear, and purposeful method of collecting information. Regular interview is relatively low-cost and low-cost.
- It is easy to extract and encode data in this method.
- This method usually has high validity and reliability.
- The order of asking the questions, the precise way of expressing them and the predetermined pattern of the questions may create this mindset in the people under study that they are not important independently but are important as a part of this study.

This issue can cause a decrease in the cooperation of the people under study [12].

Advantages and Disadvantages of Semi-regular and Irregular Interviews

Semi-regular and irregular interview is a useful method in cases where the subject of the study is relatively vague or when we want to collect deep information from the people under study. In a semi-regular interview, the interviewer can adjust the way of expressing the questions in a way that is suitable for different study subjects. For example, to express questions with different words for young and old people, or to express them more simply for people who are not familiar with the language of the questioner. Also, depending on the conditions of the interview, ask some questions earlier and some later.

- The non-standard way of expressing the questions and their non-uniform order in semi-regular and irregular interviews can lead to the collection of highly unreliable data.
- It is very difficult to extract and code answers in this type of interviews.
- These types of interviews are expensive and time-consuming.
- It is very difficult to train people to conduct these types of interviews.
- The bias caused by the influence and direction of the questioner in these interviews can be very large and fundamental to the extent that it distorts all the facts [4, 5].

The skill of the interviewer affects the quality of the answers. Standardizing the interview process from one interview to the next is the basis of increasing the repeatability of interviews. The interview should be structured with uniform phrasing, questions and non-verbal cues. The interviewer should carefully avoid the interviewer's tour. Sometimes it is necessary to ask additional questions to get the right answer. This issue is done due to the motivation of the people under study to answer the questions clearly and completely. This method is standardized by writing standard expressions in the margin of the text of each question. For example, when in response to the question "how many cups of coffee do you drink each day?," the respondent says "I'm not sure" or "every day is different." The instructions should include a series of additional questions such as "estimate as best you can" or "approximately how many cups" do you drink coffee on a normal day? The studied phenomena and variables are evaluated and measured with the help of research tools and become "data." Before collecting data, some questions must be answered. An example of these questions is given in the table below. The answer to these questions is important, but it is not fixed, and most of the answers change along with the progress of the research project and cause many elements to be revised.

Stage	Questions that are asked when collecting information, analyzing, sharing, publishing, and recording data
Information gathering	What data will be collected? How is the data recorded? Who collects the data? What is the criteria for rejecting data? What is the criteria for accepting data?
Analysis	What method is used for data analysis? Which results should be published? When will the data be released? Where are the data published?
Data storage/ recording	Which of the research records are recorded and stored? How do they store the records? How long do they keep the records? Who is responsible for data storage?
Data sharing	Which of the research records may be shared? When can records be shared? Who is responsible for making decisions about shared records?

Reliability of Research Tools

The reliability of the research tool is a function of repeatability; That is, if we measure the desired variable twice with the same instrument (under the same conditions), the results will be the same. Internal stability and correlation and agreement between observers in data collection also indicate reliability. In general, the factors affecting the reliability of the research tool are the number of questions, the range of changes in scores in the studied population, the complexity and difficulty of the questions. Types of methods for determining reliability include retesting, determining internal consistency, measurement stability of a test when it is used by different people, and equivalent forms. In the retest method, a group of people is selected and the test is presented to the people, taking into account the appropriate time interval, the same test is given to the people (with the same examiner) and then the correlation between the scores obtained is calculated to be. This method will be suitable for relatively stable variables. The time interval between the two tests should not be so short that the answers of the first time remain in people's memory and not so long that the measured variable has changed over time. The statistical techniques used are Pearson or Spearman retest. The important thing is that due to the passage of time, the correlation value decreases because the error variance increases, and the shorter the interval between two measurements, the more similar the factors affecting the error variance will be. In this test, the reliability coefficient ranges from 0 to 1, and the closer this value is to 1, the higher the correlation. A correlation higher than 0.70 for most tests and a correlation of 0.90 for cognitive domain tests is considered acceptable. In the method of determining internal consistency, the correlation between questionnaire questions is measured and is used to ensure that all questions (or observations) measure the same concept. In this method, the questions are presented to the subjects only once. Common statistical methods are Cronbach's alpha and Richardson coder. In determining the measurement stability of a test if it is used by different people, two observers will report their independent observations and then the correlation coefficient between the scores will be calculated. The statistical method used for nominal data is Kappa test, Kendall test for rank data and Pearson coefficient for range or ratio data. In determining the reliability of the research tool through equivalent forms, the stability of the results is determined in the case of using two similar questionnaires that measure the same concept. The questionnaire is presented to the subjects only once, and in cases where the use of several forms or questionnaires is desired, it is appropriate or even necessary. The statistical method used for this method will be Pearson's or Spearman's coefficient.

Validity of Research Tools

Validity is a necessary and important part of a research tool, but it is not a sufficient indicator for the completeness of that tool. Unfortunately, in many published studies, the content validity of the research tools used is not measured or reported. Determining the validity of the content is necessary for the real measurement of the required information and can improve the quality of the study. Two standard methods to ensure content validity are item sampling and test structure method. People's judgment, or the judgment (10–15 people) of specialists and subject matter experts on the contents and content of the questionnaire is one of the usual ways to determine the validity of the content. Determining relevance, clarity of questions and their simplicity along with ranking (for example, not relevant = 1, relevant but in need of basic modification = 2, relevant and in need of minor modification = 3, and relevant = 4 points) and determining the total points obtained and evaluating each question is from conventional methods [13].

Appendix C: Control of Random Errors: Issues Related to Sample Size Calculation

Abstract

Even with the most accurate and skilled study plans, when the sample size is insufficient, we will not be able to scientifically examine the research question. On the other hand, when a study is designed with a larger sample size, it becomes difficult and costly to implement. The purpose of determining the sample size is to estimate the number of members under study in the desired study. To calculate the appropriate sample size for statistical analysis, the type of analysis must be known from the beginning. It should also be noted that data type, distribution, variance, error level as well as confidence level in calculating the sample size. Calculating the sample size is a mathematical method to find an almost correct estimate of the studied members and it should be estimated at the beginning of the study design that there is a possibility of making general changes.

Introduction

In the design phase of each study, the following questions should be considered.

1. What is the required sample size to reach the desired statistical power? (for example, achieving an 80% chance of observing a clinically significant difference).
2. How can an acceptable sample size be achieved when faced with limitations such as a lack of budget, facilities, and qualified patients?

Examining these questions is usually evaluated by statistical calculation of the sample size. Determining the sample size is based on statistical relationships according to criteria such as accuracy and study power. If the sample size is evaluated with statistical criteria, it is done on the predetermined sample size, which may be small due to limitations. The main emphasis is based on the calculation of the sample size, but the application of these methods is easily possible in judging the size of the sample in advance.

In each study, the sample size is calculated based on characteristics such as type 1 and type 2 errors. For example, it is possible to calculate the sample size in such a way that the desired accuracy is achieved to achieve the desired level of confidence (or a constant type 1 error). This method is called determining the sample size with precision. One of the disadvantages of this method is the low chance of observing real differences (actually, in this method, there is no control over the statistical power of the tests). The alternative method of calculating sample size is acceptable for statistical power (type 1–2 error) and accuracy (type I error). In other words, in this method, the calculated sample size has a suitable statistical power to detect important clinical differences at a fixed level of type I error [14, 15].

H. Soori, *Errors in Medical Science Investigations*, https://doi.org/10.1007/978-981-99-8521-0

In most clinical studies, it is common to conduct a pilot study to determine the sample size. Determining the sample size based on the study of the pilot begins with examining the power function,[1] which is calculated using the information obtained in this step. In practice, the existence of contradictions in study objectives (hypotheses), study design, statistical analyzes, and sample size calculation is illogical and can cause unrealistic results to be observed. Important contradictions in this field can be caused by:

1. False test for the true hypothesis;
2. True test for a false hypothesis;
3. False test for a false hypothesis and
4. Correct test for correct hypothesis but with inappropriate power.

For this reason, it is recommended to carefully study the following steps before calculating the sample volume:

1. The goals and hypotheses of the study should be specified carefully.
2. The study design and statistical tests used are appropriate.
3. The sample size should be calculated based on the desired hypotheses and tests.

The Basis for Calculating the Sample Size

The sample size of a survey is determined by the desired confidence level, error bars, population variability, and the proportion of the population expected to exhibit a particular response. Totally, the larger the sample size, results in more accurate and precise the consequences. To calculate your sample size, use the sample size calculator or consult a statistician. When calculating sample size, it is important to consider the variability of the population, the desired confidence level, the error bars, and the expected proportion of the population that will respond in a particular way. The sample size should be large enough to provide reliable results, but not too large or too large to be practical.

The sample size is calculated based on several factors including:

1. Confidence level: The confidence level (commonly 95%) is the degree of certainty required in the statistical analysis. It is usually expressed as a percentage and represents the likelihood that the results are accurate.
2. The margin of error: The margin of error is the degree of precision required in the statistical analysis. It is usually expressed as a percentage, and it represents the amount by which the sample statistic may deviate from the true population parameter.
3. Population size: The size of the population being studied also affects the sample size calculation. The larger the population size, the larger the sample size required to achieve the desired level of confidence and margin of error.
4. Variability: Variability refers to the degree to which the data varies within the population being studied. If the data exhibit high variability, a larger sample size may be required to achieve the desired level of confidence and margin of error.
5. Type of data: The type of data being collected also affects the sample size calculation. If the data is continuous, a larger sample size may be required to achieve the desired level of confidence and margin of error compared to categorical data.

Once these factors are considered, researchers can use statistical software or online calculators to calculate the required sample size for their study. Obtaining an appropriate sample size is crucial for obtaining reliable and accurate results from the study. To reduce the error to the desired level and increase the validity of the results of

[1]The power function could be calculated as $f(x) = kx^{p}$, wherein, k and p are real numbers and k is known as the coefficient. The power function is a fixed number.

statistical analysis, an appropriate number of samples should be selected. To calculate the sample size, the type of study must be known. The type of data, distribution, variance, error level, and confidence level should also be noted.

To calculate the required sample size, it is necessary to evaluate the important characteristics and parameters in terms of study objectives in people who are eligible to enter the study, and the following steps should be performed:

1. Determining the size of the risk effect that we want to reveal in the study. For example, in a study, a researcher may want to be able to show this difference if the odds ratio of people with exposure is four times that of people without exposure.
2. The level of significance is the strength of the evidence to reject the null hypothesis. A smaller probability value means more evidence to reject the null hypothesis and as a result, the sample size becomes larger.
3. The probability of reaching the desired significance level (power of the test).

In general, there are different methods for determining the sample size:

- Determining sample size based on experience.
  In this case, the researcher determines the sample size based on the information he/she has about the possible distribution or type of data. For example, if the sample size is less than the required level, the created confidence interval may have a bigger than acceptable one, which reduces the accuracy of the estimate. Also, by selecting a bigger sample size than the required value, the cost of statistical analysis increases unnecessarily.
- Determining the sample size based on the distribution scale.
  By choosing the variance value as the measure of distribution for the estimator, the sample size can be obtained. In such a case, to achieve a smaller variance (less error) for the estimator, a larger sample size is also needed. As a result, if the objective is to determine the limits of the confidence interval, it is possible to achieve smaller confidence interval limits by choosing a large sample size.
- Determining the significance level.
  By keeping the error rate, we need more samples by increasing the confidence level or significance level. As a result, a balance must be reached between the error rate and the significance level to obtain a suitable sample. By choosing the maximum amount of error and considering the level with a suitable meaning, we will reach the minimum sample size.

Determining the sample size to estimate the proportions, determining the sample size to estimate the mean of a value, determining the sample size according to the power of the test, using tables of sample size and test power, determining the sample size using the Mead resource equation, determining the sample size in qualitative research and the sample size in stratified sampling have specific methods that are explained here and have been extensively discussed separately in different relevant sources.

Types of Errors in Statistical Tests

A statistical test can never conclude that the null hypothesis is true or false. Rather, only a sign of the strength of the evidence against the null hypothesis is revealed. When using a statistical test to decide whether to reject or accept the null hypothesis, two types of errors are revealed. Rejecting the null hypothesis when it is true and not rejecting the null hypothesis when it is false.

Therefore, there are two types of errors in statistical tests: Type I error and Type II error.

Type I error: Type I error occurs when the null hypothesis is rejected when it is true. In other words, it is a false positive result, and the researcher concludes that there is a significant difference or effect when there is none. The probability of making a Type I error is denoted by alpha (α), typically set at 0.05 or 0.01, which represents the level of significance of the test. For example, suppose a medical test is used to diagnose a disease, and the null hypothesis is that the patient does not have the disease. If the test incorrectly indicates that the patient has the disease, even though the patient does not have it, this is a Type I error.

Type II error: Type II error occurs when the null hypothesis is not rejected when it is false. In other words, it is a false negative result, and the researcher concludes that there is no significant difference or effect when there is one. The probability of making a Type II error is denoted by beta (β) and is dependent on the statistical power of the test. A higher level of statistical power means a lower chance of committing a Type II error.

For example, suppose a medical test is used to diagnose a disease, and the null hypothesis is that the patient does not have the disease. If the test indicates the patient does not have the disease, but they do, this is a Type II error.

Overall, controlling and minimizing the chances of committing Type I and Type II errors are crucial for ensuring reliable and valid statistical research results. The first one is called the first type error and the second one is called the second type error. Therefore, in a two-sided hypothesis test, when we consider the value of the first type error as 0.05, if the result becomes significant (the null hypothesis is rejected), there is a 5% probability that we have made a mistake (Fig. C.1a).

The second type of error is not rejecting the null hypothesis when it is false. This issue is shown in Fig. C.1b. The gray area is a proportion ($b\%$) of the real sample distribution that falls within the acceptance area of the null hypothesis. The probability of not committing the second type of error ($b\% - 100$) is equal to the power of the test. Table C.1 shows the occurrence modes of these two errors.

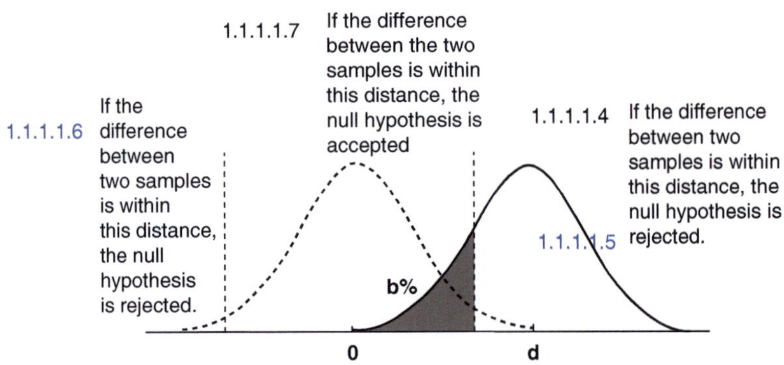

Fig. C.1 Probability of occurrence of two types of errors (type 1 and type 2 errors) in the hypothesis test with a level of 5%

Table C.1 Types of errors in hypothesis testing

Reality		
Result of a significant test	The null hypothesis is correct	The null hypothesis is not correct
The null hypothesis is rejected	Error type I Probability = significant level	Correct result Probability = power
The null hypothesis is accepted	Correct result Probability = 1 − significant level	Type II error Probability = 1 − power

Relationships for Calculating the Sample Size

To calculate the sample size for a statistical study, the following relationships are used:

1. Sample size and confidence level: As the desired level of confidence increases, the required sample size also increases. For example, a 90% confidence level requires a smaller sample size than a 95% confidence level for the same margin of error.
2. Sample size and margin of error: As the margin of error decreases, the required sample size increases. A smaller margin of error requires a larger sample size to achieve the desired level of precision in the study.
3. Sample size and population size: As the population size increases, the required sample size also increases. However, the relationship is not linear, and other factors such as the level of variability in the population may also affect the sample size.
4. Sample size and variance: A larger variance in the population data requires a larger sample size to achieve the desired level of precision. A smaller variance allows for a smaller sample size.
5. Sample size and statistical power: The statistical power of a study measures the probability of detecting a true effect if there is one. As the desired level of statistical power increases, the required sample size also increases [16].

In general, the calculation of sample size involves balancing the tradeoff between the level of precision desired, the level of confidence required, and the available resources (such as time, budget, and feasibility). It is therefore important to carefully consider these relationships and other factors when designing and conducting a statistical study. Suitable formulas for calculating sample size in general cases are given in Table C.2. This list consists of two parts. Table C.2(A) is for cases where the study aims to show a certain difference (analytical studies) and Table C.2(B) is for cases where the aim is to estimate the quantity of interest with a certain accuracy (descriptive studies, determination of prevalence or incidence), is used.

It is necessary to pay attention to this point that in cases where the comparison of two means, ratios, or rates is desired, the required sample size is calculated for each group, and by doubling this amount, the total sample size is obtained.

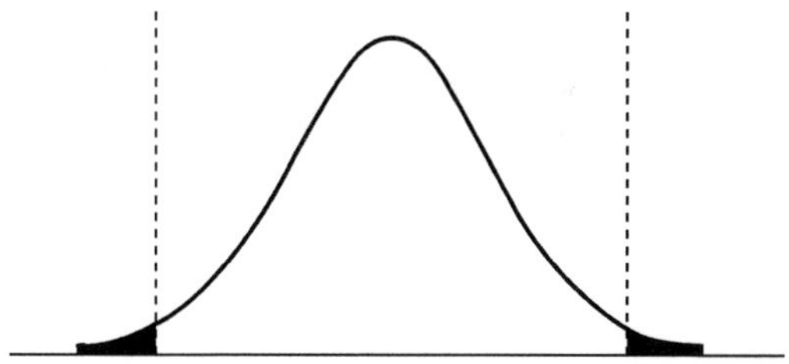

(a) Type 1 error: the null hypothesis is true and the difference between the two populations is zero. In this figure, the sample distribution curve of the difference between the samples is shown. The gray areas (5% of the area under the curve) show the probability of falsely rejecting the null hypothesis.
(b) Type II error: the null hypothesis is incorrect and the difference between the two populations (*d*) is not zero. In this figure, the curve with the continuous line shows the real sample distribution, and the difference between the samples, and the dashed line shows the sample distribution under the null hypothesis. The gray area is the probability (*b*%) that the null hypothesis is falsely rejected.

Table C.2 Calculation of the sample size: (A) studies that aim to find a significant difference; (B) studies that aim to accurately estimate the desired quantity

Study objective	Necessary information	Sample size calculation
A. Significant result		
1. Mean estimation	$\mu - \mu_0$ difference between 2 means μ μ_0	$\frac{(\upsilon + v)^2 \sigma^2}{(\mu - \mu_0)^2}$
2. Rate estimation[a]	μ rate μ_0 the value of the rate under the null hypothesis	$\frac{(\upsilon + v)^2 \mu}{(\mu - \mu_0)^2}$
3. Proportion estimation	π proportion π_0 the value of the proportion under the null hypothesis	$\frac{\left\{\upsilon\sqrt{[\pi(1-\pi)]} + v\sqrt{[\pi_0(1-\pi_0)]}\right\}^2}{(\pi - \pi_0)^2}$
4. Comparison between 2 means (sample size for each group)	$\mu - \mu_0$ difference between means σ_1 σ_2 standard deviation	$\frac{(\upsilon + v)^2 (\sigma_1^2 + \sigma_0^2)}{(\mu_1 - \mu_0)^2}$
5. Comparison between 2 rates[a] (sample size for each group)	μ_0 μ_1 rates	$\frac{(\upsilon + v)^2 (\mu_1 - \mu_0)}{(\mu_1 - \mu_0)^2}$
6. Comparison between 2 proportions (sample size for each group)	π_1 π_2 proportions $\pi = \frac{\pi_1 + \pi_0}{2}$	$\frac{\left\{\upsilon\sqrt{\left[\sqrt{\pi_1(1-\pi_1)} + \pi_0(1-\pi_0)\right]} + v\sqrt{[2\bar{\pi}(1-\bar{\pi})]}\right\}^2}{(\pi_0 - \pi_1)^2}$
7. A case-control study (sample size for each group)	π_0 the proportion of the control group with exposure π_1 the proportion of the case group calculated with $\pi_1 = \frac{\pi_0 \mathrm{OR}}{1 + \pi_0(\mathrm{OR} - 1)}$ Odds ratio $\bar{\pi} = \frac{\pi_1 + \pi_0}{2}$	$\frac{\left\{\upsilon\sqrt{[\pi_0(1-\pi_0) + \pi_1(1-\pi_1)]} + v\sqrt{[2\bar{\pi}(1-\bar{\pi})]}\right\}^2}{(\pi_1 - \pi_0)^2}$
All the mentioned cases	υ (100%-power) A percentage of the standard normal distribution corresponds to the point in the one-sided test v A percentage of the standard normal distribution that is related to the significance level of the two-sided test. For more information, refer to Table C.3	
B. Precision		
8. Mean determination	σ standard deviation	$\frac{\sigma^2}{e^2}$
9. Rate determination[a]	μ rate	$\frac{\propto}{e^2}$

Table C.2 (continued)

Study objective	Necessary information	Sample size calculation
10. Proportion determination	π proportion	$\frac{\pi(1-\pi)}{e^2}$
11. Difference between 2 means (sample size for each group)	σ_0 σ_1 standard deviation	$\frac{\sigma_1^2+\sigma_0^2}{e^2}$
12. Difference between 2 rates[a] (sample size for each group)	μ_1 μ_0 rates	$\frac{\mu_1+\mu_0}{e^2}$
13. Difference between 2 proportions (sample size for each group)	π_2 π_1 proportions	$\frac{\pi_1(1-\pi_1)+\pi_0(1-\pi_0)}{e^2}$

e Maximum acceptable standard error in all the mentioned cases
Source: Kirkwood and Sterne [14]
[a] In these cases, the sample unit is the same unit in which the rate is expressed. For example, if the rate is based on person-years, the calculated number expresses the required number of person-years

Table C.3 Different values of v for specific values of error type I (α) and υ specific values of power ($1-\beta$) and error type II ($1-\beta$)

α	Value	
	One-way test	**Two-way test**
(a) To calculate the sample size based on the selected values of error type I:		
0.1	1.28	1.65
0.05	1.65	1.96
0.025	1.96	2.24
0.01	2.33	2.58
β	$1-\beta$	υ
(b) To calculate the sample size based on the selected values of the test power		
0.50	0.5	0.00
0.40	0.60	0.25
0.30	0.70	0.53
0.20	0.80	0.84
0.15	0.85	1.03
0.10	0.90	1.28
0.05	0.95	1.65
0.025	0.975	1.96
0.01	0.99	2.33

Determining the Sample Size for Unbalanced Groups

When dealing with unbalanced groups, where the sample size of one group is significantly smaller or larger than the other group, traditional methods for calculating sample size may not be appropriate. This is because traditional sample size calculations assume that the sample sizes of both groups are approximately equal.

In cases where the sample sizes of the groups are unbalanced, other methods can be used to determine the appropriate sample size. These methods may include:

1. Power analysis: Power analysis calculates the sample size necessary to detect the desired effect size with the desired level of statistical power. Power analysis takes into account the sample size of each group, the effect size, the level of significance, and the desired level of statistical power.

2. Simulation: Simulation involves creating synthetic data sets with a known effect size and sample size, and then testing different sample sizes to determine the appropriate sample size for the unbalanced groups. Simulation allows researchers to account for the impact of sample size on the statistical power of the study.
3. Bayesian sample size determination: Bayesian sample size determination involves using prior knowledge about the population and the expected effect size to determine an appropriate sample size. This method incorporates information from previous studies or expert opinions to inform the sample size determination.
4. Bootstrapping: Bootstrapping is a resampling technique that involves randomly sampling the available data with replacement to create new data sets. Bootstrapping can be used to estimate the sample size required to achieve a desired level of precision, even with unbalanced samples.

Overall, selecting an appropriate sample size for unbalanced groups requires careful consideration of the study design and statistical analysis techniques. It is important to consult with a statistician or use appropriate software to determine the appropriate sample size for the study.

If, instead of choosing equal groups, we decide to examine different proportions of patients in each group (for example, in a case-control study, three controls for each case), the total sample size will change.

Table C.4 is the adjustment factor for use in studies where the size of the two groups being compared is unequal. In this table, factor (*f*) is used to correct the sample size of the smaller group and is equal to the sample size of the larger group is *c* equal to the sample size of the smaller group. Therefore, the sample size is smaller (*n* is the sample size in the case of an equal volume of two groups) and the sample size of the group is larger [14].

Table C.4 Adjustment factor for calculating the sample size when the sample size in the groups is not equal

Sample size proportion (larger group to smaller group)	Sample size adjustment for a smaller group (*f*)
1	1
2	3.4
3	2.3
4	5.8
5	3.5
6	7.12
7	4.7
8	9.16
9	5.9
10	11.20

Adjusting the Sample Size for Missing Cases from Follow-Ups, Confounders, and Interactions

In calculating the sample size, the possibility of non-answers or missing study members should also be taken into account and the sample size should be increased accordingly. If the effect of confounding variables is considered in the final analysis, or if the effects of subgroups are tested, these cases should also be included in the sample size calculation [17].

In many studies, participants may drop out or be lost to follow-up, resulting in missing data. When data is missing, it can reduce the statistical power of the study and impact the validity of the results. To address this issue, researchers can adjust the sample size to account for missing cases from follow-ups [16, 17].

There are different approaches to adjusting sample size for missing cases from follow-up, including:

1. Oversampling: One approach is to oversample to account for potential dropouts. Oversampling involves recruiting more participants than what is required assuming no dropouts, to ensure that the study has enough

power even when some participants are lost to follow-up.
2. Multiple imputations: Another approach is multiple imputations, which involves estimating values for the missing data using statistical models based on the observed data. This approach helps to reduce bias and increase the precision of the estimates. Once the missing data is imputed, the sample size can be adjusted to reflect the imputed data.
3. Adjustment factors: Adjustment factors can be calculated to adjust the sample size for dropout rates. These factors are based on the proportion of participants that are expected to drop out, the assumed effect size, and the variation in the data. By incorporating these factors into the sample size calculation, the correct number of participants can be recruited to ensure adequate power.
4. Sensitivity analysis: Finally, sensitivity analysis can be carried out to assess the impact of missing cases on the study results. Sensitivity analysis involves testing how sensitive the results are to different rates of missing data, allowing researchers to determine the minimal sample size required for adequate power.

Overall, adjusting the sample size for missing cases from follow-up is crucial for ensuring the statistical power and validity of a study. Researchers should carefully consider the different approaches available and select the most appropriate method based on the study design, data characteristics, and research question.

It is important to note that people who enter the study from the beginning may not be useful in the conclusion or final analysis stage. For example, the members of the sample may be unavailable, or they may not have enough follow-up, or the information on its key variables may be lost. The required sample size should be adjusted for these situations. If we assume that x is the percentage of patients who are not useful for the final analysis, then the sample size must be multiplied by the factor $\frac{100}{100-x}$. For example, if it is $x =$ % 20, then the number $\frac{100}{100-20}=1/25$ is multiplied by the final sample size, and the adjustment factor $\frac{100}{100-x}$ is missing data for $\%x$.

Once the DEFF is calculated, the adjusted sample size can be calculated as:

Adjusted sample size = sample size / DEFF

For example, suppose a study design involves households as clusters, the average cluster size is 3, and the ICC is 0.2. If we want to calculate the sample size required to detect a significant difference in a particular outcome variable with a power of 80% and a significance level of 5%, the sample size will be calculated based on the adjusted sample size formula:

$$\text{DEFF} = 1 + (3-1) \times 0.2 = 1.4$$

Adjusted sample size = sample size / DEFF

If we set the desired power to 80%, the significance level at 5%, and the effect size at 0.5 standard deviations, the sample size required without clustering would be around 64. With clustering, the adjusted sample size would be:

$$\text{Adjusted sample size} = 64 / 1.4 = 45.7$$

Thus, to achieve the same level of statistical power, we would need to recruit 46 clusters or households (assuming an average cluster size of 3).

Adjusting the sample size for cluster designs is crucial to ensure that the study has sufficient statistical power to detect significant differences and account for the clustering effect. By calculating the DEFF and adjusting the sample size, researchers can ensure that their study is adequately powered to achieve their research objectives.

You can refer to the sources [18, 19] for more details on the calculation of sample size in cluster randomized trial designs.

Real Examples

Descriptive Studies

A Descriptive Study to Determine the Prevalence

In descriptive studies, the sample size is determined based on the purpose of the study, the level of precision required, and the available resources. The sample size should be large enough to provide accurate estimates of the population parameters with a certain level of precision or confidence.

Sample size calculation in descriptive studies depends on several factors, including:

1. The desired level of precision or margin of error: This represents the acceptable level of uncertainty in the study results. It is often expressed as a percentage of the estimated population parameter or as a fixed value.
2. The level of confidence: This represents the probability that the true population parameter lies within the estimated interval. It is often set at 95%, indicating that there is a 95% chance that the true population parameter falls within the calculated estimate.
3. The variability of the population: The larger the variability of the population, the larger the sample size required to achieve the desired level of precision and confidence.
4. The nature of the population: The more homogeneous the population, the smaller the sample size required to achieve the desired level of precision and confidence.
5. The resources available: The larger the sample size, the greater the resources required for data collection, management, and analysis.

In general, the sample size in descriptive studies should be large enough to produce reliable estimates of the population parameters but should not exceed the available resources or the needs of the study design.

The World Health Organization is implementing the Vision 2020 plan to prevent, treat and reduce 80% of diseases that lead to low vision and blindness by 2020, and this plan has been accepted as a priority by the Ministry of Health, Treatment, and Medical Education. The first step in the control and prevention of diseases is to have information about the prevalence or in other words the burden of the disease in the area under study. Since there is no time and documented information about the prevalence and causes of blindness and low vision in our country. A research project was carried out in the eye research center of Shahid Beheshti University of Medical Sciences to answer this design question. In this plan, the approximate prevalence of blindness and low vision cases based on the information of the guide study that was conducted in 2013 in Karaj city, was considered to be around 15%, and according to that, the sample size was calculated as follows:

Using the above equations and considering $\pi = 0.15$ and $e = 0/004$ (the maximum acceptable standard error in the study), we have:

$$n_{\text{simple}} = \frac{0.15(0.85)}{(0.004)^2} = 7032$$

According to the study of the guide, the effect of the plan was considered equal to 1.5. According to the type of sampling design, which is a cluster sampling study with the size of 20 households in each cluster (approximately 100 people in each cluster), the total sample size is equal to:

$$n_{\text{cluster}} = (\text{Design effect}) \times (n_{\text{sample}}) n_{\text{cluster}} = 1.5 \times 7032 = 10,548$$

it will be counted, But the calculated sample only includes people with full cooperation whose information is available. Usually, in field studies, the percentage of cooperation, the number of referrals of sample members and people referred to the clinic is not complete (100%) and to adjust this issue, considering the percentage of non-cooperation equal to

25%, the final sample size was considered equal $n = \left(\frac{100}{100-25}\right) \times 10{,}548 = 14{,}064$. As a result, we need approximately 141 clusters of 20 households to achieve a useful sample size of 10,548 [20].

Descriptive Study to Determine the Incidence

Before providing a sanitary reservoir for drinking water, we would like to estimate the average number of children under 5 years of age who suffer from diarrhea throughout the year. We guess that the incidence of this complication is around 3, but we want to estimate this rate with a maximum standard error of 0.2. This means that if, for example, 2.6 complications/child/year are observed, we can infer that the actual incidence rate is between 2.2 and 4.8. In statistical terms, we want the size of the 95% confidence interval of the incidence rate to be no larger than ±0.2.

Since the length of the confidence interval is almost equal to ± 2 × se, then the standard deviation of the estimate should not be greater than 0.1. Using relation 9 from Table C.1, we have:

$$n > \frac{3}{0.1^2} = 300$$

It is important to pay attention to this point that the relationships for calculating the sample size for incidence (relationships 2, 5, 9, and 12) calculate the sample size based on the rate unit used. Therefore, in the current example, it is necessary to observe 300 children/per year. This issue is achieved by observing 300 children in 1 year or, for example, 1200 children in 3 months.

Randomized Clinical Trial

The Sample Size for Comparing Two Ratios

Comparison of the anatomical results of primary vitrectomy and scleral buckling in the treatment of retinal detachment in patients with a history of cataract surgery [21].

In this study, 44 patients who had retinal detachment and had a history of cataract surgery were randomly divided into two groups. In one group vitrectomy was performed and the other group underwent scleral buckling surgery. In the end, the anatomical condition of the retina and vision of the patients were compared at follow-up intervals (1, 2, 4, and 6 months after the operation). Equation (6) was used to calculate the sample size of this study.

In this regard, according to previous studies, approximate values π_{vitx} = % 30 (percentage of retinal detachment after 6 months of follow-up in the primary vitrectomy group) $\pi_{\text{S. B}}$ = % 40 (percentage of retinal detachment after 6 months of follow-up in the sclera buckle group) were considered. As a result, for the significance level α = 0/05 and power of test γ = % 80,we have:

$$n = \frac{\left\{\upsilon\sqrt{\left[\pi_{\text{vitx}}\left(1-\pi_{\text{vitx}}\right)+\pi_{\text{S.B}}\left(1-\pi_{\text{S.B}}\right)\right]}+v\sqrt{2\bar{\pi}\left(1-\bar{\pi}\right)}\right\}^2}{\left(\pi_{\text{vitx}}-\pi_{\text{S.B}}\right)^2}$$

$$n = \frac{\left\{0.84\sqrt{\left[0.3\times(0.7)+0.4\times(0.6)\right]}+1.96\sqrt{2\times 0.35\times(0.65)}\right\}^2}{(0.3-0.4)^2} = 125$$

That is, the number of 125 samples in each group was necessary. The actual study was completed with 126 eyes in the buckle group and 99 eyes in the vitrectomy group, in which case the real power of the test is slightly less than 80%.

The Sample Size for Comparing Two Mean

Comparison of cotrimoxazole and the classic method in the treatment of ocular toxoplasmosis [22] In a clinical trial, patients suffering from ocular toxoplasmosis were randomly assigned to two treatment groups, in one group classical treatment of toxoplasmosis (pyrimethamine) was prescribed and in the second group cotrimoxazole was prescribed. All patients were treated for 6 weeks and at the end, after 6 months of follow-up, the patients were compared in terms of changes in the size of eye lesions.

The sample size was calculated using Eq. (4), in this relation (mean lesion reduction with classical treatment) and (mean lesion reduction with cotrimoxazole treatment) and the variance of both groups was considered equal to 21. With the significance level and test power of 95%, the sample volume was calculated as follows:

$$n = \frac{(\upsilon + v)^2 (\sigma_1^2 + \sigma_0^2)}{(\mu_1 - \mu_0)^2}$$

$$n = \frac{(1.65 + 2.57)^2 (21 + 21)}{(22 - 50)^2}$$

Therefore, 30 samples are required in each group. A real study was conducted with 29 people in the classic treatment group and 30 people in the cotrimoxazole treatment group.

Case-Control Studies

Sample size in case-control studies is important to ensure that the study is adequately powered to detect a significant association between the exposure and outcome variables. The sample size calculation for case-control studies depends on several factors, including:

1. The estimated prevalence of the outcome in the population of interest.
2. The desired level of statistical power to detect a significant association between the exposure and outcome variables.
3. The expected effect size[2] or the strength of the association between the exposure and outcome variables.
4. The level of significance of the study or the alpha level.
5. The number of exposure categories.

One of the important considerations in sample size calculation for case-control studies is the ratio of cases to controls. In general, the ratio of controls to cases should be at least 1:1. However, in some cases where the outcome is rare, a higher ratio of controls to cases may be necessary to increase the statistical power of the study.

It is important to note that small sample size in a case-control study may result in a lack of power to detect a significant association between the exposure and outcome variables. Conversely, a very large sample size may lead to overpowered study results, which can lead to unnecessary expense and resource utilization. A study is designed to investigate the increased risk of death after acute respiratory infections in infants who are fed formula milk compared to infants who are fed breast milk. Mothers of the case group (mothers whose babies died as a result of respiratory infection according to the death certificate) are interviewed in terms of how they feed their babies (formula milk or breast milk). The results are compared with the data obtained from interviews with mothers who have healthy babies (control group). It is estimated that about 40% of the control group is fed formula milk. We would like an equal effect size in increasing the risk of mortality to be detectable and meaningful. The sample size of cases and controls is considered to reach 90% power. For this purpose, the following steps should be calculated.

1. Calculation, that is, the proportion of cases that are fed with formula milk [21].

$$\pi_1 = \frac{\pi_0 \times \mathrm{OR}}{1 + \pi_0 (\mathrm{OR} - 1)} = \frac{0.4 \times 2}{1 + 0.4(2 - 1)} = \frac{0.8}{1.4} = 0.57$$

[2] The side effect is a statistical measure that helps to quantify the magnitude of the difference between two groups in a statistical test. It is also known as the effect size or the standardized mean difference. The size effect is used to determine the practical significance of the statistical significance found in a statistical test.
The side effect is calculated by dividing the difference between the means of the two groups by their pooled standard deviation. In other words, it measures the size of the difference between the means in standard deviation units.

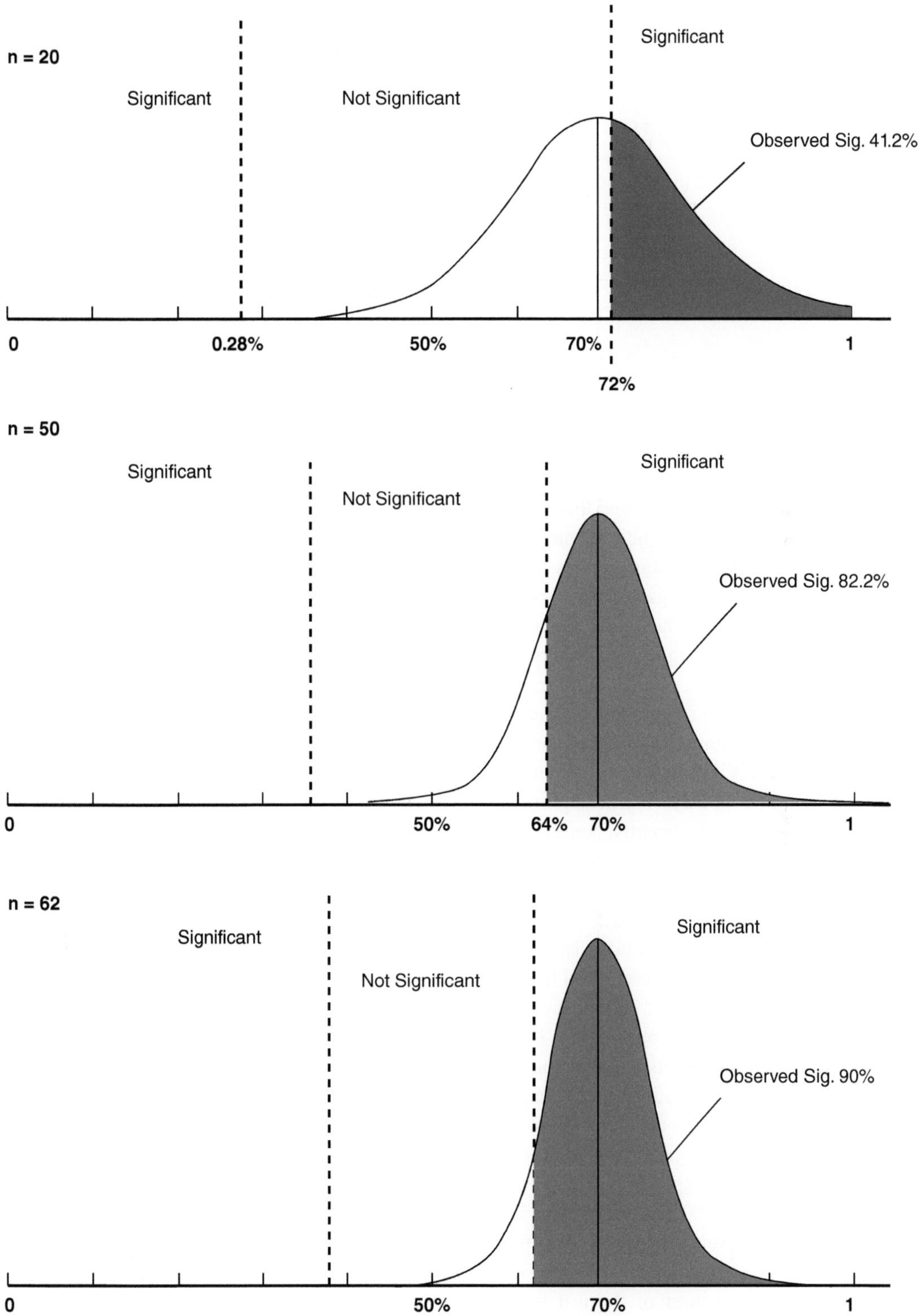

Fig. C.2 Probability of obtaining significant results at the 5% level with different sample sizes when the hypothesis is tested against the null hypothesis

2. Calculation, that is, the mean and

$$\bar{\pi} = \frac{0.4 + 0.75}{2} = 0.485$$

3. Calculation of the minimum required sample volume

$$n > \frac{\left(1.28\sqrt{(0.4\times0.6)+0.57\times0.43}+1.96\sqrt{2\times0.485\times0.515}\right)^2}{(0/57-0/4)^2}$$

$$= \frac{\left(1.28\sqrt{0.4851}+1.96\sqrt{0.4996}\right)^2}{0.17^2} = \frac{2.2769}{0.17^2} = 179.4$$

Therefore, a minimum sample size of 360 individuals is required, consisting of 180 cases and 180 controls. In relation to the interpretation of statistical tests, it is important to consider study power. To further understand this concept, please refer to Fig. C.2, which illustrates the comparison of different sample sizes for the comparison of two ratios against the hypothetical normal distribution. The figure depicts the probability of obtaining significant results at the 5% level.

Unfortunately, when researchers consider the ceiling of 5% for statistical significance and infer that any result that is not significant indicates that the null hypothesis is true, significance tests have not been used correctly. Another common misinterpretation is to interpret the probability value as equal to the probability that the null hypothesis is true. Table C.5 shows why such an idea is incorrect. This table is based on what will happen if 1000 different null hypotheses with a significance level of 5% are tested under the following assumptions. (1) 10% of tested null hypotheses are false (that is, the effect of the factor under investigation is real) and 90% of tested null hypotheses are correct. A large number of factors investigated in epidemiological studies are of this type. For example, in a study, approximately 300 risk factors for coronary heart disease were identified, but only a small number of these factors increase the risk of the disease. (2) The power of the test is 50%, which is consistent with published studies on the size of clinical trials [23]. A large proportion of these types of studies are conducted with insufficient sample sizes to investigate the research question. The first assumption is summarized in the total column of the table. In 900 tests, the null hypothesis is true and in 100 tests it is false. The ratio of the first type of error is the same as the significance level used, i.e., 5%. That is, 45 hypotheses out of 900 correct zero hypotheses have been wrongly rejected. We consider the second assumption, that is, the second type error ratio is equal to 50% (power – 100%). So, to reject 50 hypotheses out of 100 null hypotheses that are incorrect, we will make an error. As can be seen in Table C.5(A), out of 95 tests that have meaningful results, 5 tests are correct and 45 (47.4%) tests have type 1 error (false positive result). Table C.5(B) shows the details of Table C.5(A). In this table, the percentage of false positive results for different probabilities and different assumptions about the power of the test and the correct proportion of the null hypothesis are presented. For each significance level, with increasing power, the ratio of significant results, which is false positive, decreases drastically. According to this table, the probability value less than 0.001, except for the cases where the proportion of the event under investigation is very small, provides a strong reason against the null hypothesis [24–26].

Solutions and recommendations for calculating the sample size. When calculating the sample size in analytical studies, the following

Table C.5 Applications of study power to interpret statistical tests

(A) The results of statistical tests for 1000 hypotheses, when 10% of the hypotheses are false, are shown using (significance level) and 50% power

	Reality		
Result of statistical test	**True null hypothesis**	**False null hypothesis**	**Total**
The null hypothesis is rejected ($\alpha < 0.05$)	(Error type I) 45	50	95
The null hypothesis is accepted ($\alpha > 0.05$)	855	(Error type II) 50	905
Total	900	100	1000

(B) The false positive ratio in the significant results corresponds to the probability value used for significance. The power of the study and the proportion of studies where the null hypothesis is false

The proportion of studies in which the null hypothesis is fals	**Power**	$\alpha = 0.05$	$\alpha = 0/01$	$\alpha = 0/001$
80%	20%	5.9	1.2	0.1
	50%	2.4	0.5	0.0
	80%	1.5	0.3	0.0
50%	20%	0.2	8.4	0.5
	50%	1.9	0.2	0.2
	80%	9.5	2.1	0.1
10%	20%	2.69	0.31	3.4
	50%	4.47	3.15	8.1
	80%	0.36	1.10	1.1
1%	20%	1.96	2.83	1.33
	50%	8.90	4.66	5.16
	80%	1.86	3.55	0.11

steps must be done: 1) Setting null and opposite hypotheses 2) Choosing appropriate statistical tests 3) Estimating the effect size and its changes from the results of previous studies or the guide study 4) Determining the appropriate values based on the importance of avoiding type 1 and type 2 errors w Other important points that should be considered in calculating the sample size in analytical studies are: correction for non-response cases, the presence of interaction and potential confounders in the study.

- Studies in which there are nominal variables, survival analysis, cluster sampling, assimilation, modeling and multivariate analysis and special studies to examine the similarity of the subjects are the cases for which the calculation of the sample size is different from the simple cases mentioned in this chapter. And it is necessary to pay attention to specific strategies in these cases.
- The steps for calculating the sample size in descriptive studies that do not have a hypothesis are:
  - Estimation of the proportion of members with events in nominal variables and estimation of standard deviation in continuous variables.
  - Determining the desired accuracy (confidence interval length).
  - Determining the desired confidence level (for example, 95% confidence level)
- When the sample size is known according to the conditions and limitations, it is possible to calculate the minimum detectable effect size in the study or the power of the test.

- Some strategies to minimize the sample size include using continuous variables, making more accurate measurements, using a matched design, calculating the sample size for unbalanced groups, and considering more common events in the study.
- When it seems that not enough information is available to estimate the sample size, more and more detailed review of the sources, investigating the possibility of conducting a guided study or re-analyzing the data, the possibility of categorizing the variables into dichotomous variables are options that should be carefully investigated. If none of these cases are practical, realistic guesses by experienced researchers can be very helpful. Some inexperienced researchers make common mistakes when calculating the sample size, some of which are:
- Nominal variables when expressed as percentages or rates may be mistakenly considered continuous. For example, a variable such as a state of being alive (alive or dead) may be interpreted continuously when it is expressed as the percentage of the alive or the number of dead per year. Similarly, in the survival analysis, the two-mode variable under study may be interpreted continuously (such as the average survival in different months). In all these cases, the investigated response is two-mode, and in simple cases, the appropriate tests for these cases are of the Kaido-type.
- The calculated sample size should be calculated for the number of people who complete the follow-up and for whom the final responses are completed, not for the number of people who initially enter the study.

Discussion and Conclusion

The cases studied for calculating the sample size in this chapter are relatively simple cases in which the comparison of two groups is considered without any complex assumptions (such as the presence of confounders, etc.). Determining the sample size in most cases is much easier by using pre-prepared tables. Sources [27–29] contain this set of tables. Even in such simple situations, it is inevitable to have realistic ideas about the parameters of the studied society. For example, when the goal is to compare means, an acceptable estimate of the standard deviation, or in the comparison of ratios, an appropriate estimate of the size of one of the ratios in the society is required. This information can be obtained from similar studies or the study guide. In more complex situations, additional information is needed. Cases such as calculating the sample size for paired data, Bayesian methods for finding the appropriate sample size, trials whose purpose is to show the similarity between treatments, calculating the sample size for survival data, calculating the sample size when there are confounding variables or interactions are the cases that Assumptions require additional information and more complex calculations that are beyond the scope of this chapter. Readers can refer to sources [19, 20, 26–29] for more information. In many studies, it is necessary to measure and analyze various parameters of the sample members. For example, in the investigation of a disease, a wide range of syndromes, the results of diagnostic tests, and clinical examinations are collected in each patient. The number of samples calculated for a specific purpose may not be appropriate in other conditions and for other purposes. In many studies, the sample size is calculated in different conditions and for all purposes, and the final sample size is considered the largest sample size calculated in different situations; but in some studies, this method is not possible due to the cost of some experiments (measurements) or practical problems. In such cases, it is very useful to use a multi-phase sampling plan. In the first phase, certain parameters are measured for all people in the sample. In the second phase, only a subgroup of the initial sample is selected (by simple random method or other random selection methods) and other parameters are measured. This process can be developed for different phases.

References

1. Maruyama G, Ryan CS. Research methods in social relations. 8th ed. London: Wiley-Blackwell; 2014.
2. Tavakol M, Dennick R. Making sense of Cronbach's alpha. Int J Med Educ. 2011;2:53–5. https://doi.org/10.5116/ijme.4dfb.8dfd. PMID: 28029643; PMCID: PMC4205511.
3. May T, Perry B. Social research: issues, methods and process. 5th ed. London: Open University Press; 2022. ISBN 0335262104, 9780335262106.
4. Brinkmann S, Kvale S. Introduction to interview research. 3rd ed. Los Angeles: SAGE Publications; 2015. ISBN 978-1-4833-8291-3.
5. Rutterford C, Taljaard M, Dixon S, Copas A, Eldridge S. Reporting and methodological quality of sample size calculations in cluster randomized trials could be improved: a review. J Clin Epidemiol. 2015;68(6):716–23. https://doi.org/10.1016/j.jclinepi.2014.12.007.
6. Hayes RJ, Moulton LH. Cluster randomised trials. 2nd ed. Boca Raton, FL: Chapman & Hall/CRC Press; 2017. ISBN 978-1-315-15084-3.
7. Lister R. Loss of ability to drive following a stroke: the early experiences of three elderly people on discharge from hospital. Br J Occup Ther. 1999;62(11):514–20.
8. Mencap. Communicating with people with a learning disability. 2017 [cited 2023 Apr 27]. https://www.mencap.org.uk/sites/default/files/2017-11/Communicating%20with%20People%20with%20a%20Learning%20Disability.pdf.
9. Domarad BR, Buschmann MT. Interviewing older adults: increasing the credibility of interview data. J Gerontol Nurs. 1995;21(9):14–20. https://doi.org/10.3928/0098-9134-19950901-06. PMID: 7560817.
10. Emerson E. Exploring the history of learning disability. Br J Learn Disabil. 2012;40(1):69–76. https://doi.org/10.1111/j.1468-3156.2011.00710.x.
11. Karami M, Soori H, Monfared AB. Estimating the contribution of selected risk factors in attributable burden to stroke in Iran. Iran J Public Health. 2012;41(5):91–6. Epub 2012 May 31. PMID: 23113182; PMCID: PMC3468982.
12. Knott E, Rao AH, Summers K, et al. Interviews in the social sciences. Nat Rev Methods Primers. 2022;2:73. https://doi.org/10.1038/s43586-022-00150-6.
13. Streiner DL, Norman GR, Cairney J. Health measurement scales: a practical guide to their development and use. 5th ed. Oxford: Oxford University Press; 2015. ISBN 978-0199685219.
14. Kirkwood BR, Sterne JAC. Essential medical statistics. Chichester: Wiley; 2010.
15. Soori H. Uses of epidemiology. Iran J Epidemiol. 2009;5(2):1–10. http://irje.tums.ac.ir/article-1-111-en.html.
16. Suresh K, Chandrashekara S. Sample size estimation and power analysis for clinical research studies. J Hum Reprod Sci. 2012;5(1):7–13. https://doi.org/10.4103/0974-1208.97779. Retraction in: J Hum Reprod Sci 2015 Jul-Sep;8(3):186. PMID: 22870008; PMCID: PMC3409926.
17. Yi GY, He W. Analysis of case-control data with interacting misclassified covariates. J Stat Distrib Appl. 2017;4(1):16. https://doi.org/10.1186/s40488-017-0069-0.
18. Masood M, Reidpath DD. Intraclass correlation and design effect in BMI, physical activity and diet: a cross-sectional study of 56 countries. BMJ Open. 2016;6(1):e008173. https://doi.org/10.1136/bmjopen-2015-008173. PMID: 26743697; PMCID: PMC4716153.
19. Wang X, Ji X. Sample size estimation in clinical research: from randomized controlled trials to observational studies. Chest. 2020;158(1S):S12–20. https://doi.org/10.1016/j.chest.2020.03.010. PMID: 32658647.
20. Berger RL, Casella G. Statistical inference. Stamford: Cengage Learning; 2021.
21. Ramezani A, Entezari M, Banaie S, Norouzi A, Yaseri M. Mini vitrectomy as an alternative technique for intraocular pressure adjustment in non-drainage scleral buckling. Medwave. 2022;22(7):e002571. https://doi.org/10.5867/medwave.2022.07.002571. PMID: 36027575.
22. Soheilian M, Sadoughi MM, Ghajarnia M, Dehghan MH, Yazdani S, Behboudi H, Anisian A, Peyman GA. Prospective randomized trial of trimethoprim/sulfamethoxazole versus pyrimethamine and sulfadiazine in the treatment of ocular toxoplasmosis. Ophthalmology. 2005;112(11):1876–82. https://doi.org/10.1016/j.ophtha.2005.05.025. Epub 2005 Sep 19. PMID: 16171866.
23. Poulter N. Coronary heart disease is a multifactorial disease. Am J Hypertens. 1999;12(10 Pt 2):92S–5S. https://doi.org/10.1016/s0895-7061(99)00163-6. PMID: 10555607.
24. Zhou Z, Li D, Zhang S. Sample size calculation for cluster randomized trials with zero-inflated count outcomes. Stat Med. 2022;41(12):2191–204. https://doi.org/10.1002/sim.9350. Epub 2022 Feb 9. PMID: 35139584.
25. Klar N, Donner A. Design and analysis of cluster randomization trials in health research. Chichester: Wiley; 2010.
26. Dekkers OM. Why not to (over) emphasize statistical significance. Eur J Endocrinol. 2019;181(3):E1–2. https://doi.org/10.1530/EJE-19-0531. PMID: 31330499.
27. Tan SB, Tan SH, Machin D, Campbell MJ. Sample sizes for clinical, laboratory and epidemiology studies. Chichester: Wiley; 2018.
28. Machin D, Tan SH, Tan SB, Campbell MJ. Sample size tables for clinical studies. Weinheim: Wiley; 2011.

Fang JQ. Statistical methods for biomedical research. Singapore: World Scientific Publishing Company; 2021.

MIX
Papier aus verantwortungsvollen Quellen
Paper from responsible sources
FSC® C105338

If you have any concerns about our products,
you can contact us on
ProductSafety@springernature.com

In case Publisher is established outside the EU,
the EU authorized representative is:
Springer Nature Customer Service Center GmbH
Europaplatz 3, 69115 Heidelberg, Germany

Printed by Libri Plureos GmbH
in Hamburg, Germany